Medical Persuasion

Vic Velanovich

Medical Persuasion

Understanding the Impact on Medical Argumentation

Springer

Vic Velanovich
Surgery
University of South Florida
Tampa, FL, USA

ISBN 978-3-031-30370-8 ISBN 978-3-031-30371-5 (eBook)
https://doi.org/10.1007/978-3-031-30371-5

This Springer imprint is published by the registered company Springer Nature Switzerland AG
The registered company address is: Gewerbestrasse 11, 6330 Cham, Switzerland

Preface

I graduated medical school and, including my 5-year general surgery residency, have been a practicing general surgeon for 35 years. During that time, I have performed over 11,000 surgical and endoscopic procedures; and estimate that I cared for, either surgically or medically, over 15,000 patients. Since college, I have been continuously involved in various types of medical research activities, including laboratory research, clinical observational studies, randomized controlled trials, decision analyses, and meta-analyses. I have presented my work over 200 times at various regional, national, and international meetings and have published over 270 articles in peer-reviewed journals. I have been a peer-reviewer for dozens of journals, reviewing hundreds of papers submitted for publication; and I have been on, and chaired, several program committees reviewing thousands of abstracts submitted for presentation. This is the basis for my interest in persuasion. To be persuasive is to be convincing. It is to get your audience, whether it be of one or thousands, to accept your conclusions, if not outright true, then at least valid. I cannot say that I have always succeeded in persuading others. I have had many patients refuse my advice, colleagues question my judgments, and journals reject my papers. I have sat in audiences, listening to others present their research and have had the colleague to my right be in complete agreement with the presenter and my other colleague to my left completely dismiss the findings. The question then becomes: Why?

This has led me on an over 30-year study of what makes arguments persuasive. This book is the result of that study. I am not a philosopher, but I will discuss those concepts, however poorly, that may enlighten my ideas. I am not a neuroscientist or psychologist, but I will discuss those aspects of the human brain and its workings that I believe are relevant. I am not a social scientist, but I will discuss those precepts which may influence an individual to accept or reject an argument beyond the actual logic of the argument. In other words, this is a practical effort by a practicing physician to assess how medical knowledge is generated, accepted, and utilized and how medical decisions are contemplated, made, and implemented.

I will try to limit jargon and formulations in an effort to make this accessible to many who may be interested. However, sometimes precise definitions are required, and for ease, I have provided a glossary of those terms. I have made every effort that when I have given a term a specific definition, I will not use it for another meaning. I have incorporated numerous ideas and concepts from many authors much more insightful than myself. If I have misquoted or misinterpreted any, please accept my apologies and feel free to correct my errors. The errors are solely my own and should not reflect on their work. Nevertheless, I owe a great deal to these thinkers.

I would like to acknowledge the University of South Florida Morsani College of Medicine for providing a sabbatical so that I can complete this work; as well as, to my family, especially my wife Lynda, who has endured much to allow me to write this, and my colleagues near and far who have allowed me to discuss many of these topics prior to writing.

Tampa, FL, USA Vic Velanovich

Contents

Chapter 1
Introduction

1.1 A Clinical Vignette

A patient is referred to a physician with complaints of heartburn. The physician commences with the process, taught to the physician in medical school and throughout training, supplemented by the experience of medical practice, of trying to determine the cause of this symptom and what would be the appropriate treatment. Customarily, the physician would begin with the "history of present illness." This would usually include such bits of information as when did the heartburn start; is it there all the time or sporadically; if sporadically, how frequently; is it mostly at night or during the day; does anything seem to make it worse, etc. After this, the physician obtains the "past medical history," that is, any other diagnoses that the patient has had, whether still on-going or resolved. Those which are still ongoing, such as hypertension, will be assessed for any possible linkage to the patient's present complaint and perhaps their potential effects on future treatment; and those which have been resolved, such as gallstones treated by a cholecystectomy, which help narrow potential diagnoses. At this point, the physician would obtain a list of all the medications this individual is currently taking. Then, the process would continue by obtaining a "past surgical history," "family history," and "social history." The social history would include items such as marital status, employment status, and use of tobacco, alcohol or illicit drugs. This would be followed with a "review of systems," which is essentially a checklist of symptoms involving the other organ systems that were not part of the index history. After this, the physician will perform a physical examination, paying particular attention to those areas that may provide pertinent information. From this initial evaluation, a "differential diagnosis," that is, a list of possible diseases that could account for the information just gathered, would be developed.

Once the physician has the differential diagnosis in mind, they will decide whether any additional testing is needed. This could include laboratory (blood,

V. Velanovich, *Medical Persuasion*, https://doi.org/10.1007/978-3-031-30371-5_1

urine, etc.) tests, radiological images, endoscopic evaluation, and physiological tests. In this particular case, the physician opts to obtain a complete blood count, upper gastrointestinal series, high resolution esophageal manometry, and esophago-gastroduodenoscopy with placement of an esophageal pH monitoring probe. Once all these tests are returned, they will review the results. In this particular case, the patient had a normal hemoglobin level and white blood cell count. The upper gastrointestinal series showed a sliding hiatal hernia, but the remainder of the esophagus, stomach and duodenum were normal. The endoscopy demonstrated Los Angeles class A esophagitis but no other mucosal abnormalities. The pH probe demonstrated pathologic acid reflux, with a total time the esophageal pH was less than 4 of 10% and a DeMeester score of 32.2. The patient pressed the symptom occurrence button 14 times for "heartburn," and in 10 of these, the pH was less than 4. The esophageal manometry showed that the lower esophageal sphincter pressure was low at 4 mmHg and that the esophageal peristaltic pressure was normal at 80 mmHg.

With this information, a diagnosis of pathologic gastroesophageal reflux disease was made. The physician discussed all of these findings with the patient. At this point, the doctor presents the treatment options to the patient to include lifestyle changes, medications and surgery. The physician may explain their rationale for these recommendations, as well as, the risks and potential benefits of each approach. Usually, they will answer all of the patient's questions, including any questions that the patient's family may have who are present. After due consideration, the patient opts to proceed with a laparoscopic Nissen fundoplication. The physician will have the patient scheduled for that operation.

1.2 Persuasion Foundations of the Medical Encounter

The above case would be a very routine case for many surgeons throughout the world. The general outline of the encounter is familiar to all practicing physicians. However, underlying this case are dozens of arguments, many masquerading as axiomatic truths from time immemorial, that doctors have been persuaded were true, or at least, true enough, to be reliable for decision-making. The physician also presented the patient with at least two arguments: one related to how the diagnosis of gastroesophageal reflux disease was determined and the other to why the treatment options that were given were appropriate for their particular condition. The patient eventually was persuaded that a laparoscopic Nissen fundoplication was the best choice.

This book is about all of the arguments involved in the medical care of a patient and why some of these arguments are more persuasive than others. Everyone, at some time or another, tries to persuade someone of the correctness of their position. This is done by marshalling their reasons for believing in their position and communicating with their listener(s) these reasons. Just to clarify, what I mean by an argument is a language product that reaches a conclusion that the arguer believes to be true. I am going to acknowledge that this is not a very precise definition and will later (in Chap. 2) provide a discussion of argumentation. However, I want to make clear that I do not mean people having an emotional quarrel hurling slurs at one another or a simple blanket denial of the other person's position. I am going to assume throughout this book that the arguer and the listener are both persons of good will that no devious ulterior motive and are of open mind. Although I will discuss (in Chaps. 3 and 4) that people may not of as much open mind as they believe. Moreover, the arguer is not trying to fool or swindle the listener for personal gain, and the listener would be willing to accept the arguer's conclusion if, in fact, the listener was persuaded of its correctness.

I am going to establish a few "ground rules" or basic "axioms" for this purpose. I am going to assume that we are, in fact, living in what technology aficionados call "base reality." That is, what we experience in the universe we inhabit is physically real and not a simulation,[1] nor are we subjected to Descartes's "evil demon" controlling our perceptions of reality.[2] This physical universe has discoverable phenomena that behave in a consistent manner under similar circumstances. For any given repeatable phenomenon, there are potentially observable events that will reflect the underlying governing factors of the phenomenon's occurrence. These underlying governing factors may be completely deterministic, in that if x occurs, y must occur, if the circumstances are the same; or they can be stochastic, in that if x occurs, y occurs with a certain frequency, but not every time. I am also going to assume that we humans have developed a certain capacity to observe some parts of these events either directly through our senses or technologically through instruments we have invented. Although I completely acknowledge that, at times, what we observe through our senses is an illusion and does not correspond to reality, and our instruments may give us erroneous readings, for the purposes of this book, I am going to assume that we will not suffer such errors. This is for the goal of being able to focus on the reasoning of the arguer in constructing an argument for the intent of convincing a listener. On the other hand, I will deal with the problem of when such facts or premises are rejected as false or apocryphal enough to be dismissed by the listener (more on this in Chap. 3).

Although my scope here is not to expound on the philosophical issues involved in the development and confirmation of scientific theory,[3] I will say that, in my view, scientific theories are "reverse engineered" from observable phenomena to create a

---

[1] This is a topic that has received serious attention. For example, see Anil Ananthaswamy, "Do We Live in a Simulation? Chances are approximately 50–50." *Scientific American*, October 13, 2020.

[2] In *Discourse on the Method* (1637), Descartes performs the famous thought experiment imagining that he is not a physical being, but merely a mind being feed illusions by an "evil demon." He concludes that although everything he perceives may be an illusion, the fact that he can consider this at all makes him real—"I think, therefore I am." Later in *Meditations on First Philosophy* (1641), he further refines this concept into "I am, I exist."

[3] There are innumerable treatises on this topic, but for a pithy overview, see Ramus Gronfeldt Winter, "The Structure of Scientific Theories," *The Stanford Encyclopedia of Philosophy* (Spring 2021 Edition), Edward N. Zalta (editor).

model that can predict future similar phenomena. That is, scientists do not start off with a theory or model; they start with observations. They will then construct a framework such that the observations fit into a coherent model describing or explaining the phenomenon's occurrence, with the goal of being able to predict future occurrences. It is like walking around a junk yard and finding different mechanical parts and trying to put them together to create a working engine. The tools that we have to reconstruct this engine is our ability as humans to reason (more on this in Chap. 2).

1.3 Decision-Making Foundations in the Medical Encounter

With this background, let us look more closely at the clinical vignette provided earlier. The various determinations by the physician rests on multiple interlocking foundations that have been constructed over centuries of medical science and practice. Figure 1.1 shows the temporal flow of the clinical encounter coupled with the flow of information to the physician and patient in relation to the foundational paradigm of medical theory and experience. This chart will act as the basis for the analysis of the persuasiveness of medical arguments.

Let us start with how most medical encounters start, with the history and physical examination. This is the bedrock information obtained by the physician from the patient from which all subsequent decisions are made. An excellent history of the "history and physical examination" is that of H. Kenneth Walker [1], to which I refer the reader for additional details. However, for my purposes, a brief enumeration of the "crucial developments" he discusses will set the basis for how a diagnostic argument is constructed. According to Walker [1], there were ten individuals responsible for the development of physical diagnosis. I will qualify that he is referring to "Western," allopathic, "science"-based medicine; we must acknowledge that the traditional practices of Eastern medicine, indigenous peoples, folk medicine, and "alternative" medicine also have a theoretical basis incorporating versions of the history and physical examination, which we will address in Chap. 8. However, for now, let us stay with Western medicine.

These ten individuals include Hippocrates (circa 400 BCE) for establishing medicine as a rationality-based profession; Vesalius, in 1543, for conducting human dissections and producing accurate human anatomy texts; Sydeham, from 1666 to 1683, for defining "disease" in a manner which lead to nosological schema of diseases; Auenbruger, in 1760, for the discovery and development of the physical examination maneuver of percussion; Morgagni, in 1761, for correlating "morbid anatomy" to the patient's symptomatic manifestation of disease—i.e., pathology; Corvisart, in 1808, for championing and disseminating the technique of percussion in physical examination; Laennec, in 1816, for inventing the stethoscope; Louis, from 1800 to 1850, for synthesizing prior physical examination techniques and teaching these techniques widely; Mueller, from 1830 to 1900, for developing the foundations of experimental laboratory science; and, finally, Osler, in 1893, for

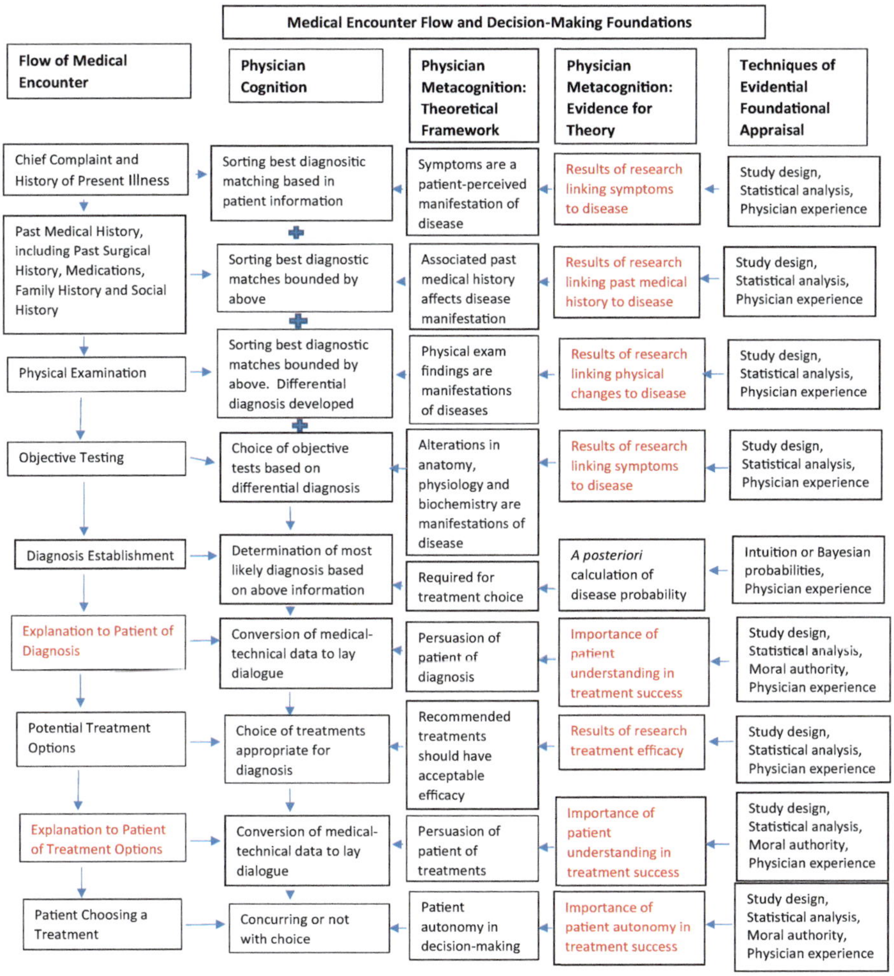

Fig. 1.1 Medical encounter flow and decision-making foundations

developing with what came before into a standardized medical curriculum. All of these individuals made observations related to their practice of medicine and then created arguments that persuaded others in their profession to adopt these new paradigms, theories and techniques.

It is now taken for granted that these techniques make up the basis of the initial information received from the patient. This model of patient evaluation has been taught and practiced for decades. This model is so ingrained that it is unlikely that any physician practicing now has reviewed the actual data and arguments made by these pioneers. It is assumed that what has been passed down in textbooks and training is true. This acceptance of this truth requires trust. That is, the physician-in-training (or, for that matter, any listener) must trust that the "facts" used in these arguments have been vetted in the past and that what is being presented is, in fact, the best method of patient evaluation. This issue of trust also is necessary for the patient to accept the arguments of the physician. In Fig. 1.1, I have highlighted in red those foundations that require trust.

Before moving on, I would like to emphasize what Walker said of Hippocrates, i.e., crediting Hippocrates for the establishment of medicine as a rational-based profession. Although what we truly know about Hippocrates's life and how much of the writings attributed to the Kos school were truly his [2], quite frankly, hashing out this history is not important for the purposes of this book. What is important is that he emphasized that rationality and reason should be the foundations of medical knowledge and practice rather than magical thinking or mysticism. That is, although it appears that the Hippocratic school emphasizes the importance of "evidence" in medical reasoning, it then becomes important for us to understand, in a more formal way, what is rationality, how is reasoning both a foundation and product of rationality, and how the techniques of logic work to support reasoning. This will be explored in Chap. 2.

Therefore, let us look at this specific encounter. We have a patient who presents with symptoms of heartburn. The physician will immediately formulate a list of possible diagnoses that can be the cause. That is, the physician starts to think. In Fig. 1.1, I call this process "physician cognition." This brings us to our first philosophical issue: What constitutes a "cause." This will be explored in Chap. 5. In this instance, one of the differential diagnoses is gastroesophageal reflux disease (GERD), among others [3]. The physician will know that GERD has an underlying prevalence in the general population. This is his *a priori* probability of disease, according to Bayes's theorem (more on this in Chap. 7). Knowing that the patient has heartburn will lead the physician to revise this probability upward, that is, the *a posteriori* probability. This revision occurs because others in the past have made the seminal observations that reflux of gastric acid into the esophagus causes heartburn [4]. This intellectual foundation is what I refer to as the physician's theoretical framework "meta-cognition" (Fig. 1.1). That is, it is the framework that bounds their thinking. It is unlikely that this physician would know that Tileston first observed "peptic ulcer of the esophagus" in 1906 and that Winkelstein in the same year first correlated the symptoms of heartburn with acid regurgitation and reflux esophagitis [4], but this knowledge has been passed down through sources that the physician trusts. Nevertheless, Tileston and Winkelstein made a series of observations in a manner which I call "techniques of evidential appraisal," that is, study design and data analysis, which produces data that was eventually published (Fig. 1.1). This is what I call the physician's "evidence for theory" metacognition (Fig. 1.1). All of these steps have had to have happened for the physician to start thinking about the patient's symptoms in the manner that they do. In addition, as the physician continues to practice, they will use their own observations and experience to further refine their metacognition basis. The physician will then continue the process of eliciting information from the patient through questioning in the history of present illness, past medical history, current medication usage, past surgical history, family history, social history, and review of systems, all the time continuing, either consciously or unconsciously, revising their *a posteriori* probabilities. The process is the same as the physical examination.

In the previous paragraph, I introduced the concepts of "meta-cognition" and "techniques of evidential foundational appraisal." I will develop the concept of "techniques of evidential foundational appraisal" in Chap. 6 and the concept of physician "meta-cognition" in Chap. 7. For now, it is only important to accept that they bound the physician's thinking (i.e., cognition) pertaining to a clinical problem.

This brings us to the physician's first major decisions—what additional laboratory tests should be obtained? Their desire is to secure the most likely diagnosis without having to perform tests that would have little impact toward this goal. The physician may or may not be aware of the testing that went into developing a specific test, but these studies have been done prior to the test being made available for clinical use. This process follows the same meta-cognition steps as the history and physical examination; however, in the case of GERD, these are much more recent developments. The tests ordered included a complete blood count, primarily to determine if anemia is present, as this could be an indicator of ulcerations associated with a hiatal hernia [5]; upper gastrointestinal series to assess for anatomic evidence of hiatal hernia [6]; high resolution manometry to assess esophageal motility [7]; and esophagogastroduodenoscopy to determine if any mucosal abnormalities are present [8] with the placement of a pH monitoring probe to determine whether pathologic acid reflux is present and its association with symptoms [9]. The accuracy of these tests has been widely studied—they have an anatomic-physiologic basis, a determined sensitivity and specificity, and many physicians have had personal experience with using these tests. These are the evidential and metacognitive basis for the physician to accept that these tests will provide useful information. Again, this basis will be explored in Chap. 6.

With this information, the physician determines that the patient's symptoms are due to pathologic GERD. In essence, the doctor places the patient into a diagnostic category. In a way, this process is an argument—the various premises (i.e., the information obtained by the physician) are marshalled in such a way as to reach a conclusion (i.e., the diagnosis). This leads to our next major philosophical issue: What is the logic used by the physician? Is it valid? Is it sound? These issues will be explored in Chap. 2.

The physician will then tell the patient the diagnosis. Although many physicians may state this as a matter of fact, most will map out to the patient how this diagnostic conclusion was reached. This is a matter of persuasion—the physician wants the patient to believe that this diagnosis is correct. The physician will explain how the disease causes the symptoms the patient is experiencing, how the diagnostic tests support this diagnosis, and what, in general, would be the natural history of the disease in this particular patient. The patient and/or family may or may not ask questions for further information or clarification. It is usually the case that the patient has little technical medical knowledge, so much of the physician's task is education. This process requires trust. As the patient cannot assess for themselves all of the premises that have gone into the physician's conclusion, they must have some modicum of trust that what the physician is telling them is true. The issue of trust in receiving information will be addressed in Chap. 3.

Next, the physician will determine the appropriate treatment options for this patient. A central issue is what is the goal of treatment? For a Western, allopathic physician, it is disease eradication. This may not be the goal of other traditional indigenous healers. A mismatch in goals my diminish from the persuasive power of the physician's argument. Going back to our physician, as with determining the appropriate diagnostic tests, this requires knowledge obtained from the various studies, texts, review articles, lectures, etc., that the physician has consumed, as well as their training and experience. For GERD, the treatment options are medical therapy with a proton pump inhibitor and "life-style" changes [10]. There are also a variety of antireflux operations available [11]. The physician will then couple their knowledge of these treatment options with the specific anatomic-physiologic pathology that the patient has. This requires a process of matching the risks, benefits, indications, contraindications, inclusion criteria, exclusion criteria as well as the physician's experience with these various options to the patient's condition. This process of determining the optimal treatment for the patient in front of the physician requires that this particular patient is substantially similar to prior patients (i.e., diagnostic category) for whom the treatments have been previously administered and their outcome known so that the physician can have enough confidence that these treatments would lead to similar outcomes is both "scientific," adhering to a logic, and "intuitive," adhering to a gestalt. This will be further developed in Chap. 7.

The physician will then present these options to the patient. Usually, the physician will enumerate the advantages and disadvantages to the patient and family, if present. They will (or should) elicit what the patient hopes to accomplish with the treatment to better match which of the appropriate treatments would achieve these goals. They will answer any questions that the patient or family members may have. This is the process of manifest rationality that will be described in Chap. 2. Again, as with the diagnosis, the operative word here is trust. However, ultimately, this is a matter of persuasion. How this is presented by the physician to the patient and how the patient receives this presentation is the culmination of the arguments that the physician has put forth. The concept of the "persuasiveness" of arguments as an interpersonal activity will be further developed in Chap. 4.

Last, the patient will make a decision as to which treatment to choose. This will be their own internal argument, which may include their family members. They will arrange the information that they have received with the way they have understood it into their own argument to try to come to some "logical" decision pertaining to their treatment. This may include several premises that have not been stated by the physician, such as financial, social, or personal priorities. Although this is a worthy area of consideration,[4] I will not address this patient-centered decision process in this book.

---

[4] There are many studies in the literature about how patients perceive medical information and how they use this information, given their own personal understanding and priorities.

1.4 Broadening the Concepts of Persuasion and Argument in Medicine

What I have presented is a fairly typical Western-style medical encounter. However, this style is not the only type of medicine practiced in the world. This then begs the question of "Are other types of medical traditions substantially different, not in content or types of practice, but in how their own arguments and persuasions are structured?" For example, traditional Chinese medicine has an extensive and well-developed theoretical foundation, many peoples throughout the world, even in "Western" communities, have indigenous and folk medical practices that are still used, and, in the West, there is new interest in "alternative and complementary" medical practices.[5] It is my contention that these medical practices were developed using the same human rationality that Western medicine was developed, with just a different set of observations which were the basis for their theoretical foundations and different premises used in their argument constructions with the aim of achieving different goals. This will be explored in Chap. 8.

Last, although the vignette given is the customary medical encounter between a human patient and a human physician, this certainly does mean that computer-based decision processes will not become increasingly important and used. Decision sciences has become its own field.[6] "Big Data" has achieved some celebrity status among the sciences. With the continuing development of artificial intelligence, in general, and its particular applications in medicine, such as IBM Watson-Health [12], the potential for "emotion-free" health care determinations is more present than ever. However, this begs the question of what logical forms are used to make these determinations. What premises are used in their logical constructions? How are patient-centered values integrated? Ultimately, will the outputs generated by these nonhuman programs be persuasive to humans? What "ethical and moral" principles will these programs use, if any? These questions I will explore in Chap. 9.

What I hope to demonstrate throughout the book are the processes by which medical knowledge is created and how it is applied to patient care. This will be primarily descriptive—i.e., how it appears, at least to me, how it is done. Although I will touch on a few normative issues—i.e., what are or should be the standards by which these enterprises should be judged—this will not be a primary focus due to the difficulty is reaching consensus as to what these standards should be. Although I will occasional address standards and techniques that can identify errors in an argument so that the conclusion should not be accepted, such as logical fallacies. The underlying thesis of this book is that humans do make conclusions based on

[5] There exists an extensive literature on all of these subjects. In Chap. 8, I will only use a few examples to illustrate my position.

[6] A very approachable history of decision sciences can be found in Leigh Buchanan and Andrew O'Connell, "A brief history of decision making." *Harvard Business Review*, January 2006.

reasons that are marshalled into an argument, whether they are aware of this process or not. My hope is that by making this process more explicit, we will be more likely to be persuaded by good arguments and recognize and reject bad ones.

References

1. Walker HK. The origins of the history and physical examination. In: Walker HE, Hall WD, Hurst JW, editors. Clinical methods: the history, physical and laboratory examinations. 3rd ed. Boston: Butterworth; 1990. p. 5–21.
2. Tsiompanou E, Marketos SG. Hippocrates: timeless still. J R Soc Med. 2013;106:288–92.
3. Bennett RD, Straughn DM, Velanovich V. Gastroesophageal reflux disease, hiatal hernia, and Barrett esophagus. In: Zinner MJ, Ashley SW, Hines OJ, editors. Maingot's abdominal operations. 13th ed. New York: McGraw-Hill Education; 2019. p. 393–422.
4. Dent J. Review article: from 1906 to 2006—a century of major evolution of understanding of gastro-esophageal reflux disease. Aliment Pharm Ther. 2006;24:1269–81.
5. Haurani C, Carlin AM, Hammoud Z, McFarlin K, Prasad M, Velanovich V. Incidence and resolution of anemia with paraesophageal hernia repair. J Gastrointest Surg. 2012;16:1817–20.
6. Levine MS, Rubesin SE. Radiology of the pharynx and esophagus. In: Richter JE, Castell DO, editors. The esophagus. 6th ed. Hoboken, NJ: Wiley-Blackwell; 2021. p. 97–147.
7. Carlson DA, Kahrilas PJ. High-resolution manometry and esophageal pressure topography. In: Richter JE, Castell DO, editors. The esophagus. 6th ed. Hoboken, NJ: Wiley-Blackwell; 2021. p. 155–87.
8. Dimou F, Gonzalez C, Velanovich V. Utility of endoscopy in the diagnosis of hiatus hernia and correlation with GERD. In: Memon A, editor. Hiatal hernia surgery—an evidence based approach. New York: Springer Nature; 2017. p. 1–16.
9. Zerbib F, Pandolfino JE. Ambulatory monitoring for reflux. In: Richter JE, Castell DO, editors. The esophagus. 6th ed. Hoboken, NJ: Wiley-Blackwell; 2021. p. 188–205.
10. Schnoll-Sussman F, Katz PO. Medical management of gastroesophageal reflux disease. In: Richter JE, Castell DO, editors. The esophagus. 6th ed. Hoboken, NJ: Wiley-Blackwell; 2021. p. 428–43.
11. Rabach L, Saad A, Velanovich V. How to choose among fundoplication, magnetic sphincter augmentation or transoral incisionaless fundoplication. Curr Opin Gastroenterol. 2019;35:371–8.
12. https://ibm.com/watson-health. Last accessed 19 May 2022.

Chapter 2
Rationality, Reasoning, Logic, Argumentation and Intuition: The Bases of Medical Assessments and Decisions

In this chapter, I will attempt to set the foundation for the physician's ability to make a diagnosis and come to a treatment decision, as well as the patient's ability to understand and critique that decision. This foundation is that both the physician and patient are rational beings, able to absorb information and to use that information for judgments and decisions. This requires that they be rational and able to use reasoning to reach a conclusion. In this sense, the doctor and patient are similar to every other human. However, then begs a few questions: What is "rationality" and what does it mean to be "rational." What is "reasoning" and how is this accomplished? How is the product of reasoning communicated with others? Why would they believe it? I will make an attempt to be both descriptive about these concepts and to a lesser extent discuss normative standards, although normative standard will not be a focus due to lack of consensus. Although I will draw on my study of philosophical writings on these issues, I am not a "trained" philosopher but have made an attempt to read what I thought would be most enlightening for a physician wishing to understand the basis of reasoning in the practice of medicine. If this seems hopelessly naïve to professional philosophers, perhaps it is. Nevertheless, I hope that any errors do not subtract materially from points I am trying to make.

I am going to start by making the basic assumption that humans are thinking beings[1] *and* can be aware that they are thinking. Although this may seem like a

[1] I freely acknowledge that humans may not be the only thinking beings on earth. All animals probably have some level of thought, as distinct from behavior driven solely by "instinct." Darwin himself believes this to be true (see *The Descent of Man and Selection in Relation to Sex*). Certainly, many animals as diverse as primates, especially great apes, cetaceans, especially dolphins and ocras, octopuses, and ravens, among others, have all shown remarkable problem-solving ability. Is this the equivalent to what humans would refer to as "thinking"? I am not in a position to say, but my guess is that we are closer to our animal brethren than what we may want to believe.

V. Velanovich, *Medical Persuasion*, https://doi.org/10.1007/978-3-031-30371-5_2

trivial assumption, stating it explicitly will be the foundation of all that follows. Aune [1] states that Aristotle acknowledged two basic forms of thinking: (1) Contemplation, which is to attain knowledge of what is, must be or may be the case, which terminates in some conclusion. (2) Deliberation, which is to make up your mind about what you may or may not do, which terminates in a decision or resolution to do that something. Aune points out that some philosophers (e.g., Plato, Aristotle, and Kant) have felt the need to appeal to the notion that humans have an "innate" ability to reason. Johnson-Laird published an article providing evidence for this position [2], and certainly the common experience of humans is that this is true. More on how the human mind evolved in Chap. 3. For Aune [1], human thought also requires an "internal language" to "conceive" the subject of the thought under a certain name or description and to attribute some characteristic(s) according to a fairly specific form of attribution. What I take from all of this is that when people think, they think in abstractions using words as the containers carrying the concepts that are being manipulated. So when one sees a bird, that individual may think about it as a bird, or woodpecker or a red-headed woodpecker, depending on the degree of specificity of language required for their thought. There is a linguistical aspect to this mental process that will be discussed later in this book. Thinking is how people make sense of the world.[2]

Since people have the capacity to think, it is crucial to understand the process of how this is done. This has been an area of great interest by philosophers, psychologists, economists, neuroscientists, and many others. This chapter certainly does not intend to summarize all of this work, in which I have no expertise. What I am concerned about has to do with how medical knowledge is generated and communicated, and how it is used to persuade. This is done by coming to conclusions pertaining to issues of importance to the physician and the patient. As the vignette in Chap. 1 illustrates, there is much that goes into determining a diagnosis, coming to a treatment decision, and conveying that to the patient from the physician's standpoint; from the patient's standpoint, there is much new information to absorb in a field of knowledge that they usually have little to no *a priori* familiarity. For this, I will describe what I feel is a practical assessment of the cognitive hierarchy (Fig. 2.1). Although, no doubt, those with expertise will find much to criticize, this at least gives us a practical framework to discuss persuasion and decision making.

---

[2] Having said this, the human brain (and probably the brains of all other animals) filters out from our consciousness all stimuli that it deems unnecessary for the task at hand. This filtering out process has helped humans survive as a species because all of the unimportant information in a person's environment will not distract from whatever is the important task. See Buzsaki G. "How the brain 'constructs' the outside world." *Scientific American*, June 1, 2022.

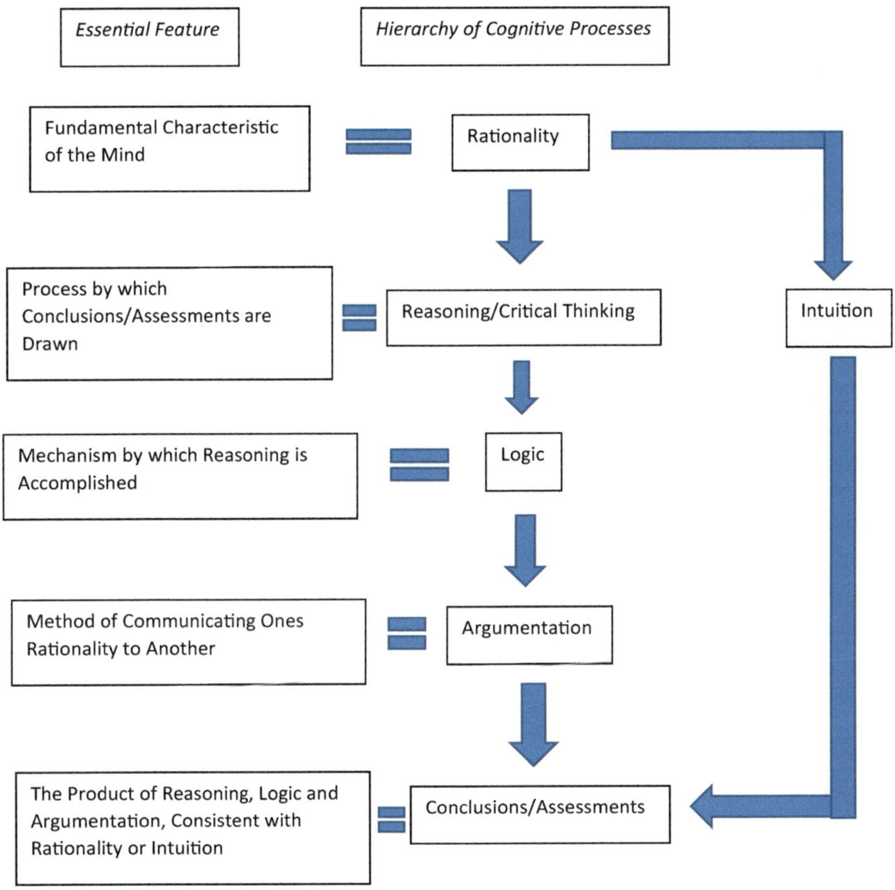

Fig. 2.1 A proposed hierarchy of cognition. Rationality, as a fundamental characteristic of the human mind, is the overarching domain. Each subsequent domain is a process by which the eventual conclusion or assessment is reached. These processes can be made overt by the arguer to the listener, by explanation or argument. The only process that lies outside the overt cognitive flow is intuition, as this is primarily an unconscious process by the individual, although, as least in my opinion, is part of the rationality domain

2.1 Rationality and Reason

2.1.1 Rationality from a Philosophical Perspective

Rationality and Reason have been the subjects of interest of philosophers since the time of Socrates and Plato in the Western tradition and perhaps before in Eastern traditions. There are numerous definitions of "rationality," being "rational," or having "reason." Although not a comprehensive list, there are a few definitions for the sake of illustration:

Reason is a mental facility or capacity in which reason might be regarded as coordinated with, but distinguished from, sensation, emotion or will. It is the power of the mind to think, understand and form judgments [3].

Reason is the capacity to consciously apply logic by drawing conclusions from new or existing information with the aim of seeking the truth [4, 5].

Rationality is the quality or state of being rational, that is, being based on or agreeable to reason [3].

Rationality is a matter of having psychological patterns that require coherence and unity[3] [6].

Rationality refers to a state of mind that could have arisen from the exercise of the faculty of reason, which is to say a coherent state of mind [7].

Rationality is connected with the analytical, systematizing and calculating functions of human reason, with an idea of method and algorithm, and thus is normative [8].

Reason is the ability to grasp, employ, or simply conform to certain principles that are usually conceived as *a priori* [9].

Rationality is both the "faculty of reason" (i.e., the ability to reason) and to a "state of mind" that could have arisen from the exercise of the faculty of reason—a coherent state of mind [10].

This list is certainly not comprehensive. They have the same general meaning, although they all differ in nuance. It is not my purpose here to analyze or debate these points (and there is still debate in the philosopher community), as I wish to approach this from the viewpoint of a practical healthcare professional. I am drawn to Shneider's theoretical model of rationality as a model of human behavior, thinking and human activity on the whole, realized in accordance with norms that find their substantiation in the procedures of analytical activity of human reason [8]. Therefore, for my intentions here, I define rationality as a *human mental framework that leads to the adoption of processes that result in well-founded beliefs and practices.* I believe that this definition requires further explanation. By "human mental framework," I mean whatever mental structure in which appropriate "processes," which can be either conscious or unconscious, such a thinking, calculating, using intuition or relying on a "gut feeling,", etc., will be recognized as a reliable method to reach accurate judgments. What I mean by "well-founded" is that a certain amount of evidence is used. The individual must believe that this evidence is either true, or close enough to true, that it is reliable enough to be used to come to a belief. The actual truthfulness or quality of this evidence is irrelevant for this purpose. By "beliefs," I mean any mental construct that the individual corresponds to some perceived or imagined phenomenon in the universe. These could be ideas, facts, theories, objects, occurrences, etc., which may or may not actually exist or have existed, but the individual believes them to exist or have existed. Last, what I mean by "practices" is that the individual will use this belief to act, or, at least, believe that

[3] I will be the first to admit that this is unsatisfactorily vague, but Kolodny does not come out with a clearly stated definition in his article [6].

they should act, in some manner, when needed. That is, because a believed phenomenon is occurring and that individual in his beliefs believes that that phenomenon requires some action on their part, then they will perform such action, or at least acknowledge that said action was needed, even if they did not perform the action. Broome [10] makes the normative statement, "Rationality requires you to intend *F* if you believe you ought to *F*." In this context, *structural rationality* is a property a person has when they have consistent beliefs and intentions, intend means to ends, etc.

Let us put this in the context of coming to beliefs and determining actions. Kolodny [6] makes the distinction between "objective" rationality, such that the rational thing to believe is whatever the evidence in fact supports and the rational thing to do is whatever the features of one's situation actually weigh in favor of doing, while "subjective" rationality tries to maintain consistency among one's attitudes. In my observations, it seems to me that people in general have a preference for subjective rationality, that is, maintaining consistency of their attitudes to protect their sense of self, over objective rationality (more on this in Chap. 3). Others make the distinction between "theoretical" reason, which involves questions that are more theoretical than practical, such as about explanation and prediction, and "practical" reason, which is concerned with matters of value and what is desirable to do, usually from a first-person point of view [11]. Aristotle proposed the concept of *phronesis*, which is practical wisdom (more on this in Chap. 7). Theoretical reason determines the truth of propositions and the reasons for beliefs. This will eventually lead to modifications of our beliefs. Practical reasons focus on the desirability or value of actions, which will then lead to a modification of our intentions [11]. From the point of view of the physician and the patient, their reason is to come to a belief (diagnosis, treatment, etc.), then to determine what best action to proceed on that belief (treatment, etc.). This action has been referred to as "instrumental" rationality [11], which requires one to take those means necessary in relation to the desired ends. For Shneider [8], any activity has a universal structure: the aim → the means → the result. Coupling this with the instrumental and structural accounts of rationality makes sense from the standpoint of medical practice. Namely, if the "ends" is the cure (or, at least, improvement) of the patient, the physician uses the best reasons they have to recommend a treatment. If this treatment fails, then the physician may determine that his reasons were wrong and may revise his beliefs. (More on this in Chap. 7.)

It is not enough for a rational individual to use reason—they must be aware that they are. Korsgaard [9] identifies "rational motivation" as the awareness that the considerations for which one acts is a reason for acting this way. For Shneider [8], an individual is rational in his actions if they are performed in accordance with some sensible reasons that make the aim pursued possible of attainment. However, this requires belief in these reasons. For Kolodny [6], rationality and irrationality apply not only the state of an individual (i.e., the set of their beliefs and processes for attaining beliefs) but also the processes that the individual uses. Specifically, we can judge a person as rational, not only by his state of mind at any given time but also by how that person transitions from one state to another. Broome [10] makes the distinction between "motivating reasons," which helps to explain why a person does something, and "normative reasons," which helps explain why a person ought to do something. What is fascinating here is that people, in general, are rational, yet they may not be consciously aware of the normative standards of what makes them rational. I suspect that this is a result of how the human brain/mind evolved.

This then leads to this issue of normativity. That is, what are the standards to judge an individual or an action is rational? As Korsgaard [9] states, when we say that an agent has a reason for what they do, we imply that there is a standard evaluation for their action and that the agent has gone some way toward meeting that standard. Kolodny [6] has the basic core requirements of rationality as such:

Positive core: Rationality requires an individual to have some belief, A, if that individual has conclusive reason to have A.

Negative core: Rationality requires an individual not to have A if that individual believes that they lack sufficient reasons to have A.

Beyond a belief, he further states that if one believes that one has conclusive reasons to do some action, *x*, then rationality requires one to at least intend to do *x* [6]. This is consistent with Broome's definition stated above. He further goes one to state that "Rationality does not *consist in* responding correctly to beliefs but it does *require* responding correctly to beliefs" [10]. The way I interpret this is that responding correctly to beliefs is not a component of the rationality structure, but in order to "act rationally", the belief must be acted upon. This begs the question of whether these reasons would be considered "good" or "sufficient" by everyone or only the individual acting on the beliefs. Because every individual most likely believes that the reasons they are using are good, then that individual would be rational, even if everyone around them thought the reasons were bad and, therefore, thought the individual was irrational. Shneider [8] does concede that the general norms that are applicable to determining the standards by which reasons and rationality are judged are imposed by the society of the individual. We will see how the predominate social culture will affect how an individual will determine what beliefs are rationally acceptable (Chap. 3). This will also affect the underlying theoretical foundations in both Western, allopathic medicine (Chap. 7), traditional indigenous medicine, and alternative and complementary medicine (Chap. 8). We will also see this rationality paradigm in medical research, as there are very strict standards in judging the validity of the results of a medical research study (Chap. 6).

2.1.2 Rationality from an Economics Perspective

Economists have long been interested in how individuals make the choice they make from the economic point of view. Communications professional are interested in this from a messaging point of view (which will be further discussed in Chap. 4). My intention here is not to provide a review of the immense economic literature on this field of study, which I am not qualified to do, but to simply highlight other theories of rationality.

In a book review, Rachlin [12] states that the standard economic theory has that the "rational" approach to a decision by an individual is to weigh all alternatives on all relevant dimensions and then to select the one with the highest weight, that is, "maximize the subjective utility." However, Rachlin [12] paraphrases Simon's 1956 article in *Psychological Review* which averred that an individual's practical ability to make the "perfect" rational decision would be too complex and take too long so as to be unworkable. So, the individual uses heuristics to make "satisfying" decisions with some less than perfect criteria, rather than a "maximal utility decision" due to constraints (e.g., of time and cognitive prowess) imposed on the individual. That is, the individual's rationality is "bounded."

In economic theory, how individuals make decisions for themselves comes under the rubric of "Rational Choice Theory." It should be said that Rational Choice Theory is not a single, fully developed theory but an amalgamation of several theories centered around the basic tenet of people making rational choices, and they do so by weighing their options on the basis of their preferences and beliefs [13]. We will see the concepts of "preferences and beliefs" being shaped by the social and cultural environment of the individual (Chaps. 3 and 4). Some examples of these theories are preference theory, game theory, expected utility theory, subjective utility theory, and so on [13]. However, all of these theories model the decision-maker as producing rational actions formulated in axiomatic terms, that is, an almost quantitative method of weighing choices and the likelihood of these choices achieving the ends desired (e.g., "expected utility" as mentioned above). However, as Herfield [13] has addressed, they all have short comings in regard to the *actual* behavior of humans. People's choices may not necessarily conform to the tenets of these theories. This may be due to limitations of cognitive capabilities (in addition to the actual intelligence of an individual, I as would add to this their cultural capabilities of what is possible, discussed in Chaps. 3, 4, 7, and 8) or incomplete information (judgments under uncertainty will be addressed in Chap. 7). People do not intuitively use Bayesian probability calculus in making probability judgments; and, for example, they may have an aversion to ambiguity. Last, none of the rational choice theories addresses why an individual has the ends they desire; that is, there is no accounting for why someone wants what they do. Moreover, there is no normative account of whether they *should* want what they do.

What this economic perspective seems to me is that understanding arguments related to decision-making cannot be made independent of human motivations. Unlike mathematics, for example, which has rules of conduct that must always be applied to perform mathematical functions properly, the "rules" of rational decision-making cannot always be determined by either the decision-maker or the critic. To truly understand someone as "rational" requires an understanding of their beliefs and preferences and how their thought is bounded by these (more on this is Chap. 3).

The difference between this view and the philosophical view previously discussed is not as great as it seems. They both rest on rationality as a structure that supports the mechanisms of decision-making. Whereas the philosophical view is satisfied if the individual is of coherent mind with respect to their beliefs and actions, the economic view tries to address how the individual determines whether their beliefs are actionable. That is, it is to say, it is one thing to believe something, but the "activation energy" to turn that into action will determine if that individual will act.

2.1.3 Rationality and Emotions

It seems contradictory to discuss emotions as a form of rationality. Much of conventional wisdom is to eliminate as much emotion as possible from rational choice. James Madison in *The Federalist Papers* wrote "...passion never fails to wrest the sceptre from reason." And Benjamin Franklin is quoted as saying "If Passion drives, let Reason hold the Reins." As true as it is that emotions may be a destructive force in human decision-making, others have proposed that emotions are essential in human rationality.

Emotions are an vital part of human reasoning. Greenspan [14] argued that "emotions are factors in practical reasoning." They do this by focusing the mind on certain "objects of thought and away from others." This then can provide "reasons for action," but still require "rational assessment and control." Kirman et al. [15] assert that "emotions can be 'useful' in making decisions" and "that they have evolved to be so" (more on this in Chap. 3). They feel that evolutionarily speaking, emotions have developed teleologically not only to trigger basic and urgent actions (e.g., fear from danger) but also to guide deliberations based on past learning and future anticipations (e.g., anxiety about what to expect). Certainly, in my experience as a practicing surgeon, the emotion of having to address newly heard "bad news" appears to focus the mind of the patient and their family. In the sense of emotion focusing the mind, as I will discuss later in the chapter in the section on intuition, how emotions can trigger the process of coming to an insight based on intuition.

It is, therefore, reasonable not to exclude human emotion from the assessment of rationality. Emotions may inspire, if not drive, other aspects of rationality, reasoning, logic, and intuition.

2.1.4 Summary of Rationality

In summary, I have made no attempt to provide a comprehensive discussion of rationality or to resolve the outstanding philosophical issues.[4] My approach for this book is that of the "instrumental" and "structural" view of rationality, applying the

[4] There are several books and treatises on rationality for interested readers, e.g., Broome J. *Normativity, Rationality and Reasoning*. Oxford: Oxford University Press, 2021, but there are many others.

normative standards of the medical profession in the Western tradition to the reasons used to determine beliefs and initiate actions. Having said that, I will acknowledge that there is a certain "black-box" nature to rationality—namely, in the way emotions and intuition function in the rational human. Rationality, therefore, holds the overarching position in the cognitive hierarchy (Fig. 2.1).

2.2 Reasoning/Critical Thinking

As with rationality, the definition of "reasoning" is difficult to find in a succinct and pithy form:

The Merriam-Webster dictionary has the definition of "1. The use of reason, especially the drawing of inferences or conclusions through the use of reason. 2. An instance of the use of reason: argument" [16].

Dictionary.com has the following reasoning: "1. the act or process of a person who reasons. 2. The process of forming conclusions, judgments, or inferences from facts or premises. 3. The reasons, arguments, proofs, etc., resulting from this process" [17].

The Cambridge Dictionary has it as "the process of thinking about something in order to make a decision" [18].

Although I find none of these definitions very precise,[5] they all essentially refer to a mental process going on in the mind of an individual trying to understand an issue. Johnson [19], in his book *Manifest Rationality* (more from this book in the Sect. 2.4 on Informal Logic and Arguments below), has reasoning as a part of a network of critical thinking, such as

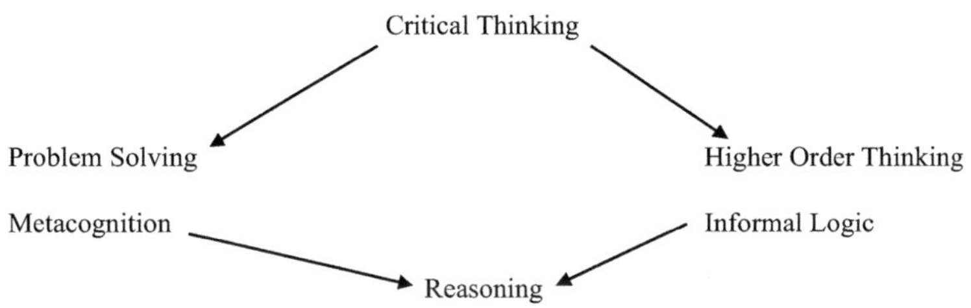

This then begs the question of what is "critical thinking"? The *Stanford Encyclopedia of Philosophy* describes it as an "educational goal" with competing definitions mostly centered on "differing conceptions of the same basic concept: careful thinking directed toward a goal" [20]. Bailen et al. [21] claim that critical thinking has three salient features:

[5] Interestingly, *The Encyclopedia of Philosophy* and *The Stanford Encyclopedia of Philosophy* do not have entries specifically addressing "reasoning" as a topic.

1. It is done for the purpose of making up one's mind about what to believe or do.
2. The person engaging in the thinking is trying to fulfill standards of adequacy and accuracy appropriate to the thinking.
3. The thinking fulfills the relevant standards to some threshold.

The "components" of the process are said to include observing (one notices something) and feeling (one feels puzzled or uncertain about something. Note how this is related to how emotions may function in rationality), wondering (one formulates a question to be addressed. Emotions, yet again), imagining (one thinks of possible answers), inferring (one works out what would be the case if a possible answer were assumed), knowledge (one uses stored knowledge of the subject matter to generate possible answers. This seems to be related to abductive logic, discussed below), experimenting (one designs and carries out an experiment or a systematic observation), consulting (one finds a source of information, gets the information, and makes a judgment on whether to accept it), identifying and analyzing arguments (one notices an argument and works out its structure and content as a preliminary to evaluating its strength), judging (one makes a judgment on the basis of accumulated evidence and reasoning), and deciding (one makes a decision on what to do or on what policy to adopt) [20].

If this sounds similar to the qualities of rationality, well, it does to me as well. Therefore, as with rationality, a specific definition of "reasoning" appears to be wanting.[6] That being said, the qualities and characteristics described above are certainly acceptable and would be familiar to most people who are trying to come to some conclusion or decision. For Walton [22], reasoning is what is done before you argue and your argument expresses your best reasoning. He provides a useful list of the types of reasoning:

Monolectical—a single individual reasoning alone to come to some conclusion.
Dialectical—two or more people reasoning together. (This allows for immediate criticism to improve the argument.)
Alethic—denoting modalities of truth, such as necessity, contingency, possibility and impossibility.
Epistemic—related to knowledge and the degree of its validation.
Practical—related to everyday affairs.
Theoretical—related to theoretical issues not directly related to everyday affairs.

Obviously, there is some overlap among these types of reasoning, but it does give a good account of the breadth of reasoning.

[6] I must confess that I struggled with "rationality" and "reasoning." The concepts are so familiar that they almost seem like common sense. However, when I delved into more specific information to obtain some level of precision in definitions, much was what was written appeared to me circular. That is, many of the definitions of "rationality" include description using the words "reason," "reasoning," "logic," etc., and similarly for "reasoning," including the words "rational," "reasons," "logic,", etc. Although my definitions are perhaps sophomoric by philosophers' standards, I believe that they will serve the intentions of this book.

Therefore, for the purposes of this book, I define reasoning as a process by which well-founded beliefs and practices are drawn to be consistent with my definition of rationality. That is, as a matter of practicality, it is an inferential process that takes as inputs some attitudes of a subject and yields as output the formation or modification of other attitudes [11]. Therefore, although I again acknowledge that all this is not as precise as we would like to be in medicine, I assert, as others have, that reasoning is required for rationality (Fig. 2.1).

I have used the term "reason" in two ways. The first is as a synonym of "rationality." The second is as a proposition related to some fact, bit of evidence, idea, item, observation, situation, intention, etc., to be used to infer some conclusion or belief. From heretofore in the book, reason will only take on the second meaning. Rationality will be used only in the sense defined previously. In addition, in colloquial English, "reason" can also be used to denote a "cause." I will later discuss causation more in Chap. 5. Needless to say, in this book, reason is never used as a synonym for cause.

Last, the preceding discussion was intended to be descriptive in nature, rather than laying out any normative standards. It is obvious that to achieve conclusions that are as close to approximating the observed phenomena, "good" reasons (i.e., the closest to the truth) would be more likely to achieve a reliable conclusion than "bad" reasons. However, this is dependent on the individual actually wanting to achieve that type of approximation (more on this in Chap. 3).

What I hoped to establish in the foundation that both the physician and the patient have the capacity and the mechanisms to come to conclusions about diagnoses and decisions about treatment options. Making explicit what these mechanisms are is the subject of the next section.

2.3 Logic[7]

Everyone believes that they are "logical." However, what is logic? In a broad sense, logic is simply a mechanism of reasoning. From a more academic sense, logic investigates and classifies the structure of statements and arguments, both through the study of formal systems of inference and through the study of arguments in a natural language, but is not concerned with the psychological processes connected with thought or emotions [23]. Hodges [24] prefers to define logic as the "study of consistent sets of beliefs," acknowledging that others "define logic as the study of

[7] The history of logic extends over many centuries over many regions. Although a narration of this history is beyond the scope of this book, it is worth noting that in the Western civilization tradition, the study of logic has been traditional thought to have started with Aristotle and passed on to medieval Europe through Islamic philosophers, especially Al-Kindi and Avicenna. There was a robust study of logic in the classical Islamic world, India and China. For the interested reader, see Lejewski C, Staal JF, Graham AC, Reschar N. History of Logic. *The Encyclopedia of Philosophy,* Vol. 4, pp. 513–571.

valid arguments." I do not necessarily see a conflict between these definitions, and, I believe, they do describe what is actually done by logic. Therefore, I assert that rational individuals who reason use logic, although this may not be the overt, formal logic that modern logicians use.

As previously mentioned, logic is a method of constructing propositions or premises such that conclusions can be reached. It is also a method of analyzing arguments to determine if they are valid and sound. Although someone with explicit training in logic can use this training to construct their arguments, this training is not necessary, as it seems most humans have an intrinsic capacity to understand logical construction in a natural language [2]. From the analysis aspect, it is hoped that "deconstructing" arguments can relieve the logical structure used and, therefore, determine if the conclusion is valid. Therefore, it has a normative function. Clearly, from the point of view of the physician and the patient, being able to understand arguments is essential in determining the best treatment option.

Having defined what logic is in a general sense, are there "types" of logic? If so, what are they? And, which are the most useful for our purpose? Not surprisingly, there has been much effort expended by philosophers on this issue. It is beyond the scope of this chapter to discuss all types (or even most); however, for the sake of reference, Table 2.1 lists the types of logic I could determine exist and a brief description of each. Logic, in general, tries to reduce the subjects (i.e., premises or propositions) of an argument to abstract or universal variables so that it can specify the essential universal relationships that make arguments sound. The weakness, which is recognized by proponents of "relevance" logic, is that the specifics of the variables are essential in understanding the relationships between the variables (more on this later).

Although I do not intend to try to explain all of the types of logic listed in Table 2.1, a few do deserve expounding. *Deductive logic* is probably the one with which most people are familiar. If properly constructed, if the premises are true, then the conclusion has to be true. This is best shown with an Aristotelian syllogism:

If all A are B
And all B are C
Then, all A are C

Another way to think of this is that deduction goes from the general to the specific. That is, if we accept the facts pertaining to all items in a class stated in the premises, then we must accept the fact of the specific item that is a member of the class.

Inductive logic was introduced to account for premises that are not absolutely true or false, that is, having some probability of being true. In fact, this is the realm in which most medical arguments happen. For example:

Ninety percent of patients with acute appendicitis will present with acute right lower quadrant pain.

This patient had acute right lower quadrant pain.

This patient has a 90% chance of having appendicitis.

Table 2.1 Types of logic

Type	Description
Abductive	A type of inference which creates a proposition which "explains" observed phenomena, without knowing if such a proposition is true. A process which suggests the something "may be" true.
Combinatory	Branch of mathematical logic that analyzes certain processes, such as substitution, which are associated with variables.
Deductive	A type of logical inference such that if the premises/propositions are true, the conclusion *must* be true. That is, following from the general to the specific.
Deontic	"Logic of obligation": the formulation and systemization of principles as that nothing can be obligatory and forbidden at once and that whatever we are committed to do by what is obligatory is itself obligatory.
Formal	The abstract study of propositions, statements, or assertively used sentences and of deductive arguments into the structure they embody.
Inductive	A type of logic inference such that the premises/propositions are not known to be absolutely true, but perhaps probably so, so that the conclusion is not guaranteed to be true but is probably so. Also a process of deriving reliable generalizations from observations so that the premises of an argument are believed to support the conclusion, but not necessarily so. That is, following from the specifics to the general.
Informal	A logic to be used in improving "real-life" thinking, reasoning, and arguments by combining accounts of argument, evidence, proof and justification with an emphasis on the usefulness of the analysis in "real-life" arguing.
Intuitionistic/ constructive	A system of symbolic logic that differs from the systems used for classical logic by using the notion of constructive proof, which is a proof that demonstrates the existence of a mathematical objects by providing a method for creating the object.
Many-valued	Logic in which there are more values to a proposition than "true" and "false" (i.e., rejection of the law of the excluded middle).
Modal	The logical features of necessity, possibility, impossibility and related concepts.
Predicate	Analyzes simple sentence forms and sentence connectives, as well as quantifiers.
Propositional/ sentential	A logical system in which formulae representing propositions can be formed by combining atomic propositions using logical connections and a system of proof rules that allow certain formulae to be established by theorems.
Relevance	A kind of non-classical logic that requires the antecedent and consequent of an implication to be relevantly related.
Symbolic	Uses symbolic abstractions that capture the formal features of logical inference. Usually associated with formal and deductive logic.

Note, we are not saying that the patient has appendicitis, only that they have a 90% chance. Another aspect of inductive logic has to do with making general principles from individual observations. This is also very common in the generation of medical knowledge (more on this in Chap. 6). To use the above example pertaining to appendicitis, physicians have made innumerable observations of patients with acute right lower quadrant abdominal pain. They noted that approximately 90% of these patients have appendicitis as a cause. Therefore, as a general principle, if a patient presents with acute right lower quadrant pain, appendicitis must be considered in the differential diagnosis.

Abductive logic was first proposed by C. S. Pierce in the nineteenth century [25]. In this type of logic, which some consider a type of inductive logic, a person infers an explanation for observations. Let us return to the example of appendicitis as a cause of abdominal pain. In Chap. 1, we mentioned that Morgagni developed the insight that the "morbid anatomy" he was observing in deceased, ill patients was somehow related to the illness from which these patients were suffering [26]. In 1886, Reginald Fitz coined the term "appendicitis" and recommended appendectomy as the cure [27].[8] That is, he recognized the inflamed appendix as the best explanation for acute right lower quadrant pain, hence, abduction.

Last, there is *informal logic*. This is distinct from formal logic in that formal logic rejects ambiguities in propositions and defines each proposition as being either true or false, reducing the logical analysis to the logical structure of the propositions and the conclusion [24]. While informal logic accepts that not all everyday argumentation can be reduced in such a manner without losing nuance and meaning. Its task is to develop nonformal normative standards, criteria, procedures for the analysis, interpretation, evaluation, criticism, and constructions of argumentation in everyday discourse [19].

Although these descriptions are useful in categorizing the types of applications in the analysis of arguments, there is some obvious overlap among the concepts of these logical types. In addition, it is apparent that none of these logical analytical techniques should be dismissed because some techniques would certainly be more useful for some problems than others. This is also the position of Govier [28].

Let us start by stating that any logical analysis of arguments using natural language[9] is to determine exactly what is meant by the words in the sentence and the sentence as a whole. Let us return to our vignette from Chap. 1. The patient comes into the office with a chief complaint. They express what that complaint is. Some individuals are very good at expressing what they are experiencing, while others have difficulty finding the right words. In this instance, the patient complains of "heartburn." It is then the physician's job to determine if what the patient means by "heartburn" is what the physician understands heartburn to be. This is crucial, as the differential diagnosis of heartburn includes esophageal disease other than GERD, nonesophageal disease such as cardiac ischemia, and upper abdominal disease such as peptic ulcer disease or biliary colic (i.e., pain from the gallbladder). This is where the physician through questioning on the character of the symptom comes to understand what the patient means by the symptom. In this manner, the physician is trying

---

[8] Interestingly, the first appendectomy recorded was performed by Claudius Amyand on an 11-year-old boy who had an inguinal hernia with a fecal fistula in the scrotum. The appendix was located in the hernia and was perforated by a pin [21]. It is interesting that the first appendectomy was not for appendicitis. The term "Amyand's hernia," meaning an appendix in an inguinal hernia sac, is still used to this day.

[9] I am going to limit my discussion to natural language logical structures. There is a very large body of literature on logic that foregoes actual words for symbols. In Table 2.1, these logics are the formal, symbolic, predicate, intuitionistic, combinatory, and others I may not have mentioned. Having said this, I will use some symbolic forms to express some points.

to eliminate ambiguity in the patient's statement. As Hodges [24] points out, ambiguity can either be *lexical* (having to when a word has more than one meaning) or *structural* (when a phrase can be interpreted in more than one way). A particular problem is ambiguity in predicates (i.e., descriptors of nouns used in declaratives statements, especially having to do with number) may affect that soundness of an argument. Overall, the physician's cognitive process is narrowing the differential diagnosis (see Fig. 1.1).

Although there are multiple ways to do a formal logical analysis, for the sake of example, I will try to follow the method as espoused by Hodges [24], which is clearly deductive in nature. In his method, he starts by defining a "declarative sentence as a sentence which can be put in place of '*x*' in the sentence, 'Is it true that *x*.'" Using a medical example, the statement 'blood is red' is a declarative statement since we can ask 'Is it true that blood is red.' Declarative sentences are true in certain situations and not true in other situations. For example, the sentence 'blood is neon orange' is a declarative sentence that is not true. For Hodges, *phrases* refer to things in certain situations. The truth or untruth of a sentence commonly depends on the references of its parts, which may change from one situation to another [24]. This may seem tediously elementary, but it is important to be precise with our definitions.

Additionally, for Hodges [24], declarative sentences are either true or false—there is no middle ground.[10] Therefore, each sentence has a "truth value." Moreover, any argument is a set of sentences that can be tested for consistency of the statements and the validity of the argument. One of the methods is the "semantic tableaux" method. I will not go into the details of this method (the interested reader can find a discussion of it in Hodges), but the "branches" of the tableaux are closed when an inconsistency is reached. If all of the branches are closed, then the argument is said to be inconsistent. If one or more branches are open, then the argument is said to be consistent. An argument is then said to be valid if there is no possible situation in which the premises are all true and the conclusion not true. This is referred to as *reduction ad absurdum.* Although this method works in the mechanical sense, for long, complex arguments, it rapidly becomes unwieldly. I, for one, cannot see its practicality in a medical encounter.

A second method Hodges [24] describes is "truth-tables." To do this more efficiently, we can substitute sentence variables, e.g., using the Greek letter ϕ, for the phrase "blood is bright red when oxygenated." Therefore, for example, the sentence "blood is bright red when oxygenated, but dark purple when deoxygenated" can be simply written as "ϕ but ψ." This will then yield the following truth table:

[10] This notion of statements being true or false is the concept of the "law of the excluded middle", which dates to Aristotle. This law is specifically rejected by proponents of "many-valued" logic. There are also potential difficulties when applying it to statements of probability. For example, given the circumstances, the sentence "This patient has an 80% chance of appendicitis," would be a true statement, but anyone hearing would understand that the patient may not have appendicitis. Therefore, its truthfulness may not help in decision-making.

ϕ	ψ	ϕ but ψ
True	True	True
True	False	False
False	True	False
False	False	False

That is, the statement is only true when both sentence variables are true. Hodges [24] does make the caveat that not all sentences have truth tables and some also have incomplete truth tables. Again, although it is possible to create truth tables for any sentences used in an argument, it does become quite apparent that this method will become quite impractical for more complex arguments.

In fact, the method may be misleading. Hodges [24] uses "interpretation substitutes" for declarative sentences by substituting a capital letter for the sentence. (He acknowledges, however, that this can lead to hidden inconsistencies, but I will not address that here.) Let us return to the clinical vignette in Chap. 1. Our patient had heartburn. Let us substitute "Patient has heartburn" with H. In the history of the present illness, the patient could have had a myriad of other symptoms, e.g., regurgitation, dysphagia, chest pain, abdominal pain, cough, wheezing, pyrosis, and weight loss, among others. If these symptoms are taken as conjunctions, i.e., heartburn (H), regurgitation (R), dysphagia (D), chest pain (P), abdominal pain (A), etc., we can obtain a symbolic logical sentence of:

$$(H \wedge R \wedge D \wedge P \wedge A \wedge \ldots)$$

$$\text{where} \wedge \text{means ``and.''}$$

Certainly, a truth table can be created on whether the patient does have these symptoms. Similarly, the physical exam findings, as well as the laboratory, images and physiological studies, can be added to this "as" well. The physician then makes the diagnosis of GERD, such that:

$$(H \wedge R \wedge \ldots \wedge M) \rightarrow G$$

$$\text{where} \rightarrow \text{means ``entails.''}$$

Where M would stand for, say results of the pH monitoring and G for GERD. This would be read such that if whatever was within the () was present, then GERD would be entailed. Now, I will completely acknowledge that I may have the logical structure of this wrong, and a trained logician would laugh at my errors. Nevertheless, it certainly appears to me that this is blatantly not the way that physicians come to a diagnosis; and, if they did, it certainly would not guarantee the truthfulness of the diagnosis. That is, it fails both in a descriptive and normative sense. Hence, the use of formal logical analysis is both impractical and, most likely, unreliable for the purposes of analyzing how medical arguments are actually constructed. This is not to say that formal deductive logic (or any of the other more formal or symbolic logics identified in Table 2.1) is not useful for certain purposes. For example, mathematically based investigations, decision sciences, Boolean-based computer algorithms, and artificial intelligence, to name a few, are no doubt dominated by formal deductive logic (some of this will be explored in Chap. 9) and rightfully so. Nevertheless, what I am addressing here is more everyday human-to-human communication about their thinking.

It may be that the fundamental issue with the use of formal logic for complex, naturally expressed arguments is similar to the issue of reductionism in biology. The concept of reductionism is that the behaviors of more complex systems can be reduced to understanding the smaller scale systems that make up the more complex system [29]. For example, explaining the physiology of an organism by the quantum mechanical predictions of its constituent atoms. Logical structures are relationships among semantic items (words/phrases). There is a difference between these connotations and the actual physical relationship that these phrases denote. For example, the actual relationship between blood flow into and out of the spleen through arteries and veins, especially given the variability of flow from time to time as opposed to static logical relationships of semantic variables in propositions used in symbolic form. Similarly, Govier [28] lodges a similar criticism of deduction for real-world arguments—namely, deductivism (formal logic) obtains its rigorousness at the cost of being applicable to real arguments. That is, it is nearly impossible to translate all the nuanced points of real arguments into the formal structure of symbolic logic without losing at least some of the meaning of these points. It, therefore, seems to me that the more fruitful approach to the analysis of real medical arguments would be with informal logic.

2.4 Informal Logic and Argumentation

This is section I will discuss argumentation, the construction of arguments, their analysis with informal logic and why this would better reflect both how actual reasoning is done in medical practice and as a way to assess the validity of such arguments. That is, I will address both descriptive and normative aspects of medical discourse. Much of what follows comes from Johnson's manifest rationality [19], which I found to be quite helpful in thinking about argumentation and persuasion. I also owe some of the more practical aspect of argument as a discourse among participants from Weston's *A Rulebook for Arguments* [30].

Let us start with more precise definitions. I contend that argumentation is a fundamental method of communicating the rationality of one's position to someone else. Actually, that someone else can even be yourself, as you try to reason though a problem. Johnson's [19] definition of an *argument* is an "intellectual product that seek to persuade rationally." This definition is somewhat different than mine in that I assert that an argument can be used to come to a "truth" whether you persuade someone else or not. However, this is consistent with Johnson's view that argumentation is a public discourse.

2.4.1 Arguments Versus Explanations

Let us start by distinguishing between an "argument" and an "explanation." One may feel that this distinction is a rather trivial one. Nevertheless, they actually share a very important function. What is this function? Again, let us start with definitions. We have already defined what an argument is, but what of explanation? Generally, an "explanation" is a language-based description of sequences in the occurrence of a phenomenon. This is usually merely recounting what is known about the phenomenon. It does not purport to claim new information is being generated, although the information may be new to the listener of the explanation. It is an attempt to make something clear or understandable.[11] For example, in the vignette recounted in Chap. 1, when the physician speaks to the patient on the relationship between acid reflux and the patient's heartburn symptoms, this is an explanation. The physician is making no new discoveries. An argument, on the other hand, is a sequence of propositions culminating in a conclusion. This conclusion purports to have created new information, not only to the listener but, perhaps, the rest of humankind. Although these distinctions between argument and explanation are real and important, they can also share a similar purpose—namely, persuasion. The physician, by explaining the disease process to the patient, is also hoping to persuade the patient who he has the disease. Therefore, I will sometimes refer to explanations such as arguments as tools of persuasion.

2.4.2 Arguments as a Method of Deriving New Truths

I am going to make the distinction between arguments that are used to arrive at a new truth or expand the corpus of knowledge of a subject from arguments merely trying to persuade an individual to change their beliefs or take on some action, although, of course, these arguments asserting new truths hope to persuade others as well. Much of the literature on argumentation addresses the latter, but in the realm of science, including medical science, the former is the stock-in-trade of scientific or medical investigators. In particular, these issues will be further discussed in Chap. 6.

Johnson [19] has created the following network to proceed from reasoning to argument (the reader will remember the network he created from critical thinking to reasoning in the Sect. 2.2):

---

[11] From a philosophical point of view, an explanation is actually more complicated than this. This centers around an explanation as an elucidation of causation. There is controversy between those taking a "realist" position of a literal description of external reality and those of an "epistemic" position of the processes or entities described in an explanation that do not necessarily exist in any literal sense but are simply useful for organizing the human experience (see Mayes GR. Theories of explanation. In: *Internet Encyclopedia of Philosophy*. https://iep.utm.edu, last accessed June 7, 2022). For my purposes, these different viewpoints are not important.

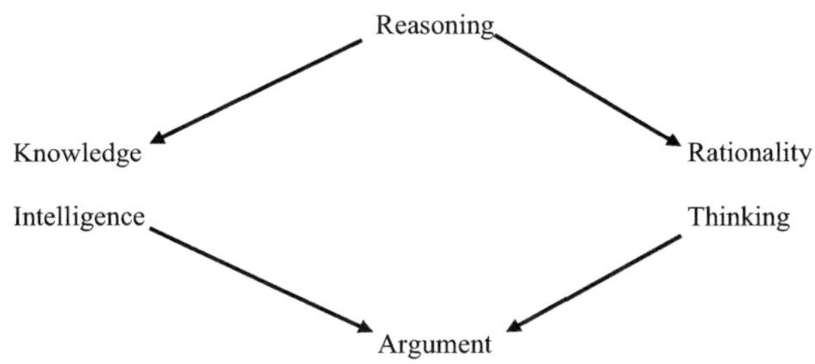

As noted previously, as with much of the writing on rationality and reasoning, there is some circularity in the network. Nevertheless, it serves as a basis for obtaining the ability to develop an argument.

I am not going to address Johnson's greater theory of argumentation, although this is interesting, it is beyond the purpose of this book. Nevertheless, Johnson's position that an argument is more than just the construction of premises to a conclusion. This, he refers to as the illative core. His view is more of a public dialectic; it includes the initial presentation of the illative core, a "dialectic tier" of objections, criticisms and responses, and finally "manifest rationality" where the whole process of the argument and its revisions produces a public agreement of the conclusions. This is a useful framework to assess argument both for the sake of generating new knowledge and in the process of the physician presenting a diagnosis and treatment options to the patient. Moreover, this is exactly how a medical research article is generated, submitted for publication, peer-reviewed, revised and resubmitted (more on this in Chap. 6). However, for now, let us address the illative core.

My view of the basic structure of the illative core is illustrated in Fig. 2.2. In this model, there are a series of premises that are related in some way that can be logically defined, the sum of which leads to a conclusion. In my view, the mechanisms of the relationships can be deductive at times (i.e., completely deterministic), inductive at times (i.e., stochastic) and what some informal logicians call conductive at times (i.e., the weight or preponderance of evidence), depending on the premises and what would produce the most sound argument. Although I do not want to address specific issues pertaining to conductivism, for the sake of clarity, Johnson [19] quotes Goveir [28] that

> A conductive argument is "that sort of reasoning in which (1) a conclusion about some individual case (2) is drawn nonconclusively (3) from one or more premises about the same case (4) without any appeal to other cases."

Although arguments are constructed to reach a conclusion, these premises may not necessarily be arranged sequentially. That is, the conclusion by be stated before the premises, or other such arrangements to maximize it persuasiveness. With this background, let us look more closely at the illative core.

There are three basic structural components to an argument: the premises, the relationship among the premises, and the conclusion. For Johnson [19], the premises of an argument must satisfy three criteria: they need to be relevant, sufficient

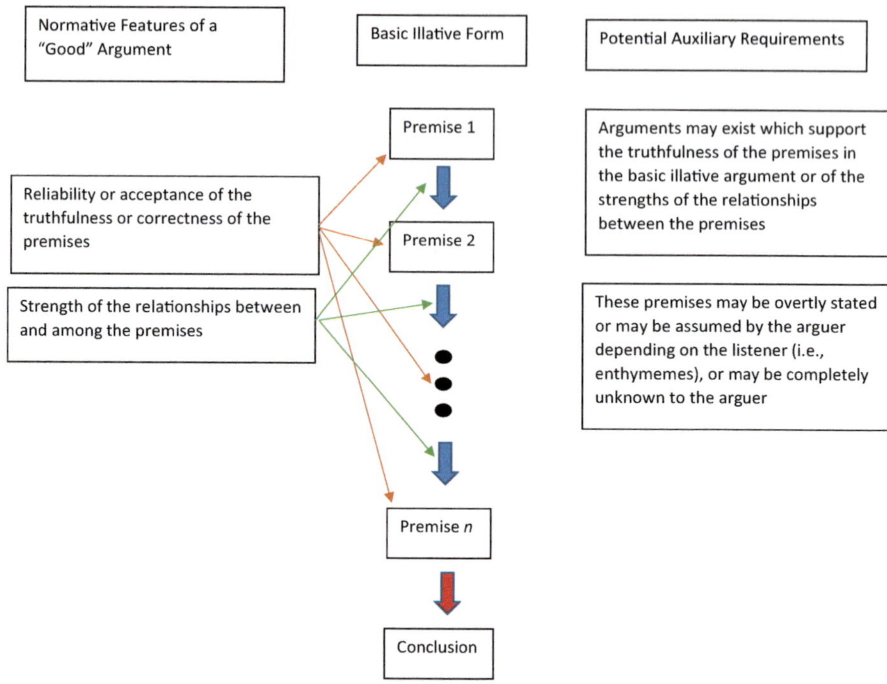

Fig. 2.2 The basic illative form of an argument. The basic form is that of premises having some relationship with each other that creates a logical structure, leading, either deductively or inductively, to a conclusion. This structure is independent of the truthfulness of the premises and the strengths of their relationships. Therefore, a "good" argument requires that the premises be reliably true, or true enough, and that the relationships are strong enough that the connections between the premises can form a logical structure. Sometimes, these premises may be the result of prior arguments demonstrating their truthfulness, in which case, these arguments will have to be agreed upon by the listener. Some premises are considered so basic, as there is no need to state them; these are enthynemes in the parlance of logicians. However, there are some relevant premises that are unknown to either the arguer or listener, such that the material truth of the conclusion would be in doubt even if they are unaware of it

and acceptable. The *relevance* criteria is a basic requirement. For a premise to be relevant to an argument, it must have some tangible connection to the topic in question. This is a pragmatic property not related to semantics or syntax, but it should be acknowledged that the normative criteria for a premise to be relevant have not been well developed [31]. Nevertheless, it seems to me from a practical standpoint that the propositions made in an argument should have some relevance to the topic of the argument. Johnson [19] expounds on its characteristics. One is that relevance can apply to an individual premise, a set of premises or the entire collective of premises. Another is that it is a matter of degree—some premises would be more relevant than others. Last, it is a "dialectical" property; that is, it is something decided upon by the arguer and the listener. The *sufficiency* requirement is that the premises must provide sufficient support for the conclusion. It is a pragmatic property of the premise set. Like with relevance, it is a matter of degrees. Finally, the *acceptability* criteria are based on whether the listener finds that premises acceptable for the argument. Johnson [19] makes the point that acceptability is that of *rational acceptance* rather than acceptance based on some inchoate belief (although this is, no doubt, how many individuals will determine whether a premise is acceptable, as will be discussed in Chaps. 3 and 4). Acceptability applies to each premise individually and is also a dialectical criterion with the interaction between the arguer and the listener. Having established these criteria, how are they applied to the illative core?

Returning to Fig. 2.2, the column to the left states the normative features of a "good" argument. The top box states that in concordance with Johnson's criteria on premises, reliability or acceptance of the truthfulness or correctness of the premises is a main feature. Whether the premises are true may be important with respect to whether the conclusion is physically true but may be irrelevant as to whether the argument is persuasive. The column to the right of the basic illative form states the potential "auxiliary" requirements for the premises. Namely, the premises used in this argument were at one time conclusions of another argument that established their truth. In medical research articles as well as professional discourse among physicians, reference to published articles supporting their argument is nearly universal. Another feature of a good argument is the strength of the relevance among the premises and the conclusion. Govier [28] suggests that the strength of the connections between the premises and the conclusion of an argument is on a spectrum of degrees of no connection whatsoever to an unassailable linkage. As with the premises, these relationships may have been previously established, acceptable to the arguer and listener, or completely contested. Last, some premises may be assumed by the arguer and even the listener (i.e., enthymemes), which require no overt expression, or they may be assumed (ignored or unknown) by one but not the other and will, therefore, lead to confusion. Nevertheless, agreement between the arguer and listener on the relevance, sufficiency and acceptability of the premises and their relationships may actually produce wrong conclusions from the standpoint of what is the actual situation in the universe.[12] Specifically, arguments can be internally consistent and sound with valid conclusions from the standpoint of the illative form but still be materially (i.e., with respect to what actually occurs in the universe) wrong due to missing premises (i.e., relevant facts/premises either unknown by the arguer or unknown to humankind), which will change the logical relationships and relevancy of the premises used. Nevertheless, this does not necessarily mean it was a bad argument.

Having said this, Johnson [19] does provide his view of the properties of a "conclusive" argument:

1. Its premises would have to be unimpeachable or uncriticizable.

[12] What I am speaking about here is an argument, usually through some type of research, where a conclusion is made about some phenomenon in the universe. The argument is constructed with words and grammar, which reflects a mental model corresponding to the observed universe. Then, of course, there is the actual universe that proceeds unhindered by the mental models of humans.

2. The connections between the premises and the conclusion would have to be unimpeachable or the strongest possible.
3. A conclusive argument is one that can successfully and rationally resist every attempt at legitimate criticism.
4. The argument would be regarded as conclusive by the listener(s).

Having said this, an argument does not have to be conclusive to be a good or an effective argument.[13]

2.4.3 Arguments as a Method to Come to a Decision

In the previous section, I discussed arguments as a method to come to new knowledge; in this section, I will discuss arguments as a means of coming to a decision, specifically, a decision to act in some way. What I mean by "act" is some activity that will produce some real-world consequences for the one who acts and those whom the act may affect. Additionally, I am addressing actions that are not those that are "morally" obligatory, rather those that lead to some perceived tangible benefits. This comes under the rationality rubric of one "ought to do" of Kolondy [6], the aims-means-results view of Shneider [8], the "enkrasia" principle of Broome [10], and the "instrumental rationality" of Wallace [11].

Let us take as an example inguinal hernia repair. Although the details and nuances of inguinal hernia are not particularly relevant for this discussion, what should be known is that an inguinal hernia is a defect in the transversalis fascia in the inguinal canal either through Hesselbach's triangle (for "direct" hernias) or the internal inguinal ring such that the abdominal wall is unable to retain the abdominal viscera. This can lead to pain or discomfort for the patient, a visible bulge, and, rarely, the devastating consequence of bowel incarceration and strangulation. Therefore, these are frequently repaired.[14] For the surgeon, the instrumental rationality of this problem is clear: the aim is to restore the patient to normal anatomic function, the means are with some type of operation, and the result is elimination of the hernia defect. In 1989, I published a paper reviewing the arguments used to recommend specific operative hernia repairs in surgical textbooks published from 1889 to 1986 [32]. There were three different types of arguments found in the textbooks: description of procedures without justification, description of procedures with justification based on anatomically based arguments, and description of procedures with justification based on results of the published operations. Of the articles references in these

[13] A major area of study in informal logic is the study of fallacies. One definition of a fallacy is an argument which ought not persuade a rational person of its conclusion (see Kahane H. *Logic and Contemporary Rhetoric: The Use of Reasoning in Everyday Life, 6th ed.* Belmont, CA:Wadsworth, 1992). I will not address the issues of fallacies as it is beyond the scope of this book, but I will discuss why fallacies may be believed by some people in Chap. 4.

[14] The interested reader can find chapters on inguinal hernia and its repair in every standard surgical textbook.

textbooks pertaining to inguinal hernia repair, there were five different types of arguments: justification based on an anatomically based argument, justification based on the results of a single case report, justification based on a single observational cohort of patients with a particular type of repair, justification based on a comparison of two or more observational cohorts, and justification based on a comparison of two or more repair types in a single study.

The anatomic argument more or less follows this basic reasoning. Let us use the Bassini repair as an example. In a Bassini repair, the hernia sac (which is the lining of peritoneum protruding through the defect) may or may not be excised, and the transversus abdominis aponeurosis (the broad tendon of the third most inner layer of the lateral abdominal wall) is sutured to the inguinal ligament (the tendon of the outer most muscle of the abdominal wall at the inferior aspect of the Hesselbach's triangle), covering the defect in the transversalis fascia (the inner most layer of connective tissue adherent to the peritoneum) Fig. 2.3 shows the before and after illustrations of the defect and repair. The basic form of an anatomic argument would be

To restore functional anatomy, the hernia defect must be covered by strong tissue.

The most available strong tissue is the transversus abdominis aponeurosis.

To fix this tissue over the hernia defect, it must be sutured to the inguinal ligament.

Therefore, an effective inguinal hernia repair is suturing the transversus abdominis aponeurosis to the inguinal ligament.

This is a fairly straightforward deduction and certainly follows the illative form illustrated in Fig. 2.2. However, a critic (in Johnson's sense of an argument being a public dialectical process) would say the problem with this argument is that the hernia will be repaired at the end of the operation, but it may not stay repaired for the life of the patient. Note that this criticism does not attack the soundness or validity of the argument, it proposes that the argument has missing premises. This is where the second type of argument adds additional relevant premises to the first, which is the case report:

A patient's inguinal hernia was repaired with the Basini technique

The patient recovered from the operation without incidence

The hernia had not recurred at the last follow-up of x years since repair.

Therefore, an effective inguinal hernia repair is suturing the transversus abdominis aponeurosis to the inguinal ligament.

This now addresses a missing premise that would have been identified by a critic—namely, how good is the repair? However, another critic may say that is all well and good for this patient, but what of others? Hence, the third type of argument of an observational cohort,[15] again adding premises to the argument.

y number of patients had their inguinal hernias repaired with the Bassini technique

After x years, only z patients had recurrence of their hernias.

Therefore, an effective inguinal hernia repair is suturing the transversus abdominis aponeurosis to the inguinal ligament.

[15] Previously, this would be referred to as a case series.

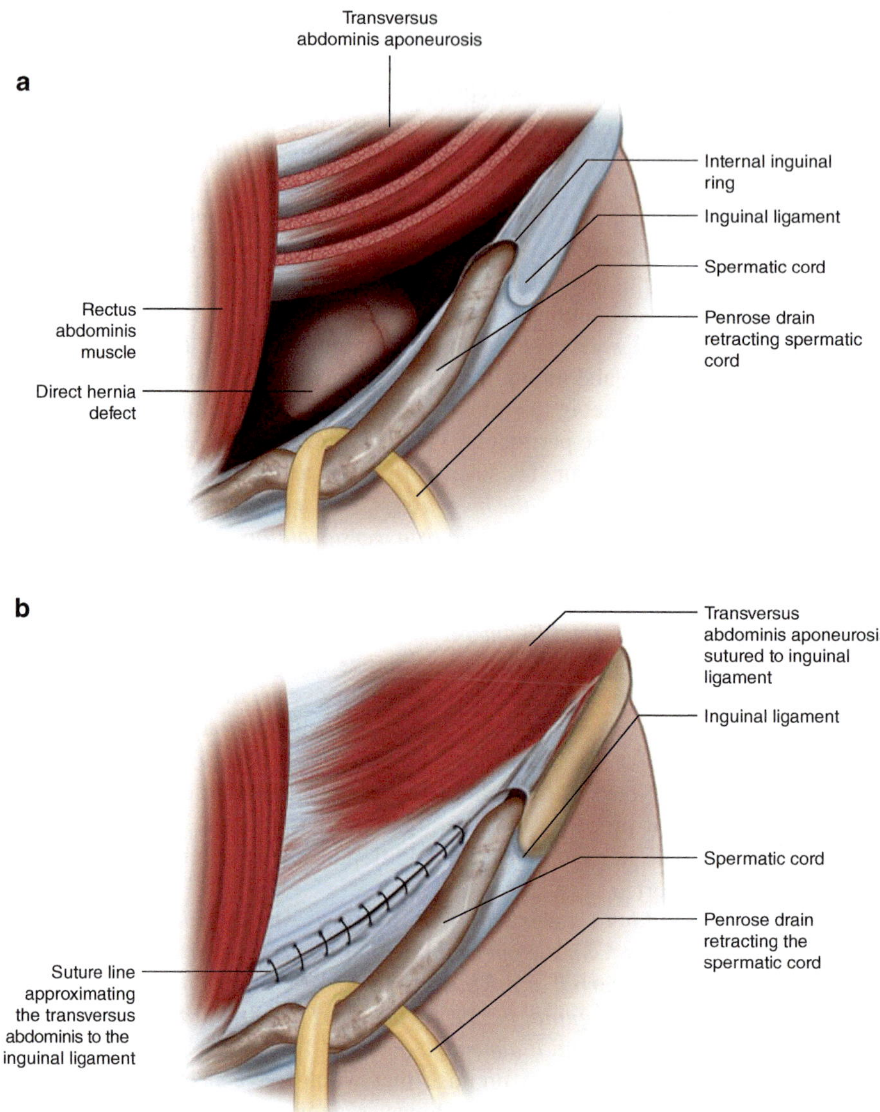

Fig. 2.3 (**a**) An illustration of the anatomic defect involved with a direct inguinal hernia. (**b**) An illustration of the Bassini repair whereby the aponeurosis of the transversus abdominal muscle is approximated to the inguinal ligament with suture

Therefore, this type of argument does show that this type of repair is good for more than a single patient. However, again, a critic would point out, but is this better than another type of repair, say, the Shouldice repair? This is where the fourth type of argument was used—namely, comparisons of the results of different types of hernia repairs.

y_1 number of patients had their inguinal hernias repaired with the Bassini technique

y_2 number of patients had their inguinal hernias repaired with the Shouldice technique

After x_1 years, z_1 number of Bassini repair patients had a recurrence of their hernias

After x_2 years, z_2 Shouldice repair patients had hernia recurrence.

$z_1/y_1 > z_2/y_2$, that is, there was a higher frequency of recurrence in the Bassini patients

Therefore, Shouldice repair is a more effective inguinal hernia repair.

This addresses the criticism of another type of repair better. However, the advocate of the Bassini repair may retort, these are different repairs, by different surgeons, on different patients, at different times—are they truly comparable? This brings us to the structure of the final type of argument, the cohort comparisons (at the time of the study, there were no randomized trials of hernia repair cited in the textbooks, but the argument illative structure is similar).

y_1 number of patients had their inguinal hernias repaired with the Bassini technique by the same surgical group.

The y_2 number of patients had their inguinal hernias repaired with the Shouldice technique by the same surgical group.

After x_1 years, z_1 Bassini repair patients had a recurrence of their hernias.

After x_2 years, z_2 Shouldice repair patients had a recurrence of their hernias.

$z_1/y_1 > z_2/y_2$; that is, there was a higher frequency of recurrence in the Bassini patients.

Therefore, Shouldice repair is a more effective inguinal hernia repair.

What is important to note is not the details of the repairs and the reports, but what has changed is what constitutes a persuasive argument based on the inclusion of all relevant premises leading to the conclusion. The aim has remained the same. Although each argument meets the illative form from the standpoint of structure, they do not necessarily meet the dialectical requirements of premise and relationship relevance, sufficiency and acceptability. Understanding these arguments will help surgeons make inguinal hernia repair treatment recommendations.

The examples also illustrate other aspects of informal logic in argumentation. All of the arguments for inguinal hernia repair at various times were reasonably good arguments at the time. However, none of these arguments would one consider conclusive. One can have a good argument that is not conclusive [19]. One can also have good arguments for or against a particular thesis, but these arguments need to be thought of more in terms of their purpose (in what we are speaking here is decision-making), rather than their structure, and, as previously mentioned, be able to withstand some modicum of criticism. Inconclusive arguments can still be persuasive if the listener judges that the preponderance of evidence is sufficient for, at least, provisional acceptance.

A second opinion from another physician is another fine example of good arguments that may come to different conclusions based on the same propositions. A physician's opinion may differ from another's opinion based on several factors. First, one physician may be in possession of additional information that materially changes the illative core of the argument. That is, additional premises are added, and perhaps others are deleted. One physician may judge aspects of the patient's situation differently than the other; that is, some aspects of the relevancy, sufficiency and acceptability criteria are different. An example of this is the relative effects on reasoning and conclusions of reducing or eliminating information variables. Specifically, for a patient, *A*, with disease *x*, who has associated medical conditions, $y_1, y_2, \ldots, y_n$, the extant information on *x* does not consider these associated conditions. How will this information be applied to any reasoning or argument formation with regard to *x* in *A*? Perhaps one physician believes that certain associated conditions are relevant and others not, based on their own personal observations or experience (see the "Techniques of Evidential Foundational Appraisal column" of Fig. 1.1). Another possible conflict is in the application of previously observed long-run frequencies on estimates of near future individual probabilities as point estimates. What is meant here is if past studies show a 5-year hernia recurrence rate of 10%, what that actually means is 10% of the patients from that study had a recurrent hernia at 5 years. This group of patients is what I refer to as a "bounded" population, which is defined as the population from which a sample size is obtained. The question then becomes a relevancy question for the physician for a particular individual patient. If circumstances for this particular individual patient are different than the original conditions in which the long-run frequency was observed in other patients, this would question the reliability (in terms of relevance and acceptability) of these frequencies as point probability estimates for this particular patient (more on issues of long-run frequencies used at future probability point estimates in Chap. 6).

Therefore, for arguments generated for a decision, the ultimate result weighs heavily on the process. The dialectical process of attempting to identify missing premises and judging the relevancy, sufficiency and acceptability of the premises and the relationships among them are at the core of the process.

2.4.4 Arguments to Persuade

Persuasiveness is probably the most important function of an argument. I will explore this more in Chap. 4. I have used the words persuade, persuasion, persuasive, persuasiveness, etc., frequently in this and the preceding chapter, yet I have not given it a formal definition. The Merriam-Webster dictionary defines "persuade" as "to move by argument, entreaty or expostulation to a belief, position or course of action" [33]. For the purposes of this book, I believe that this is a fairly precise definition of what I am trying to convey.[16]

---

[16] Of course, there is a long history of persuasion in rhetoric, such as an oration or public debate (e.g., see Rapp, C. Aristotle's rhetoric. In: *The Stanford Encyclopedia of Philosophy* (Spring 2022 edition), Zalta EN (Ed.). https://plato.stanford.edu/archives/spr2022/entries/aristotle-rhetoric/). However, the orator's purpose in his rhetoric is to persuade, but not necessarily believe the position they are taking themselves. This is not my purpose here, for I have assumed that the arguer truly believes their position and is trying to persuade someone else with a cogent, committed argument.

The persuasiveness of an argument is related to, but not the same as, the structural validity and propositional soundness of the argument. There are other aspects of what people believe and want to believe (more on this in Chaps. 3 and 4). The arguer, therefore, needs to understand their listener. For example, whether the premises are true may be relevant and important to whether the conclusion is physically true (i.e., actually corresponding to a phenomenon in the physical universe) but may not be relevant to whether the argument is persuasive. In another aspect, an educated audience, e.g., physicians, may be so well aware of the topic that they will be able to naturally fill in the relevant premises even if the auger does not explicitly state them, giving the auger more time and space for other aspects of the argument. Therefore, I agree in general with Johnson [19] that we should change the conception of an argument from that of a "proof" to that of a dialog. This is argumentation from a pragmatic viewpoint—a dialectical process that includes a response by a critic, the arguer's response to the critic, modification of the argument, further criticism, etc. Last, in medicine, you do not have to prove that something is absolutely true, all you need is to prove that it is "true enough"—either as a probability or reliability—to act, especially in the face of time constraints.

In sum, argument for persuasion not only requires a sound illative core but also an understanding of the listener's potential objections to the premises and how to adjust the argument, perhaps in a semantic and syntactical sense, to meet these objections.

2.5 Intuition in Medical Decisions

The notion of "intuition" has probably been around from as long as humans have recognized their ability to perceive and think. The Merriam-Webster dictionary defines intuition as "a: the power or faculty of attaining to direct knowledge or cognition without evident rational thought and inference. b: immediate apprehension or cognition" [34]. Intuition has been recognized and, at least among the general public, accepted as a cognitive phenomenon among humans, with its most renowned example probably being a "mother's intuition."[17] However, it is recognized in all manner of human activities, and it has received quite some attention.

I like to understand intuition as a recognition of a nonobvious phenomenon. However, there are many other ideas as to what intuition is. For example, Kutsch states that "intuition can be thought of as an insight that arises spontaneously

[17] It is unclear when and how the concept of "mother's intuition" or a "mother's instinct" as such came about. Marga Vicedo, in her book *Mother Love and Human Nature: A History of the Maternal Instinct,* traces the concept from the nineteenth century. There are, of course, numerous examples of mothers having "eyes in the back of their heads," etc., and "sensing" some adverse event related to their child; nevertheless, it is curious to me that there are not very many documented instances of this intuition or instinct being wrong. I suspect the times when the intuition is right gets much attention, and when the intuition is wrong, it is simply forgotten.

without conscious reasoning" [35]. Geigerenzer and Gaissmaier [36] view intuition as a form of unconscious intelligence that is grounded in heuristics. Malewska describes intuition as a "quick and automatic process that accesses the many deep resources of experience and knowledge that people have gathered over the course of their lives" [37]. Dijksterhuis and colleagues [38] place intuition under their rubric of "deliberation-without-attention." Klein [39] believes that it is part of a "naturalistic decision making" movement where highly experienced individuals tend to compare patterns and then determine how the situation would play out, which enables them to make relevant decisions quickly and competently. The Noble laureate, Daniel Kahneman, proposes that humans have two kinds of thought—fast and intuitive and slow and reasoning. He states that the fast and intuitive is more prone to error, while the slow and reasoning is less susceptible to producing bad decisions [40]. Wescott understands intuition as "the ability to reach sound conclusions from minimal evidence" [41]. I can continue enumerating other definitions, but what they all seem to have in common is that the process of coming to an insight or decision does not involve conscious, deliberate reasoning but rather just "appears" into the person's mind. How and why this happens in unexplainable, sometimes even by the person who has the insight.

I am going to make an aside to make a distinction of our topic of intuition from its erstwhile synonyms. Occasionally, one here's someone say, "My *instinct* was to do…" I have heard physicians use these exact phrases innumerable times. This use of "instinct" is not in the biological sense of an animal's behavior being innate and unlearned, such as, for example, a bird's instinct to migrate to a particular location at a certain time of the year. Truly what the speaker means here is their intuition. That is, they unconsciously assessed the situation, and a course of action came to them. One will hear as well, "I was *inspired* to do…" When one hears an artist speak of inspiration, they mean an agent or influence having an animating or exalting effect leading to a creative endeavor. However, intuition has a similar effect, and certainly, many solutions to these conundrum problems prescribed by intuition can be creative. I have certainly witnessed and participated in many exceptionally creative solutions to perplexingly difficult surgical problems that can only be referred to as inspiring (I have a saying to the surgical trainees—"You're not going to find this in the doctor books."). One can also say the same of words like *hunch, gut feeling, sixth sense,* etc. When such words are used to describe a leap into an insight, they will fall under what I am discussing here as intuition. In Fig. 2.1, I have placed the pathway of intuition from rationality to conclusions/assessments, effectively bypassing reasoning and argumentation, as there is no overt, conscious reasoning or argument construction as previously described. Nevertheless, in the subsequent sections, I will promote the concept that there is a covert, subconscious rationality to intuition. Similarly, there are no boxes in Fig. 1.1 containing intuition; however, I will contend that intuition functionally operates from a physician's experience.

2.5.1 Intuition in Medicine

Intuition has been and is a subject in the practice of medicine. There are books pertaining to medical intuition [42] and surgical intuition [43]. My basic thesis is that intuition as used in medicine is a subconscious generator of insights. It is dependent on knowledge, experience, practice, and keen (often unconscious) observation. I want to emphasize that I am not referring to the "medical intuitive practitioner," who is someone who claims to be able to make diagnoses or treat illnesses on the basis of their feelings and "intuition" rather than grounded in specialized education, training, or scientifically evaluated experience as a form of alternative/complementary medicine [44].[18]

There is a perceived tension between those who claim that there is a role for intuition in medical practice and those for whom it is irrational and prone to error [45]. Nevertheless, intuition can "fill in the gaps" where objective, specific information or knowledge is lacking. Adler [46] also notes that medicine is particularly prone to difficulties in applying a general rule to a specific case represented by an individual patient. The use of intuition is the physician's attempt to bridge this gap. Much of what follows I owe to the insights of Abernathy and Hamm [43]. They rightly point out that decision analyses based on scientific evidence may be appropriate in a global sense when pertinent data are available, but that data are not always available and are not always good (more on this in Chap. 9). Guidelines based on the "best evidence" are only applicable if the patient meets the criteria of the guidelines (more on this in Chap. 7).[19] Intuition does not insert itself into normal, everyday "routine" care, such as the vignette presented in Chap. 1; it comes to the physician when the case is perplexing and not consistent with what they would expect. The use of intuition has been studied in family physicians [47], nurses [48], hospital specialists [49], internal medicine, family medicine and emergency room physicians [50] and radiologists [51].

Intuition is different from other types of thinking, that is, from rational, analytical, logical thinking. It is thought, without analysis, such that the answer springs from the mind's unconsciousness [52]. Abernathy and Hamm [43] make the clear distinction between "everyday" routine thinking and intuition. Although their focus is the intuition of the surgeon, what they say can be applied to other physicians as well, as will be demonstrated below. For them, surgeons have extensive knowledge and often use it intuitively as a natural consequence. Experts make comprehensive, accurate judgments so rapidly and automatically that they cannot easily say how they did it. Master physicians are able to use intuitive judgments for complex cases

[18] The *medical intuitive* is an alternative medicine practitioner. Apparently, this is a somewhat burgeoning field. There exists an "Academy of Intuition Medicine," where one can further develop their intuition in this realm (https://intuitionmedicineonline.org, last accessed June 13, 2022).

[19] We also in the United States have to contend with insurance companies' coverage policies based on guidelines and best evidence, which may be appropriate for the vast majority of diagnostic and treatment decisions but can be too rigid when a particular patient has circumstances that require another approach.

that do not easily fit into routine, "guideline" recommendations. A key here is "extensive knowledge" and "experience." This actually corresponds quite well to the "10,000 hour" rule of intensive practice to achieve mastery of complex skills [53].[20] Others have observed the same. In a study of family physicians, more experienced physicians reported more "gut feelings" than less experienced physicians [47]. In addition, those physicians experiencing "good feedback" (i.e., feedback that leads toward better insight into their intuitive process) will lead to good intuition, whereas those experiencing poor feedback will not [54]. I have an aphorism that most of my trainees and junior faculty have heard: "Experience only counts if you're paying attention." That is, experience is not just performing a task, it is to pay attention to how the specific task one is performing is being done, so that later, when the result of the task is known, the physician can go back and assess which of the maneuvers of the task process most likely lead to the outcome. In a way, this is a form of inductive logic—that is, going from the specific (the results of this individual task) to the general (what is the likelihood that if this particular task is done the same way, the same result will occur). Over the course of years of focused practice of many patients registering many tasks and outcomes, supplemented by education by reading books and journals, attending medical conferences, and discussions with other physicians, the physician's bank of knowledge and experience will have a substantial number of deposits from which to draw.

Intuition in medicine appears to have certain patterns. As mentioned previously, a vast corpus of knowledge, personal experience and attentiveness is essential. However, there are other requirements. Attention to one's own feelings and emotions is vital [43]. I have previously mentioned that emotions can be a very useful component of rationality. I believe that this is where it becomes evident. Even in passing conversations with physicians about patient matters, one would frequently hear phrases such as "this patient made me nervous," "I'm truly worried about this patient," "something is not right here," "things aren't adding up," or other such phrases confessing anxiety or dread. Others have identified this as "judging intuitively is an emotional process whereby the judging is felt" [47] or as a "metacognitive feeling of unease with conflicting information" [55]. Woolley et al. [47] identified three types of intuitive decision processes in a study of family physicians: (1) "Gut feelings" whereby the physician senses something is not appropriate. They equate this with the "slowing down" process observed in surgeons who realize that they need to be more deliberate in the conduct of the operation but do not know why [56]; (2) "Recognition" whereby the physician uses a heuristic approach of pattern

[20] I realize that the "10,000 hours" rule has come under some scrutiny, e.g., see Macnamara BN, Maitra M. The role of deliberate practice in expert performance: Revisiting Ericsson, Kramps & Tesch-Romer (1993). Royal Society Open Science, 21 August 2019, https://doi.org/10.1098/rsos.190327. However, for the general purpose that it requires quite some time (whatever that may be) of focus practice and attention (whatever that may be) to attain a certain level of expertise and mastery is undoubtedly true. In addition, certainly if you ask most physicians and medical educators (not to mention patients), those physicians with more experience and a more complete regimen of updating their knowledge would qualify as experts and masters.

recognition based on salient features and simple rules [57]; and (3) The "insight" that they feel is related to the "incubation" period after failed analytical thinking. In some ways, this "insight" type has similarities with abductive logic. Vanstone et al. [50] identified four patterns: (1) "Sick/Not Sick," which a broad categorization, usually instantaneous, made with confidence. (2) "Something Not Right," which is accompanied by worry, along with its subcategory of "Mismatch," which is a discrepancy between the physician's subjective appraisal of the patient and objective evidence (i.e., the patient looks "sicker" than what the objective findings would indicate). (3) "Frame-shifting," which is a flash of insight that suggests a new diagnosis or course of action. (4) "Abduction," which is a logical leap to a specific diagnosis without sufficient evidence; and its subcategory of "Eureka," which the diagnosis is achieved, while skipping a number of usual steps. I am not going to debate whether Woolley, et al.'s or Vanstone, et al.'s types are better, rather the importance is when intuition tends to occur and occur most effectively, it is in the more experienced physician, who is intensely focused on a patient, who clinical presentation is not routine.

So what is it that the physician observes or senses that leads to a determination that the particular case they are addressing is not routine. In the clinical vignette in Chap. 1, the information obtained from the patient was through verbal communication and the physician's physical examination. As this was a routine, everyday clinical case, in the sense of Abernathy and Hamm [43], this was more than adequate time to start the deliberated, reasoned diagnostic proceed. However, every physician can tell you that there is much more to what is being communicated than the words being spoken. The tone of voice, cadence of speech, interruptions with what appear to be spasms or moans of pain, the facial expressions, not only of the patient but also of the family, the posture in the chair, examination table, or stretcher, and the "sense in the room," among many others are all analogue "data points" that the physician observes, either consciously or unconsciously, which will affect their "feeling" about a case and, most likely, their intuitive response. In this way, the thoughts of experts, whether applied routinely in familiar situations or intuitively in challenging situations, can encompass more knowledge at once than an explicit analysis can [43]. The experienced physician will make distinctions between essential versus coincidental symptoms, test data, and signs and will do so intuitively. This ability to judge importance and relevance comes to be embodied in one's perception. That is, while observing the patient, the expert physician "sees" (or, rather, "senses") only the relevant and important features [43]. In essence, the experienced physician, either consciously or unconsciously, is able to determine which of the "premises" to use in their argument toward a diagnosis and treatment should be included.

However, I would caution that if intuition is an unconscious process based on the physician's "bank of knowledge and experience," then it is only the deposits from that bank from which they can withdraw. Let me expand on this thought. In general, our thoughts about a topic are bounded by what we know about the topic. Although it is true that we can develop completely novel ideas (e.g., Newton and gravity; Einstein and relativity), these are exceptionally uncommon events. When confronted with a perplexing situation, most people will fall back on what they know or throw up their hands and proclaim “I don’t know.” Therefore, one’s intuition must be bounded by the physician’s knowledge and experience. Therefore, intuition is not infallible; and, just as with a mother’s intuition, we tend to celebrate when our intuition is right but, perhaps, not confess to when it was wrong.

In summary, intuition as it is used by medical practitioners is generally used occasionally, in perplexing, nonroutine cases, usually by more experienced physicians. It is not a reasoned argument toward a diagnosis or treatment decision. Because, however, the application of “medical science” may not be appropriate for all the myriad of patients who a physician encounters, intuition will probably always have some role in medical practice.

2.6 Conclusions

What I have attempted to do in this chapter is to lay the foundation for a physician’s rationality and the mechanics by which they reason, or access their intuition, if appropriate. I have tried to describe these mechanisms using examples from medical practice. I have laid down the foundation for future analyses of how physicians may persuade patients and how researchers may persuade other professionals.

References

1. Aune B. Thinking. In: Edwards P, editor. The encyclopedia of philosophy, vol. 8. New York: MacMillan Publishing Co., Inc. and The Free Press; 1967. p. 100–4.
2. Johnson-Laird PN. Mental models and human reasoning. Proc Natl Acad Sci U S A. 2010;107(43):18243–50.
3. Warnock GJ. Reason. In: Edwards P, editor. The encyclopedia of philosophy, vol. 7. New York: MacMillan Publishing Co., Inc. and The Free Press; 1967.
4. Proudfoot M, Lacey AR. The Routledge dictionary of philosophy. 4th ed. London: Routledge; 2009.
5. Reschar N. In: Honderich T, editor. The Oxford companion to philosophy. 2nd ed. Oxford: Oxford University Press; 2005. p. 791.
6. Kolodny N. Why be rational? Mind. 2005;114:509–64.
7. Broome J. Reasons and rationality. In: Knauff M, Spohn W, editors. The handbook of rationality. Boston: The MIT Press; 2021. p. 129–36.
8. Shneider VB. What is it to be rational? Philosophy Now. www.philosophynow.org. Last accessed 2 Jun 2022.
9. Korsgaard CM. Rationality. www.people.fas.harvard.edu. Last accessed 2 Jun 2022.
10. Broome J. Reasons and rationality. In: Knauff M, Spohn W, editors. Handbook of rationality. Boston: The MIT Press; 2021.
11. Wallace RJ. Practical reason. In: Zalta ED, editor. The Stanford encyclopedia of philosophy; 2020. https://plato.standford.edu/archives/spr2020/entries/practical-reason. Last accessed 3 Jun 2022.
12. Rachlin H. Rational thought and rational behavior: a review of bounded rationality: the adaptive toolbox. J Exp Anal Behav. 2003;79:409–12.
13. Herfield C. The diversity of rational choice theory: a review note. Topoi. 2020;39:329–47.

14. Greenspan P. Practical reasoning and emotion. In: Mele A, Rawlings P, editors. Rationality. New York: Oxford University Press; 2002.
15. Kirman A, Livet P, Teschl M. Rationality and emotions. Philos Trans R Soc B. 2010;365:215–9.
16. “Reasoning.” Merriam-Webster Dictionary. https://www.merriam-webster.com. Last accessed 3 Jun 2022.
17. “Reasoning.” Dictionary.com. https://www.dictionary.com. Last accessed 3 Jun 2022.
18. “Reasoning.” The Cambridge Dictionary. https://dictionary.cambridge.org. Last accessed 3 Jun 2022.
19. Johnson RH. Manifest rationality: a pragmatic theory of argument. New York: Routledge; 2012.
20. Hitchcock D. Critical thinking. In: Zalta EN, editor. The Stanford encyclopedia of philosophy; 2020. https://plato.stanford.edu/archives/fall2020/entries/critical-thinking/.
21. Bailin S, Case R, Coombs JR, Daniels LB. Common misconceptions of critical thinking. J Curr Stud. 1999;31:269–83.
22. Walton DN. What is reasoning? What is an argument? J Philos. 1990;87:399–419.
23. The basics of philosophy-logic. https://philosophybasics.com/branch_logic.html. Last accessed 20 May 2022.
24. Hodges W. Logic. 2nd ed. London: Penguin Books, Ltd.; 2001.
25. Douven I. Abduction. In: Zalta EN, editor. The Stanford encyclopedia of philosophy; 2021. https://plato.stanford.edu/archives/sum2021/entries/abduction/.
26. Morgagni GB. In: Clendening L, editor. Source book of medical history. New York: Dover Publications, Inc.; 1960. p. 240–53.
27. Streck CJ Jr, Maxwell PJ IV. A brief history of appendicitis: familiar names and interesting patients. Am Surg. 2014;80:105–8.
28. Govier T. Problems in argument analysis and evaluation. Dordrecht: Foris; 1987.
29. Velanovich V. Reductionism in biology and medicine: the implications of fractal and chaos theory. Theor Surg. 1994;9:104–7.
30. Weston A. A rulebook for arguments. 5th ed. Indianapolis, IN: Hackett Publishing Co., Inc; 2018.
31. Woods J. Sunny prospects for relevance? In: Johnson RH, Blair JA, editors. New essays in informal logic. Windsor, ON: Informal Logic; 1994.
32. Velanovich V. The logical basis of efficacy determination: arguments of inguinal hernia repair. Theor Surg. 1989;4:140–6.
33. Persuade. Merriam-Webster Dictionary. https://merriam-webster.com. Last accessed 9 Jun 2022.
34. Introduction. Merriam-Webster Dictionary. https://merriam-webster.com. Last accessed 13 Jun 2022.
35. Kutsch L. Can we rely on our intuition? Sci Am. 2019.
36. Gigerenzer G, Gaissmaier W. Heuristic decision making. Ann Rev Psychol. 2011;62:451–82.
37. Malewska K. Intuition in decision-making—theoretical and empirical aspects. Bus Manag Rev. 2015;6:23–31.
38. Dijksternuis A, Bo MW, Nordgren LI, van Baaren RB. On making the right choice: the deliberation-without-attention effect. Science. 2006;311:S1005–7.
39. Klein G. Naturalistic decision making. Hum Factors. 2008;50:456–60.
40. Kahneman D. Thinking fast and slow. New York: Farrar, Straus, & Giroux; 2011.
41. Wescott MR. Toward a contemporary psychology of intuition. New York: Holt, Rinehart & Winston; 1968.
42. Braude HD. Intuition in medicine: a philosophical defense of clinical reasoning. Chicago: The University of Chicago Press; 2012.
43. Abernathy CM, Hamm RM. Surgical intuition: what it is and how to get it. Philadelphia: Hanley & Belfus, Inc.; 1995.
44. Medical Intuitive. The Free Dictionary. https://medical-dictionary.thefreedictionary.com/medical+intuitive/.
45. Habermann E. Intuition—a two-edged sword. Theor Surg. 1991;6:85–96.

46. Adler I. The medical gap: intuition in medicine. Med Health Care Philos. 2022; https://doi.org/10.1007/s11019-022-10081-4.
47. Woolley A, Kostopoulous O. Clinical intuition in family medicine: more than first impressions. Ann Fam Med. 2013;11:60–4.
48. Melin-Johansson C, Palmqvist R, Ronnberg L. Clinical intuition in the nursing process and decision-making—a mixed-studies review. J Clin Nurs. 2017;26:3936–49.
49. Van den Brink N, Holbrechts B, Brand RL, et al. Role of intuitive knowledge in the diagnostic reasoning of hospital specialists: a focus group study. BMJ Open. 2019;9:e022724.
50. Vonstone M, Monteiro S, Colvin E, et al. Experimental physician descriptions of intuition in clinical reasoning: a typology. Diagnosis. 2019;6:259–68.
51. Patel SH, Itri JN. The role of intuitive cognition in radiologic decision making. J Am Coll Radiol. 2022;19:669–76.
52. Gross K, Lorenz W. Intuition in surgery as a strategy of medical decision-making: its potency and limitations. Theor Surg. 1990;5:54–9.
53. Gladwell M. Outliers: the story of success. New York: Little, Brown & Co.; 2008.
54. Hogarth DM. Educating intuition. Chicago: The University of Chicago Press; 2001.
55. Thompson VA, Prowse-Turner JA, Pennycook G. Intuition, reason and metacognition. Cogn Psychol. 2011;63:107–40.
56. Molton CA, Regehr G, Lingard L, et al. Slowing down to stay out of trouble in the operating room: remaining attentive in automaticity. Acad Med. 2010;85:1571–7.
57. Schmidt HG, Rikars RM. How expertise develops in medicine: knowledge encapsulation and illness script formation. Med Educ. 2007;41:1133–9.

Chapter 3
The Human Mind: Relationship of Evolutionary Imperatives on Discerning Truth

Chapter 2 treated rationality, reasoning, logic, argumentation and intuition as free-standing, independent entities from the human mind. What I mean by this is that they have been treated as if in isolation from the human mind and the foibles of human nature, just like a building's existence is independent of the person seeing the building. They appear to have their own normative and descriptive framework, structure, features and mechanisms all to their own. This is not true. The concepts of "rationality," "logic,", etc., are inventions of the human mind. They do not exist in nature—humans have imposed it on their perceptions of nature. They are merely descriptions of how the human mind processes information (or ought to process information) obtained through the senses of the human, with some individuals (philosophers, economists, psychologists, neuroscientists, etc.) trying to both describe the mental processes associated with reasoning and argumentation and/or impose normative standards so that this process can lead to as reliable beliefs and decisions as humanly possible. That is not to say that there are some areas of human thought that do have very strict normative standards. For example, mathematics is such a field. The "rules" and "procedures" of mathematics, both theoretical and applied, are explicit and uniform. It matters not who is performing the math or, moreover, if even a human is performing the math. However, the same cannot be said of human rationality.

Human rationality is part of the function of the human mind, and the human mind is inseparable from the human brain. The average human brain contains approximately 2×10^{11} neurons, 1×10^{12} glial cells, 400 miles (700 km) of blood vessels and 100,000 miles (160,000 km) of axons, comprising the neuropil [1]. This brain receives approximately 11 billion bits of information per second through the human sensory system, with conscious mind processing of only 16–50 bits per second [2]. Even "willed" movement is preceded by neuronal activation 1–8 s prior to our consciousness actually "deciding" to physically move [2]. In fact, as I will discuss later, the conscious mind accounts for only a very small part of the activities of the human brain (Fig. 3.1). Some say that 95% of the human brain is dedicated to

V. Velanovich, *Medical Persuasion*, https://doi.org/10.1007/978-3-031-30371-5_3

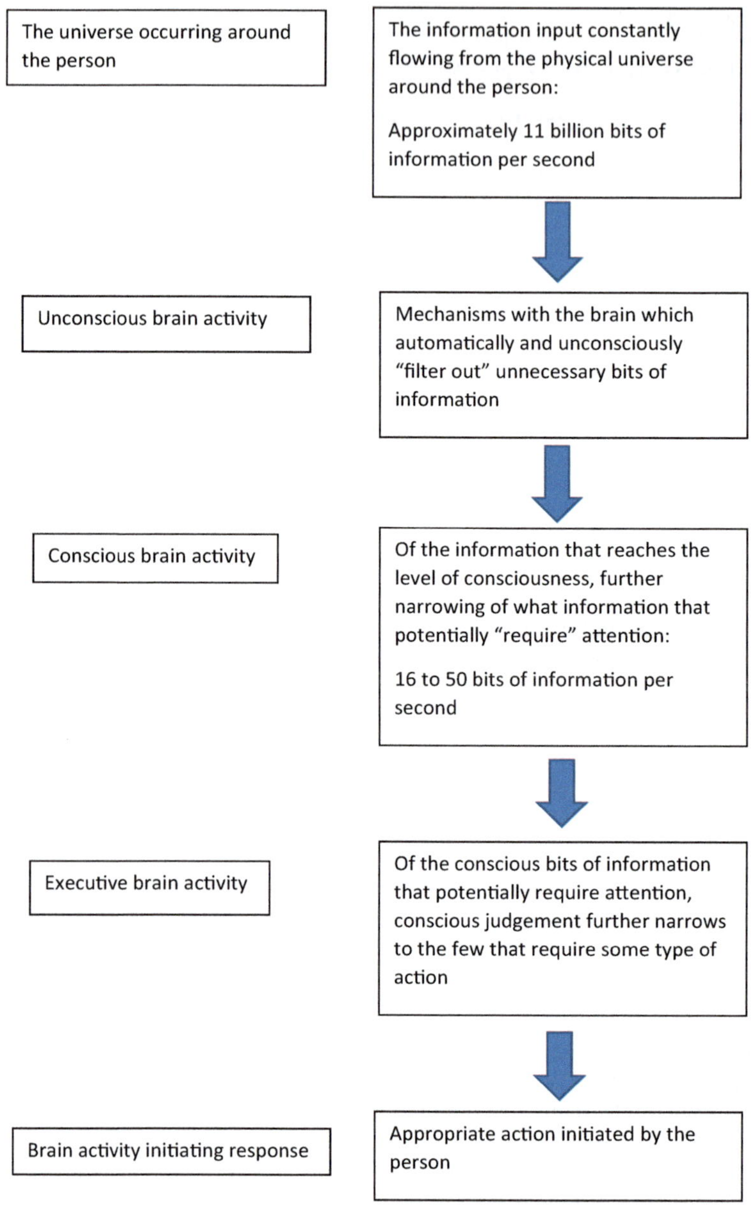

Fig. 3.1 A schematic representation of how sensory input from the individual's surroundings is processed into conscious awareness and potential need for action. Blue arrows show the direction of information flow

the unconscious[1] processing of information input, as well as control of physiological activities and internal brain maintenance, while only 5% is actual conscious thought [3, 4] (Fig. 3.2). A natural question is: How did it get this way? Therefore, we cannot understand the function of the mind without understanding the function of the brain.[2] Moreover, for the purposes of this book, we cannot understand how people (patients, physicians, healthcare professionals, scientists, etc.) can be persuaded without understanding how the mind functions. What I hope to show in this chapter is how our evolutionary imperatives shaped our brain function, which, in turn, shaped the function of our mind. My overall thesis will be this: *The human mind evolved to survive; it did not evolve to discern truth*. Therefore, what becomes important in the mind of humans is "How will what I am thinking about help me to survive?" This is a rhetorical evolutionary teleological statement; I do not mean that our ancestors consciously asked themselves this question. It also leads to my second thesis: *Determination of survival benefit is at most an unconscious appraisal based on our evolutionary imperatives during the millennia of human existence prior to*

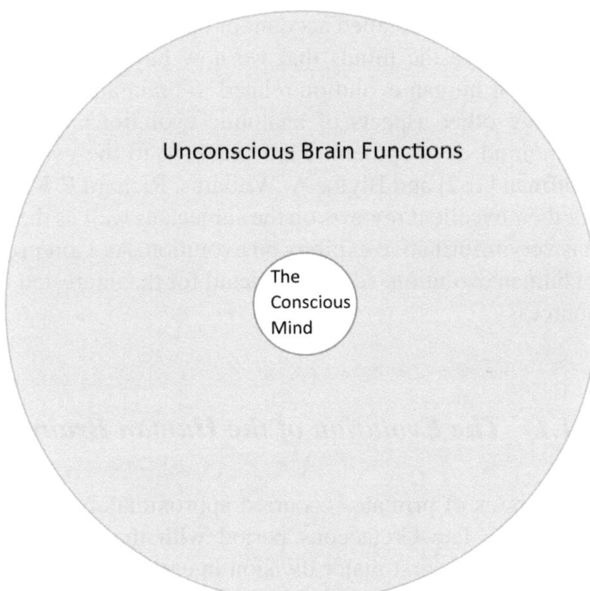

Fig. 3.2 A schematic representation of the relative components of the conscious and unconscious activities of the human brain. This is not meant to be a "to scale" depiction but to convey the general sense that the preponderance of activity, perhaps up to 95% or more, is unconscious

[1] I am going to refer to all brain/mind activity that is going on unawares of the individual as "unconscious" activity. I will make no distinction with what some psychologists refer to as "subconscious" activity. Perhaps there is a nuanced difference between unconscious and subconscious, but for my purposes, it is not a crucial difference, and I would like to keep my terms as consistent as possible.

[2] I understand that, at present, neuroscience certainly does not have a complete account of the function of the brain particularly as it pertains to consciousness and thought. I will use some of the information available on this topic, understanding this is an immense field of research and I am touching on only a small sample of it. Nevertheless, I believe that the statement is an accurate one, despite our present state of understanding of the brain.

civilization. These archetypal, "background," unconscious imperatives are used as a normative standard for what humans choose to believe and how they are persuaded.

3.1 A Brief Review of Primate Evolution to Anatomically Modern Humans

All living organisms (at least on Earth) have the same biological imperative: to survive long enough to reproduce. Every other imperative is subordinate to this—finding food and water, avoiding predation, finding mates, etc. This is all in an effort to ensure as much as possible that the organism's genes will continue to be in the pool of genetic material in the universe. This is what Richard Dawkins refers to as "the selfish gene" [5]. The present version of humans, *Homo sapiens* (subspecies *sapiens*), is referred to in the literature as "anatomically modern humans." When I use the word "human(s)," I am referring to anatomically modern humans. This is not intended to be a detailed account of human evolution but to provide a foundation of how we have the minds that we now have. Therefore, I will only discuss those aspects of human evolution related to brain anatomy and function while generally ignoring other aspects of anatomic evolutionary changes, unless it is related to brain/mind development. I am indebted to the evolutionary accounts of Michael Hoffman [1, 2] and Blythe A. Williams, Richard F. Kay and E. Christopher Kirk [6] for their excellent reviews on the subject, as well as the Smithsonian Institute, which has very informative exhibits on evolution. As I am providing the barest of outlines of human evolution, additional detail for the interested reader may be found in these sources.

3.1.1 The Evolution of the Human Brain

The origins of primates occurred approximately 83 to 70 million years ago (mya) during the late Cretaceous period with the waning of the non-avian dinosaurs (Fig. 3.3). The first major division in early primates that we can ascertain from the fossil record occurred during the Palaeo-Eocene Thermal Maximum period at approximately 55 mya, which raised global temperatures approximately 6 °C and lasted approximately 200,000 years [1]. This led to a divergence between the strepsirrhines ("wet-nose" primates), which would eventually include lemurs and lorises, and the haplorhines ("dry-nose" primates), which would eventually include tarsiers, monkeys and apes [1, 6]. These primates were primarily arboreal inhabitants of the canopies and were small and nocturnal. In this environment, the ability to see branches, judge distances, and handle objects were survival advantages; therefore, this fostered the development of stereoscopic vision and a corticospinal tract for the manual manipulation of objects. In the brain, the granular cortices of the caudal

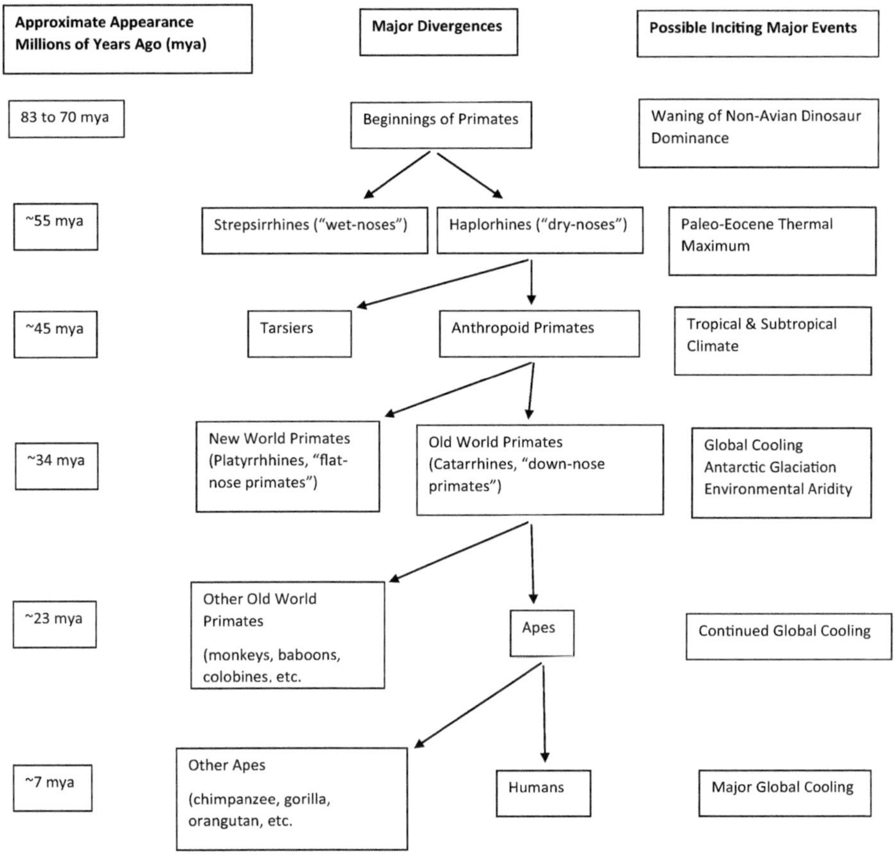

Fig. 3.3 A flow diagram of the major events of primate evolution from the first appearance of primates to humans, with the generally accepted dates of divergence and the proposed major geo-climatic activity in which the divergences occurred. This obviously is a very rudimentary and only meant to convey that the present human brain (with its associated mind) developed as a result of meeting a broad array of evolutionary challenges

prefrontal cortex of layer 4 of the 6-layer mammalian brain continued to enlarge.[3] In this environment, the plesiadapiforms (stem primates) developed increased fronto-parietal circuitry for working memory. Teleologically, working memory allowed for knowing and remembering trees and branches that these primates inhabited for effective, safe movement in their environs. This working memory later becomes an essential feature of the human mind for reasoning and persuasion [1, 2].

During this time, the primate brain approximately doubled in size compared to their contemporary mammalian counterparts by the end of the Paleocene period

[3]The six layers of the mammalian brain from outer to inner are layer (1) The molecular layer; (2) The external granular layer; (3) The external pyramidal layer; (4) Internal granular layer; (5) Internal pyramidal layer; and (6) Multiform layer.

(approximately 60 to 25 mya), which may be related to an increase in high-quality foods as well as responding to social challenges of group living [2]. Group living, presumably, was a response to predation (primates were certainly not at the top of the food chain, but were on the menu of many predators) [1, 2]. That is, the group allowed for improved survivability of the individual (and hence, a better chance at passing on genes). Approximately 40 mya, there is evidence that grooming emerged among primates, with the consequences of improved group cohesion [1], which benefitted the members of the group as a whole. This becomes a key feature of primates, and eventually, in humans, there was an evolution into "vocal grooming" and then language (more about language later) [1]. The divergence between the anthropoid primates and the tarsiers occurred approximately 45 mya during a period predominated by a tropical and subtropical climate [1, 6]. Williams et al. [6] suggest that recent evidence may point to more than one location of these divergences, as well as the divergence of the new and old world primates. Moreover, at approximately 50 mya, the Tethys Ocean, which allowed for a more equatorial circumvolution current, and the extant tropical and subtropical climate, closed due to plate tectonic movement of the continents [1]. This led to a period of global cooling, which accelerated approximately 34 mya by the formation of the Antarctic ice sheet.[4] At this time, the divergence of platyrrhines ("flat-nose" or new world primates) and catarrhines ("down-nose" or old world primates) occurred [1, 6]. The importance of how climate drove this evolution cannot be overstated.

As the climate cooled, this led to more environmental unpredictability. The anthropoids developed a new prefrontal granular cortex, leading to a more rapid ability to learn and thus fewer errors in foraging, which was a survival advantage [1, 2]. There was further development of other brain regions, including the ventral prefrontal cortex (improved auditory and visual input), the dorsal prefrontal cortex (ability to sequence actions), the dorsomedial prefrontal cortex (enabled choosing and evaluating actions based on previous experience) and the polar prefrontal cortex (sometimes referred to as the frontopolar cortex), which is associated with analogical reasoning, making inferences and adaptation to novelty [1, 2]. These allowed the anthropoids to adapt to new situations by learning quickly, sometimes to just a singular event, which offered a survival advantage [1, 2]. This ability to learn becomes a *sine qua non* feature of humans.

During the period of continued global cooling, the divergence of apes occurred from the other old world primate at approximately 23 mya [1]. These apes eventually developed into small apes (hominoids), such as gibbons and hylobatids, and great apes (hominids), such as chimpanzees, gorillas, orangutans, and bonobos [1]. There appeared to be the development of the capacity to differentiate oneself from others, and an increase in sociality with the development of the dorsomedial prefrontal cortex and presupplementary motor areas [1]. These were key features for

[4] It is beyond the scope of this book to delve into the causes of the changes in climate over this evolutionary period. These include the variations in the shape of Earth's orbit around the sun, the changes in the tilt of the axis of Earth's rotation, as well as the wobble of the axis of Earth's rotation (Milankovitch cycles); geologic activity; shift in tectonic plates; sun cycles, and so forth.

social learning. The important development of social learning in humans will set the stage for our social and cultural evolution.

Other important brain developments, including the superior temporal gyrus, were associated with gaze-specific and facial recognition. This will become in humans a crucial feature for the development of nonverbal communication, which affects persuasion. These neurons are very "spinous," allowing for vastly increased connections with other neurons, resulting in a more complex brain connectivity [1] and, presumably, brain function and mental activities. Eventually, humans (hominins) diverged from the other apes approximately 7 mya during a period of greater global cooling and increased aridity [1]. The important point of this summation of primate evolution to humans is the way the brain enlarged and became more interconnected, eventually allowing for human thought communication and societal development [1]. That is, the social imperative of group living has become embedded in the human mind. The importance of this in human persuasion will be discussed later in the chapter.

Human evolution did not proceed in an orderly, stepwise pattern, although much early renditions of ape to human evolution gave that impression [7]. A "missing link" as a common ancestor of both apes and humans has yet to be discovered. In fact, there have been many hominin species that were not in the direct ancestral line to *Homo sapiens* [7]. Many human species actually coinhabited the world together simultaneously [7]. All of these appear to stem from possibly the three earliest known hominins—*Sahelanthropus tchudensis* (found in present day Chad), *Orrorrin tugensensis* (modern day Kenya), and *Ardipithecus kadabba* (modern day Ethiopia). The first species of the genus *Homo* was *Homo habilis* (a.k.a., "handy man") who lived from 2.4 to 1.4 mya [8]. The next most prominent species was *Homo erectus*, which lived from 1.89 million to 110,000 years ago. They have been, to date, the longest living of the human species. There is evidence that they used the hand axe and appeared to care for their old and weak. These were the first human species to migrate out of Africa [8]. *Homo heidelbergensis* lived from 700 to 200 kya and was the first human species to live in a cooler climate. There is evidence that they used spears and built simple dwellings from wood and rock [8]. They appeared to have developed an additional granular prefrontal cortex, which increased learning by imitation (mirror neuron system stage 3) and mental time travel (i.e., foreseeing a future state, such as imagining an action before taking it) [2]. These abilities become an essential feature of human reasoning and social development. Some believe that the following two human species evolved from this species, although the evidence is not conclusive [9, 10]. *Homo neanderthalensis* lived from 400 to 40 kya and overlapped considerably with *Homo sapiens.* They are modern humans closest extinct relatives but were not ancestors to modern humans. There is evidence that they controlled fire, lived in shelters, made and wore clothing, were skilled hunters, ate plants as well, and perhaps buried their dead and marked their graves [8]. There is DNA evidence that points to interbreeding between the Neanderthals and modern humans [7]. *Homo sapiens* appeared 300 kya and is the only surviving species of humans. They evolved during a period of dramatic climate change, and their mental abilities were crucial to their survival. By 30 to 15 kya, all other hominin species became extinct [7]. Culturally, the discovery and development of agriculture and animal husbandry approximately 12 kya was possibly the most profound change that a single species conferred on the Earth [8]. What follows is a very brief and broad account of the seminal changes in the human brain that allowed for this. As with human evolution in general, there is not a strict timeline of the occurrence of these developments but, rather, just an enumeration of them. I owe this account to Michael Hoffman's excellent books on the subject [1, 2] and its extensive references.

As with the description of brain evolution from primates to hominins, the following is simply a sketch of (primarily) the brain evolution of early hominins to humans. There is no fossil record found to date of the presumed evolution of hominoids to bipedal hominids (one of the so-called "missing links," the other being the common ancestor of apes and hominins), which presumably occurred between 14 and 6 mya [1]. However, bipedalism is a key occurrence in hominoid evolution, even though it is thought to have occurred millions of years prior to brain enlargement [1]. Approximately 10 to 5 mya, the occurrence of the "African Valley Rift," as a result of continuous plate tectonic movement, led to a particularly unstable climate, promoting hominid evolution to hominins [1], that is, selecting for the brain/mind function of learning and innovation. The "Pulse Climate Variability" hypothesis proposes that this led to an extended East African arid period with interspersed wet periods, correlating with hominoid brain growth, speciation and dispersals [1]. There is a hypothesis that further evolution occurred in a littoral setting where early hominins waded in shallow water in search of shellfish and other aquatic food [1]. This allowed for additional sources of high-quality foods.

Although there is evidence that pounding of rocks with other rocks to produce flakes occurred at approximately 2.6 mya, *Homo erectus* appeared to have consistently produced stone tools and hand axes at approximately 1.9 mya[5] [1]. This correlated with improvements in procedural memory and conceptual thought [1]. Making of a stone hand axe requires planning (a conception of the future product, i.e., mental time travel) plus the ability to judge how each strike on the stone progresses to the end product. In addition, *Homo erectus*, being an obligate bipedal creature, appears to have predominantly slept on the ground, with its consequential increase in predation risk—and need for group cohesion. They also appeared to have used fire and cooked their food, which supported increased sociality and group size [1]. Their praxis circuitry for toolmaking may have formed the basis for the eventual neuronal circuitry for language development [1]. That is, the embedded neuronal activity for tool-making was further developed into language making.

In hominoids, cerebral reorganization occurs before an overall increase in brain size [1]. An essential development was the "mirror neuron system" [11]. This development is proposed to have occurred in seven stages:

1. Grasping
2. Mirror system for grasping

[5] Interestingly, there did not appear to be an innovation on the stone hand axe for approximately 1 million years.

3. Simple imitation
4. Complex imitation
5. Protosign
6. Protospeech
7. Modern language

This development is considered crucial in the survival of hominins through increased sociality and group cohesion because of the ability to imitate others in the group and, eventually, speech communication. This allowed not only enhanced group cohesion against predation but also cooperation in other activities, such as foraging and hunting.

In conjunction with the mirror neuron system, episodic memory developed. This allowed for the mind to perform the previously mentioned mental time travel, that is, imaging future scenarios, being aware of "time-stamping" events (i.e., how one occurrence was temporally related to an occurrence of another event), and contemplating the past and future [2]. This was all necessary for rationality in both the philosophical and economic senses of rationality discussed in Chap. 2. With this, the "episodic buffer" is the principal route by which the central executive brain functions retrieve long-term memories [2] (I will later address the importance of memories in persuasion in the next chapter). This allows for "thought experiments" (i.e., contemplating how a series of actions could possibly unfold) followed by real-time trials of those actions [2]. This ability to recall memories allows for mental simulation of future events, which can have survival advantages. We will see later how this may be the biological basis for the "mental models" theory of human reasoning. From the standpoint of persuasion, this is also essential. An individual must be able to "see" in their mind's eye what can potentially happen to be persuaded. Learning and memory probably coevolved with recursive language to share episodic knowledge with conspecifics and in conjunction with emotional intelligence [2]. The frontal polar cortex further developed for the ability to switch between internally and externally oriented thoughts [2]. That is, to be able to realize that what you are thinking is not going to be automatically known to anyone else, and if you want someone else to know what you are thinking, you will have to communicate it.

Approximately 164 to 75 kya, there appears to have been catastrophic ice age conditions causing the reduction in the extant human population to perhaps a few hundred to a few thousand individuals living along the southern African coast [1]. During this time, there appears to be an unexplained difference in the emergence of anatomically modern humans (approximately 200 kya) and the modern human mind (approximately 50 kya) [1]. It does appear that the parietal lobe started to enlarge approximately 150 to 100 kya, which is associated with the analysis and elaboration of sensory input, visuospatial working memory function, number, time, and space computations [1]. Eventually, other parietal lobe functions will include cross-modal sensory proficiency that enables language comprehension, metaphor interpretation, symbolism conceptualization, abstract thinking, language, and prospective memory function [1].

As previously mentioned, enhanced working memory was essential for the development of the modern human mind, occurring from 77 to 30 kya [1]. This increased human abilities for a visuospatial "sketchpad" (e.g., innovation, modeling, and simulation of future states), phonologic storage capacity (e.g., facilitating modern language), and episodic buffer augmentation (e.g., creativity). This allowed for the progression of the mirror neuron system to stage 7 (chimpanzees, on the other hand, only have achieved stage 2) [1]. Enhanced working memory upgrades from stage 6 to 7 of the mirror neuron system appear to have occurred approximately 50 kya with the development of abstract thought, improved behavioral flexibility, creativity and "theory of mind" (which is the ability of an individual to take the perspective of someone else and understand that they can have different intentions, desires and knowledge than oneself) [1]. It is believed that the final enhancement to working memory occurred approximately 30 kya [1]. There is no ability to reason without working memory.

The modern human brain achieved its current size approximately 200 kya, but the modern cerebellum size was reached approximately 28 kya [1]. This was associated with escalations in corticocerebellar connectivity [1]. These expanded corticocerebellar functions were possibly associated with speech, tool-making and tool use, with the cerebellar contribution to these abilities being improved human cognitive efficiency and as a component to working memory. Verbal working memory and the cerebellum may have been instrumental in language evolution, such as inner speech, and coupling speech and language [1]. Brain circuitry was evolutionarily repurposed for reading, arithmetic/mathematics, and art [1]. Part of the hominin's solution to predation included color vision[6] and sociality within the group [1]. Other brain circuitry in humans that further developed included "mind-reading" (i.e., anticipating what another individual in the group is thinking), intentionality, and eventually "social" emotions—fear, anger, happiness and sadness [1]. All of these evolutionary developments were in response to the enhancement of survival. Any one individual's chances of surviving to reproduce were improved by staying within the group. Moreover, many of these social imperatives appear to be embedded into the brain's structure. That is, it is the human brain's "default" setting. The importance of this cannot be overstated—human rationality (in the sense of the prior chapter) is not imposed on a "blank slate" of a human's mind by education; there is already in place a brain circuitry that conforms rationality to it. I will discuss this further below with social and cultural evolution.

The earliest evidence of modern brain executive function appeared approximately 18 kya [1]. Executive brain function includes a wide array of cognitive abilities, including temporal organization of information, motivational and intentional aspects of behavior, empathic and socially appropriate behavior, impulsivity and compulsivity control [2]. These appeared primarily in conjunction with activities requiring socialization in humans. The ability to process and store information and

[6] The tri-chromatic vision of the apes has been hypothesized to be an evolutionary selection advantage to identify venomous snakes.

pass on this information to others within the group has become a fundamental feature of humans [1]. Humans not only appeared to learn but also appeared to like to learn. Perhaps because epistemic curiosity is connected to the hedonic reward centers of the brain [2]. That is, we, as humans, derive pleasure from learning. This ability to learn and pass on to others in our group was a survival advantage. Humans developed a "social brain." This social brain was essential for the survival of our ancestors. It appears to be ingrained in human brain and mental functioning. In addition, our ancestors may have reinforced it through their own selection process.

3.1.2 Human Self Domestication/Emotional Plasticity

Customarily, when we think of evolution, we think of external "selection" pressures on organisms, such that those organisms that have the genetically produced phenotypes best able to survive and reproduce in that environment will become successful in that niche, while those organisms that have phenotypes that are maladapted to that environment will die out and become extinct. Certainly, in the broad sketch of human brain evolution elucidated in the previous section, this was how the stage was set—successful defense against predation, improved foraging/hunting of high-quality foods, successful rearing of offspring to sexual maturity.

However, a recently proposed, albeit controversial, hypothesis has garnered attention. In 2014, Wilkins et al. [12] proposed the "domestication syndrome" to explain the relatively rapid socialization of humans based on neural crest cell behavior and genetics. Wrangham [13] later published a book to suggest that this process of "self-domestication" led to humans being both less (toward members of their own group) and more (toward conspecifics of other groups) violent. Briefly, the basic features of this hypothesis that human group cohesion was so vital to the survival of the members of the group, that any individuals who disrupted this cohesion, primarily because of uncontrolled violence or other undesirable behaviors, were either outright killed before they could reproduce or were ostracized from the group and presumably died in the wilderness without the group's support. On the other hand, "proactive (or premeditated)" aggression, aimed at members of other competing conspecific groups who may have threatened the index group, was encouraged as a way of protecting the group, allowing for survival and reproduction of members of the group. Wrangham [14] reviewed nine proposed mechanisms for self-domestication, and he favors the "language-based conspiracy" theory, which is a form of "collective intentionality." Briefly, the development of sophisticated language allowed for males of low fighting prowess to cooperatively plan and execute the elimination of a physically aggressive male. In small groups, this mechanism is referred to as a "leveling" mechanism and was possibly accelerated by group-structure cultural selection. Clearly, this hypothesis has great implications for the selection of an underlying desire to stay within the group and closely adhere to the group's behavioral norms and mores. It also has implications for what further became "human universals" discussed later in the chapter.

It is well known that the process of domestication led not only to an increase in the docility of the animals being domesticated but also to physical changes. Not surprisingly, Darwin made some of the first observations of domestication in the context of evolution [15]. Biologically, domestication of animals appears to be based on functional alternations in the neural crest cells, which can account for both the brain function changes and physical changes associated with domestication [12]. Therefore, basic support for the theory of human self-domestication would be evidence that such alterations occur. Obviously, it is impossible to return in time and study the neural crest of humans during their supposed self-domestication process. However, other indirect evidence is available. Williams-Beuren syndrome is a genetic anomaly that is phenotypically expressed with craniofacial dysmorphisms (facial reduction and retraction) and cognitive/behavioral characteristics (pronounced friendliness and reduced reactive aggression) [16] that are typically associated with domestication. Zanella et al. [17] studied neural crest cells from Williams-Beuren patients and showed changes in the 7q11.23 chromosome region and 28 gene deficits that caused neural crest cell-related craniofacial dysmorphisms and cognitive/behavioral characteristics. They claim that these changes are consistent with the hypothesized neurocristopathy mechanism for the self-domestication changes of the modern human face, in conjunction with reduced reactive aggression.

This self-domestication hypothesis is not without its critics. Shilton et al. [18] take umbrage with the term "self-domestication." They point out that many of the traits of domesticated animals are not traits of humans; therefore, it is not appropriate to use the term "domestication" in reference to the social evolution that occurred in human groups. For example, they point out that in domesticated animals, docility to their domesticator was of primary importance; however, for humans, the requirement was for condition-dependent prosocial behavior among group members, but highly aggressive behavior, if needed, toward conspecifics of other social groups. They argue that what underlies human social evolution was a selection for socially mediated emotional control and plasticity. The first stage of this evolution was the development of mimetic (i.e., the practice of representation or imitation of the real world) communication, which required socially mediated emotional plasticity and was accompanied by new social emotions. The second stage was language communication with which group members could instruct others in their group and relied on more extensive emotional plasticity and culturally learned emotional control [18]. Certainly, in the previous section on brain evolution, there is evidence of the brain's increase in size and connectivity, which would allow for this to occur [1, 2]. As this process continues, late human evolution was dominated by selection for intragroup pro-sociality over aggression, the so-called "survival of the friendliest" [19]. I will discuss more on social and cultural evolution in the following section.

I will not engage in this debate about whether humans were "self-domesticated" or simply developed "emotional plasticity and self-control." Frankly, to me, the debate seems more of a matter of semantics. However, the important point, with which both viewpoints tacitly agree, is that *after* the appearance of *Homo sapiens*, this species continued to develop a physical and behavioral phenotype of prioritizing group cohesion over individualism. This process, in my view, has resulted in humans that have an embedded tendency to default to their group's accepted norms and perceptions. I will have more to say about this later in discussing what I will refer to as the *social umwelt*. However, for now, what I had hope to show by the prior sections is that the human mind was evolutionary positioned for social and cultural evolution.[7] This social/cultural evolution is the foundation upon which human rationality, and the ability to be persuaded, rests.

3.2 Social and Cultural Evolution Emphasizing Group Cohesion

In the previous section, I provided an outline of human brain anatomic and functional evolution as a foundation for understanding the importance of social and cultural evolution in the context of a survival and reproductive imperative of staying within your group—that is, group cohesion. There is no group cohesion without individuals finding value in the group (whether consciously, unconsciously or instinctively). This is done through social bonding.

3.2.1 The Social Brain

As previously mentioned, the apex imperative that any living organism has is to survive long enough to reproduce. Every other imperative serves this apex one. Evolution is the result of genetically modified organisms succeeding or failing in this imperative. Although there is no "rationale" to evolution, understanding evolutionary changes teleologically can provide clarity as to why some phenotypes have succeeded.

Humans have large brains relative to their corporeal size. There have been many hypotheses proposed to address how this came about. Dunbar and Shultz [20] have reviewed several of these hypotheses. They point out, as others have [1, 2], that large brains are energetically costly [20]. In fact, there are only a few animal species other than primates that have large brains, e.g., cetaceans. So why is this so? They aver that animals can solve their "fitness" limiting problems[8] individually (e.g., by trial and error learning or insight) or socially (by the presence of several individuals explicitly cooperating for the necessary solution to be effective). They point out that their fitness-limiting factors can be direct (i.e., acquisition of food or mates) or

[7] I completely understand that physical phenotype human evolution overlapped temporally a great deal with social and cultural evolution. I have separated them for the purposes of this book for clarity.

[8] The way this is phrased is clearly teleological. No individuals ever decide in what direction their phenotype will evolve. However, speaking of evolution in terms of "problem solving" does add clarity to why a genetically altered phenotype survives and reproduces.

indirect (e.g., insuring group coordination to manage an exogenous threat to survival or fertility) [20]. They reviewed several explanations, which they put into a figure that I have adapted (Fig. 3.4). I have adapted their figure to emphasize the capacities engendered by a larger brain, leading to what type of capabilities, responding to which types of environmental or social challenges, ultimately conferring what type of advantages to the individual.[9] And, by implication, how these capabilities were woven into the fabric of the human brain and mind.

For primates, as previously mentioned, one of their primary challenges was predation. This threat was from both actual predators and other competing conspecific groups. Primates "solved" this problem by forming groups [1, 2, 20]. These were stable, coherent, coordinated groups that were socially bonded [21]. Living in groups, although beneficial, was extremely costly for the individual in other ways. Increasing group size unavoidably increases competition and costs in terms of the time required for foraging, travel and social bonding. For females, there were significant physiological costs because of the impact of social stress on fertility [20]. There were two types of relationships to manage: those based on direct interactions and those inferred from third-party interactions [20]. This was quite cognitively demanding. This required a theory of mind, as previously discussed, and the ability to model the social world in a virtual mental space, with the ability to foresee the consequences of their actions [20]. That is, they had to create a propositionally structured description of the world to mentally manipulate prior to action—in a

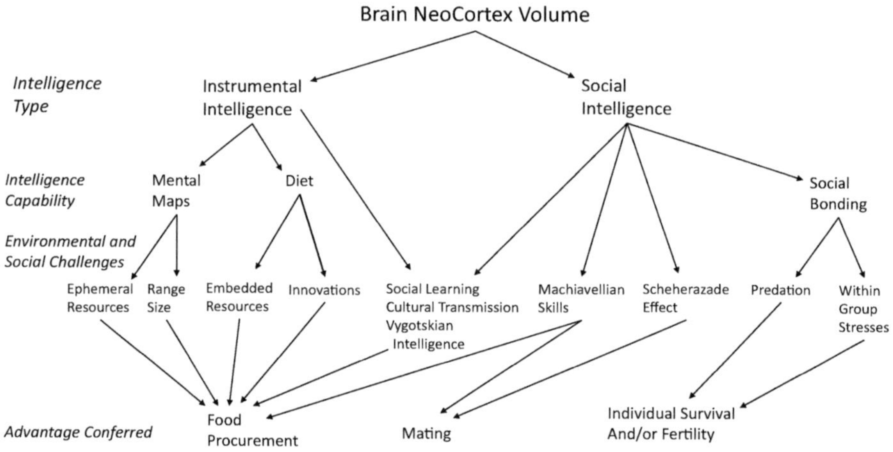

Fig. 3.4 A hierarchical diagram of capacities and abilities under the control of brain neo-cortex volume (adapted from Dunbar and Shultz [20]), with the presumed survival and procreative advantages conferred. Although Dunbar and Shultz's purpose was to assess the various hypotheses proposed for the enlargement of the primate brain, my purpose is simply to illustrate the various challenges primates face in their evolutionary development and the brain functions that have developed

[9] I certainly hope I have not done too much of a disservice to Dunbar and Shultz by manipulating their figure in a way that it was not originally meant.

word, plan. Managing third-party relationships is especially demanding because of the need to discern "strong" from "weak" relationships [21]. Therefore, intense dyadic relationships (i.e., "friends") formed that alleviated stresses that arose by living in close physical proximity to others and could not be escaped by simply leaving the group (without dire consequences). This may be why grooming in primates leads to endorphin release and social interactions in humans leads to oxytocin release, both "feel good" neurotransmitters, to reinforce social bonding and group cohesion.

Humans have developed a brain circuitry to process social interactions. We have developed over 10,000 facial expressions, a subtle but expansive body language, nuanced intonations in our speech, the ability to process visual and sound information, and manners of personal touch, all of which communicate to another individual or groups of individuals [1]. For my thesis, in addition to actual rationality and argumentation, this may be why in-person or seeing someone visually, for example, on television, may be more effective methods of persuasion than reading just the words.

Returning to Fig. 3.4, although much is self-explanatory, other aspects of the figure require a more in-depth explanation [20]. Instrumental intelligence is the mental ability to determine what to do to survive. This includes having a "mental map" of environs in which the individual lives. This is necessary as the resources upon which the individual depends may change over time (i.e., they are ephemeral) and the extent of the territorial range it inhabits so as not to expose itself to undue dangers. The individual is limited by their diet, requiring intelligence relating to their foods (i.e., embedded resources) and perhaps an ability to innovate in foraging. Social intelligence is the mental ability that interacts with other conspecifics. Vygotskian intelligence is the social aspect of intelligence related to collaboration, communication and teaching. This form of intelligence is considered a "phase shift" in both how social life is organized and the kinds of cognitive demands placed on the mind [22]. This type of intelligence may be necessary for the management of larger-scale human societies [20]. The Machiavellian effect is related to the proposition that some members within the group will behave in a selfishly competitive way and, if left unchecked, can lead to group fragmentation. The Scheherazade effect is related to the effects of managing mate fidelity in sexual selection. This may influence pair-bonding. Again, although Dunbar and Shultz's [20] main purpose of their study was to determine the strength of evidence of each of these hypotheses on brain size, and certainly none of these hypotheses can be considered conclusive, they all speak to some level of abilities that lead to individual and species survival.

In summary, the human social mind is an evolutionarily embedded function of the human mind. This creates the environment to transition from phenotypic evolution to cultural evolution. This is where humans ceased to evolve physical traits but evolved social structures to enhance survival and reproduction. Moreover, these social imperatives have evolved to be the default setting of the human mind. Overcoming this default setting will require both education and a certain amount of self-discipline.

3.2.2 *Other Minds*

Cultural evolution requires some level of transfer of ideas, thoughts, feelings, etc., from one individual to another. This requires that the transmitter of the idea have some belief that the receiver of the idea is both capable of understanding what is being transmitted and did not already have the idea. This has been referred to previously as "theory of mind." In philosophy, it is often referred to as "Other Minds" [23]. The question reduces to this: How much do we truly understand of how someone else truly thinks and feels? This is not an inconsequential question in general, and for medicine, it is vital. As a physician, when someone tells me they are in pain, how is it I can know what the pain their experiencing is? This has immense implications for how I will therefore treat the patient.[10]

Unfortunately, there is no satisfactory answer to this question. A rudimentary answer is an argument from analogy. As Shorter [23] explains, if a given phenomenon A has been found to be associated with another phenomenon B, then any phenomenon similar to A is very likely to be associated with a phenomenon similar to B. Therefore, since I am human (phenomenon A) and I think and feel (phenomenon B), then another human, say $A^{\prime}$, (very similar to me as a human) very likely thinks and feels, say $B^{\prime}$ (very similar to the way I think and feel). Going back to my example of treating a patient in pain: I know how I act when I am in pain, when I see a patient act in the same way, then I know the patient is in pain. The problem with this is that we cannot assure the correctness of this argument. There is no way to independently and objectively measure my thought and the other individual's thought so see if, in fact, what I think that they are thinking is, in fact, what they are thinking. The other is that I have only myself as the single source of reference. That is, I am making myself the "gold standard" from which to judge what another person is thinking. Once again, we end up with a lack of objectivity.

This all may be an issue of precision. That is, although we may never know what exactly the other person is thinking, because all we know is what we think they are thinking, evolution has equipped humans with a social brain that allows for communication (in its various forms) so that thoughts and feelings can be understood by another human being in a satisfactorily close enough approximation to allow for effective cooperation. That is, our exchanges can be meaningful, even if they cannot have the experience that another person has. Hence, we can use our communication for cultural evolution.

---

[10] There are many studies in medicine where the management of pain has been the subject of physician bias. For example, see Hoffman KM, et al. Racial bias in pain assessment and treatment recommendations, and false beliefs about biological differences between blacks and whites. Proc Natl Acad Sci USA 2016;113:4296–4301. In a way, this is a problem of "other minds," that is, not truly understanding the experience being recorded in another individual mind.

3.2.3 *Evolution of the Cultural Framework*

In the previous section, I outline how the mental capacities of modern humans formed such that one of the primary qualities of the human mind is the strong imperative is to live in a group and be social within that group. Over some period of time, the norms and mores of the group eventually coalesced into a *culture*. The Merriam-Webster dictionary gives six definitions of culture, the first of which (containing four parts) is relevant for my purposes:

(a) The customary beliefs, social forms, and material traits of a racial, religious, or social group.
(b) The set of shared attitudes, values, goals, and practices that characterizes an institution or organization.
(c) The set of values, conventions, or social practices associated with a particular field, activity, or societal characteristic.
(d) The integrated pattern of human knowledge, belief, and behavior depends upon the capacity for learning and transmitting knowledge to succeeding generations [24].

All of these definitions are useful in a common sense way of understanding culture. However, from the standpoint of understanding how *cultural evolution* has superseded genetic evolution in modern day humans, I believe the definition put forth by the Cultural Evolution Society is more precise: “Information capable of affecting individuals’ behavior that they acquire from other members of their species through teaching, imitation and other forms of social transmission” [25]. As a result, as Rosaldo puts it, “If people think and feel differently about the world, they are not demented or stupid. Instead, they simply are making different assumptions and using different categories to make sense of the world they inhabit and find meaning in it” [26]. For this society, cultural evolution “is that cultural change constitutes an evolutionary process that share fundamental similarities with—but also differs in key ways from—genetic evolution” [25].

I am going to acknowledge that the word “culture” has some controversy. For example, there are some in the social anthropology field that assert that “culture” cannot be separated from “nature” [27]. Quite frankly, I am not equipped to comment on this debate, nor, for the purposes of this book, do I necessarily think it is relevant. I am more inclined to agree with Rosaldo [26] that culture “became a term which was primarily used in an anthropological sense of a ‘way of life’ of distinct human groups to something of shared values and beliefs of social groups.” In this sense, “social groups” could mean just about any collection of humans that are associated with one another. There is a burgeoning cottage industry dedicated to improving “organizational culture” for businesses, for example. In this sense, Rosaldo [26] further goes on to say that “there is not a single, eternal definition of culture, but rather provisional definitions that will be revised as debates unfold through time.” Therefore, from the standpoint of my thesis, I will adopt the definition of the Cultural Evolutionary Society [25] because it acknowledges the importance of the members of the group imposing the cultural beliefs and norms onto others in their group.

It is uncontroversial that humans learn. It is also uncontroversial that they can learn in a variety of ways. In general, learning can be categorized as "individual learning" and "social learning" [28]. Social learning, in Henrich's [28] definition, is the learning that occurs when an individual is influenced by other conspecifics. Individual learning is the learning that occurs in situations in which individuals learn by observing or interacting with their environment. As appealing as these definitions are, social and individual learning are not exclusive. As Henrich [28] points out, the least sophisticated form of social learning occurs simply as a byproduct of being around others and then engaging in individual learning. Moreover, the environment created by the individual's ancestors has laid the foundation of what can be learned and how [29]. As I interpret this, over the course of generations, the group has developed processes to acquire and apply knowledge that has led the group to survive as a group. This acquired knowledge is passed down to the succeeding generations, some of which is perpetuated, some of which is modified, perhaps consciously, perhaps unconsciously. Over time, young members of this group simply absorb this knowledge and processes as part of living in their world.

The *Homo sapiens* diaspora over the last 300,000 years has lived in pockets of communities scattered across six continents. It is certainly easy to understand how these disparate groups developed different norms and mores, in sum, cultures, to adapt to the environments in which they found themselves. What is less obvious is the number of "universals" that all humans seem to share [30]. According to Brown [30], human universals are "those features of culture, society, language, behavior and mind that, thus far as the record has been examined, are found among all peoples known to ethnography and history." These universals can be grouped into the following categories, although many have overlap among groups:

Cultural: myths, legends, daily routines, rules, concepts of luck and precedent, body adornments, the use and production of tools, etc.

Language: grammar, phonemes, polysemy, metonymy, antonyms, inverse ratio between the frequency of use and length of words, etc.

Social: division of labor, social groups, age grading, the family, kinship systems, ethnocentrism, play, exchange, cooperation, reciprocity, etc.

Behavior: aggression, gestures, gossip, facial expressions, etc.

Mind: emotions, dichotomous thinking, wariness around or fear of snakes, empathy, psychological defense mechanisms, etc.

He further goes on to say that many of these universals almost certainly have distinctive, even dedicated, neural underpinnings [30]. Certainly, in the previous sections, I put forth the narrative that human brain evolution has, in fact, produced a brain with the neural, glial and neuropil mass to be able to encode beliefs and behaviors similar to these.

Brown [30] further states that some of these features are overtly or consciously recognized by the group (*emic* features), while others are in the group's culture but not recognized (*etic* features). Many universals have a collective rather than an individual referent. For example, all cultures have music, but not all individuals are musical. The important point here for my purposes is that there will be influences on an individual's thought based on cultural features influencing them. This has profound implications for persuasion.

Finally, Brown [30] categorizes universals into kinds:

Absolute: found in all peoples at all times.
Near: Some few known or suspected group exceptions.
Conditional: If a particular condition is met, then the trait in question always accompanies it.
Statistical: Not absolute, but occurs in unrelated societies at a rate that seems higher than chance.
Universal Pool: a limited set of options exhausts the possible variations from one society to another.

Therefore, in other words, some "universals" are, in fact, universal—everybody has them. On the other hand, other universals have some variation in penetrance; that is, a certain number of people in a certain number of groups at some particular times in history will display these universals. This is most likely related to the causal processes that led to the universals to be developed initially. According to Brown [30], there are a surprisingly small number of such causal processes:

1. The diffusion of ancient and useful cultural traits.
2. The cultural reflection of physical facts.
3. The operation, structure and evolution of the human mind.

Ultimately, Brown [30] concludes that whatever is constant through all human societies must be due to something that goes with people wherever they go. However, the observed variation in culture is entirely compatible with a "panhuman" design of the mind. What I conclude is that there are bedrock universal mind and behavioral characteristics that all humans have; however, there is culture-specific variation that can affect how individuals may hear and understand an argument. Moreover, quite of bit these cultural characteristics are not immutable, that is, they can be changed.

3.2.4 Are There Unconscious Influences on How Humans Receive Information?

What I have tried to show in the previous sections is that the human brain evolved to produce a mind that is highly social, in need of being within a group, and absorbs the cultural priorities of the group, at least some, if not much, is etic. So this then begs the question: Are there certain ideas that have great, albeit unconscious, meaning to humans?

Brown [30] identified that all human groups have their own myths and legends. These are passed down as stories, initially spoken or sung, but now written. Are there commonalities among these myths and legends? Could those commonalities be exploited for persuasion? Carl Jung, an early twentieth century psychologist, developed a theory of the "collective unconscious" [31]. Part of this theory was the notion that all humans, through their collective unconscious, harbored certain "archetypes" that represented specific notions related to understanding the world. Although it has fallen out of favor from the standpoint of a psychological theory used to treat mental illness, the concept of archetypes that are found in all forms of art is still valuable. My purpose here is not to enumerate or analyze these archetypes but note the consistency of the notions of "human universals" with archetypes that may unconsciously be very influential to humans. I will have more to say about this in the next chapter, especially with respect to storytelling as an instrument of persuasion.

3.3 The Idea of the Social Umwelt, or Although Seeing Is Believing, Sometimes We See What We Believe

3.3.1 Introducing the Concept of the Social Umwelt

In 1909, the biologists Jakob von Uexkull introduced the concept of the *umwelt* as it pertains to the way animals perceive the world [32]. Briefly, all animals have senses that take in information of the world around them. Their brain (and mind[11]) processes this information, and they behave accordingly. Therefore, for humans, evolution has provided us with five senses: vision, hearing, smell, taste and touch. Specifically, we have tricolor vision, which can see colors in the "visible" (to humans) spectrum.[12] Wavelengths and frequencies outside this spectrum are completely invisible to us. Our hearing covers an "audible" frequency[13] and within this range and is also related to the "loudness" of the sound, which we measure in decibels. Sounds outside this audible spectrum or softer than the loudness can carry are completely silent to us. Our olfactory organ can react to a number of chemicals[14] that stimulate the organ to recognize an odor when the chemicals reach a sufficient concentration. Chemicals outside of these or at lower concentrations will be completely odorless. Our tongue has five regions of particular taste that respond to

[11] I am not going to get into the issue of whether or not animals other than humans have a "mind" in the sense that we believe that humans have a mind. I will reveal that my view is that they do have a mind, consistent with their umwelt, but I have no proof to support this assertion.

[12] The typical visible spectrum for the human eye is wavelengths from ~380 to ~750 nm, or 400–790 THz frequency.

[13] The audible frequency spectrum is between 20 and 20,000 Hz, but with some variation among individual humans.

[14] The number of odors that humans can distinguish is thought to be more than one trillion.

chemicals in contact with the tongue, the combination of which leads to the flavor we experience when we put something in our mouths. Our skin has a variety of receptors that respond to pressure, temperature and a spectrum of noxious stimuli. Last, although not considered a "sense" in the same manner as the above senses, we also have the sense of proprioception, that is, we know where our body parts are in space, even if we cannot see them. In combination, this is our umwelt—it is how we perceive the world. Moreover, save for the instruments that allow us to perceive the parts of the world that we cannot (microscopes, telescopes, sonars, etc.), this *is* our world.

However, it is not how all other animals perceive their worlds. For example, many birds and insects can perceive colors outside of our visible spectrum. To them, flowers, plants, other birds or insects, inanimate objects can look very different to them than to us. Bats and dolphins have sonar capabilities; that is, they create a sound and are able to perceive the return echo, which they use for "echolocation" purposes, usually for prey. For bats, the sound they produce for echolocation is at a frequency that is out of the range audible for humans. Pit vipers have infrared sensors in their pits to sense the body heat of prey. On the other hand, all snakes lack hearing; theirs is a world of silence. Many fish are able to sense the electrical field generated by other marine organisms. Dogs and bears have relatively poor vision (bichromatic) compared to humans but exceptional olfaction for both the range of chemicals that can be resolved into specific smells and the concentration of chemicals that can elicit a smell. By virtue of these different sensory capabilities, these animals perceive the world differently than humans. In essence, the world for them *is* a different place than it is for humans.

By analogy, I am proposing that humans have a *social umwelt*. That is, because of the culture they inhabit, their perceptions of the world are different. Moreover, what counts as a perception worth registering is a function of this social umwelt. In fact, this social umwelt is the culmination of human biological, social and cultural evolution. Evolution has produced a species that better survived as a group to avoid predation; the human brain evolved to be well suited to being aware of the social conditions of their group; brain chemicals—such as endorphins and oxytocin—are used by the brain to reinforce social interactions as pleasurable for humans; there is evidence that humans removed from their midst individuals who did not adhere to norms of the group—especially aggression to group conspecifics; with the advent of language, the ability to educate other members of the group as to the norms of the group developed; these norms, perhaps through stories and art,[15] have become embedded as human universals, which also vary to a greater or lesser extent from cultural group to cultural group. In summary, the "default" setting for humans is to maintain the social cohesion of their group by adhering to these norms, which, in

[15] The fact that there are paintings found in caves created by our ancestors thousands of years ago and that all known human cultures have some type of oral tradition of stories speaks forcefully for the immense importance of these forms of communication in the cultural indoctrination of humans into their groups. These forms of communication are probably the most effective forms of persuasion (although not necessarily the most likely to arrive at truth).

essence, becomes their world view. Recently, there have been several proposals of what these world views are and how they affect how humans perceive and understand the world. What follows are only a few examples simply to illustrate the point.[16]

3.3.2 *Primal World Beliefs*

Primal World Beliefs was a concept introduced by Jeremy D. W. Clifton and his colleagues in 2019 [33]. These "beliefs" are considered by the authors as "environmental" beliefs having to do with the overall character of the world. Although it is beyond the scope of this book to review or critique this theory, I will provide a brief description. These authors assert that every person has a "subset of beliefs specific to the overall character of the world," that is, "beliefs about everything" [33]. This theory has been distilled into 26 primal beliefs about the world [34]:

Primary Primal: Good vs. Bad
Secondary "Primals": Safe vs. Dangerous, Enticing vs. Dull, Alive vs. Mechanistic
Tertiary Primals Related to the Secondary Primals:

> Related to Safe vs. Dangerous: Pleasurable vs Miserable, Regenerative vs. Degenerative, Progressing vs. Declining, Harmless vs. Threatening, Cooperative vs. Competitive, Stable vs. Fragile, Just vs. Unjust
>
> Related to Enticing vs. Dull: Interesting vs. Boring, Beautiful vs. Ugly, Abundant vs. Barren, Worth Exploring vs. Not Worth Exploring, Meaningful vs. Meaningless, Improvable vs. Too Hard to Improve, Funny vs. No Funny
>
> Related to Alive vs. Mechanistic: Intentional vs. Unintentional, Needs Me vs. Does not Need Me, Interactive vs. Indifferent
>
> Unrelated Tertiary Primals: Acceptable vs. Unacceptable, Changing vs. Static, Hierarchical vs. Nonhierarchical, Interconnected vs. Separable, Understandable vs. Too Hard to Understand

Again, I am in no position to judge how well this theory assesses, in fact, how well people actually feel about the world,[17] my interest in it is as an example that some researchers recognize that humans indeed have a world view that then affects how they perceive the world and what type of information will influence their judgments about the world. For example, someone who views that world as a "dangerous" placed will be more inclined to believe in the credence of information compatible with this view. Persuading this person of something that places the world in a "safe" light may be difficult.

---

[16] The inclusion of these theories in this book does not imply that I endorse any of these theories. They are included only as examples of how a world view affects ones thinking.

[17] One can actually take the survey for oneself on their website; see Ref. [34].

I also find it curious that in this particular theory, all of the primals are dichotomous, and, as Brown [30] previously established, dichotomous thinking is a human universal. Whether these "primals" are an innate, inborn character of the individual person or whether they are acquired during life is an area of research in this field, which, again, is beyond the purposes of this book.

3.3.3 *Moral Foundations*

Another theory as to how human evolution led to innate and culturally developed modes of perceiving and responding to the world is the Moral Foundation Theory [35]. This was initially a theory to explain the pluralism of morality norms among human cultures but now hopes to explain the reactions of humans to various situations [36]. These authors report basing this theory on what is known about human biological and cultural evolution. They then try to determine the psychological mechanisms for why people and groups hold divergent moral values and beliefs [35]. These authors claim that the human brain has evolved so that there is an innate "first draft" of the "moral mind," which is organized prior to any experience that the person may have [35]. Certainly, from the prior discussion about human biological evolution of the mind [1, 2], the human mind has evolved neural structure and function to allow for this. Others, such as Brown with his ideas of "human universals" [30] and Jung with his ideas of archetypes [31], suggest this as well. Moreover, Moral Foundation Theory claims that the human mind is organized biologically "in advance of experience" such that "it is prepared to learn values, norms, and behavior related to a diverse set of recurrent adaptive social problems" [35]. They create a brain model containing "modules" for the acquisition of "cognitive competence" [35]. Because there were many recurrent social challenges in human groups, several, if relatively few, moral foundations developed [35]. As humans spread across the globe, these moral foundations fostered specific cultural structures to address the unique challenges faced by those groups.

These authors claim that humans have six basic moral foundations [36]:

1. Care/Harm Foundation. Because human evolution led to large brains and subsequently fewer children per pregnancy and because these children would not survive without at least maternal care for an extended period of time, humans have also evolved an innate sense to care for children, then for others in the group. That is, humans place a moral value of caring for others, at least in their own group, and find those who are not morally offensive. Certainly, this corresponds to the "self-domestication" theory previously discussed [12–18].
2. Fairness/Cheating Foundation. As humans evolved to live in cohesive groups, a premium was placed on cooperation with others in the group. Again, this is also consistent with the self-domestication theory previously discussed. Reciprocity also became valued, as Brown [30] enumerates as a human universal. Those who did not cooperate or did not reciprocate were not an asset to the group. This then developed into the foundation of "fairness" to others within the group, while

those who tried to "cheat" (i.e., enjoy the benefits of group living without contributing to the group) were morally offensive.

3. Loyalty/Betrayal Foundation. As primates evolved into groups, hierarchies developed. Both primate evolution [1, 2] and human social evolution [20, 21] provide evidence of this. Group cohesion required recognition and acceptance of this hierarchy. This developed further into loyalty to the group and its members (and, secondarily, its leaders). This then led to the moral foundation of being loyal to your group, while those who betrayed it would morally repugnant.
4. Authority/Subversion Foundation. Primate hierarchy imposes the authority of more dominant individuals over weaker individuals. The initial mother-child relationship is such an authority relationship. This extended to other relationships in the hierarchy such that weaker individuals (however, "weaker" is defined) submit to the authority of "stronger" individuals (however, "stronger" is defined). Those that subvert such established authority can damage group cohesion.
5. Sanctity/Degradation Foundation. During their evolutionary process, primates were exposed to a variety of pathogens and other environmental risks. Although, obviously, the causative agents of such risks were not initially identified (science later did this), items known to be associated with such risks were avoided, e.g., foul smelling food, or, as Brown [30] notes, snakes. This further evolved into these items eliciting a sense of disgust—what the authors call the "behavioral immune system." Conversely, behaviors that avoided disgusting items were sanctified. This then extended to other behaviors outside the accepted spectrum of behaviors for that group.
6. Liberty/Oppression. Even within groups, there is a constant struggle for dominance. Those who must submit to the dominance of the hierarchy develop feelings of reactance and resentment toward those who dominate them and restrict their liberty. Those who find affinity to this foundation often find themselves at odds with those who value the Authority/Subversion foundation.

Again, I make no endorsement of Moral Foundation Theory's correctness, although it appears to me that there is more than a modicum of truth in it. More importantly, this is another example of researchers trying to understand how both biological and social/cultural evolution have worked to construct the social umwelt that humans live in.

I feel at this point, a clarification is in order. I have previously discussed in this chapter that humans are born into groups and that their brain has evolved to believe that there is a survival advantage of staying within the group. Human cultures have evolved for the primary purpose of maintaining group cohesion in the face of threats—first from predation and then from conspecific groups. However, it is blatantly untrue that all humans in a group will think the same. Although the social umwelt may impose some type of structure, there is a certain amount of variation to a greater or lesser degree.

3.3.4 Motivated Cognition

The theory of *motivated cognition* is the idea that people seek to deflect threats to their identities and roles assigned by their cultural norms, which may be contested by others, especially others in an "outside group" [37]. Daniel Kahan and his collaborators have studied this phenomenon extensively. They explain that motivated cognition is a form of information processing that promotes individuals' interests in forming and maintaining beliefs that signify loyalty to important affinity groups [38]. The basic premise is that group membership can affect how people process information about nearly all categories of stimuli in the social world [39]. In this view, individuals tend to adapt the beliefs common to members of their "in-group" and resist revision of those beliefs even when contrary evidence is presented, particularly when this evidence originates from members of the "out-group," who are likely to be perceived as less trustworthy [40]. This theory is consistent with what I presented previously on human biological, social and cultural evolution.

This leads to several consequences with respect to an individual's ability to appraise an argument and the possibility of them being persuaded. In Kahan et al.'s [38] study of the "white-male effect," an observation that white males are less risk adverse than women or members of other ethnic groups demonstrated that white males are more likely to hold anti-egalitarian and individualistic attitudes, which are woven into their cultural world view. These individuals are disposed to accept or dismiss risk claims in a manner that expresses their cultural values [38]. This is especially true when they are confronted that activities integral to their social roles as constructed by their cultural commitments are attacked as societally damaging, especially from members of the out-group. That is, it is a defensive response to their cultural identity [38]. This extends to other groups as well. In another study, Kahan et al. [41] found that individuals who have the skills necessary to evaluate quantitative data will selectively interpret culturally affirming data favorably and dismiss culturally discordant data [41]; that is, they will make the data support their side. These responses are consistent with what has been previously presented with respect to human biological, social and cultural evolution. The imperative to stay within your group for many overrules, most likely unconsciously, dispassionate critical thinking. That is, Kahneman's "fast-thinking" system, which is more ingrained, is the default over the "slow-thinking" system [42].

The implications for persuasion are obvious. If the listener is predisposed to believe that the arguer is either a member of their group or not, their willingness to be persuaded by the argument can be greatly affected. A key feature here is trust. That is, the listener must trust that the arguer's premises are true and that the arguer has the listener's personal and cultural interests at heart. Obviously, this can create conflict if the listener does not perceive this, despite the logical strength of the illative core of the argument.

3.3.5 Self-Deception

Humans are prone to a certain amount of self-deception. Mijovic-Prelec and Prelec [43] studied human self-deception. In their view, there are three levels of belief:

1. Deep Belief—this is what drives actions, including overt statements of beliefs.
2. Stated Belief—what the individual states as their belief.
3. Experienced Belief—This determines the emotional state following a statement of belief.

When a stated belief does not match the deep belief, these authors define this as a potential act of self-deception. If the experienced belief (i.e., the emotional response) matches the stated belief, then the attempt at self-deception was a success. The attempt falls short if the experienced belief discounts the stated belief. That is, if an individual states that x is true but their deep belief (perhaps consciously, perhaps not) is that x is false **and** the individual emotionally reacts to the statement *as if* they believed it to be true, then this constitutes self-deception. On the other hand, if the individual reacted to their statement in a way that belies the truth of x, then even though they stated that x were true, they know that it is not. That is, the individual knows that they are trying to fool themselves.

These authors contend that some deep beliefs are "inaccessible," meaning that the individual may not be consciously aware of them [43]. Again, this appears consistent with biological, social and cultural evolution. However, these statements have "self-signaling" value. That is, there may be motivation for self-deception to provide some type of value to the individual. The incentives for this self-deception (say, cultural coercion) and self-knowledge (actually being consciously aware of the deep belief) jointly determine whether the self-deception is successful. The authors further go on to present experimental evidence of their theory of self-deception as self-signaling game theory based on Bayesian calculations (some of this in the next chapter) [43]. Ultimately, however, self-deception is an external, public activity rather than an inward, private one. That is, the individual is trying to prove something (i.e., a signal or a shibboleth) to others in their group.

The philosopher Quassim Cassam in his book *Self-Knowledge for Humans* tries to work out how humans are aware of the things they know [44]. Much of the book explores the philosophical theories trying to address "trivial" self-knowledge (e.g., "My belief that I am now wearing socks") to "substantial" self-knowledge (e.g., "How do I know I am a good person"), making pointed comparisons of real *Homo sapiens* to the hypothetical *Homo philosophicus* and *Homo economicus*. Although interesting in its own right and not without its critics,[18] my purpose is not to elaborate on his views but to bring up his observations related to self-deception. These include belief-perserverance, self-ignorance and attitude recalcitrance. *Belief perse-*

[18] For example, see the book reviews by Richard Moran, "Review of Cassam, *Self-Knowledge for Humans*," *Times Literary Supplement*, July, 2015 and Peter Carruthers, "Self-Knowledge for Humans," *Notre Dame Philosophical Reviews*, April 16, 2015.

verance refers to the extent to which people will hold on to their beliefs despite evidence that their beliefs are not true [45]. Nesbitt and Ross suggest that part of the reason for this is *confirmation bias*; that is, people tend to seek out, recall and interpret evidence in a manner that sustains their beliefs [45]. What modern journalists now refer to as "echo chambers." This is certainly consistent with what I previously said about the social umwelt and studies having to do with motivated cognition and cultural identity. *Self-ignorance* essentially comes in two flavors: not knowing *what* your beliefs are and not knowing *why* you have those beliefs [44]. In the first, you may have beliefs, you are just not consciously aware that you do or do not have them, while in the second, you know you have a belief, you just do not know how it came about that you have that belief. Once, again, this is consistent with biological, social and cultural evolution of humans—perhaps also consistent with a few human universals. Last, *attitude recalcitrance* is that you *know* that you do not have a particular good reason to have the belief, but you have the belief nevertheless [44]. Cassam [44] discusses two types of attitude recalcitrance: judgment insensitive and judgment sensitive. He gives the example of judgment-insensitive attitude recalcitrance of fear of harmless spiders—you know that the spider cannot harm you, yet you are afraid of it anyway. In judgment-sensitive recalcitrance, you do have the ability to consciously appraise evidence for and against your belief, and despite evidence against, you hold on to the belief. You simply do not recognize that your belief has been discredited, which Harman [46] calls *clutter avoidance*. The point here is that humans have an underlying capacity to fool themselves. This is a consequence of how human evolution produced the human mind it did. This is consistent with my overall thesis that the human mind evolved to survive, not to discern truth.

3.3.6 Susceptibility to Logical Fallacy

Logical fallacies, which were only mentioned in passing in the prior chapter, as accepting as sound arguments that are logically invalid.[19] These mental mechanisms that evolution has produced predispose humans to logical fallacies. Gilovich [48] attempts to explain why so many people hold untrue beliefs. He states that people hold questionable beliefs not because they are not exposed to reliable, relevant evidence, nor because they are stupid or gullible. Humans' erroneous beliefs, Gilovich writes, are derived primarily from the misapplication or overutilization of generally valid and effective strategies. Many apocryphal beliefs are due to our mental ability to process good data, while others are due to the data themselves being incomplete or "messy" [48]. He emphasizes specific fallacies:

[19] For example, Johnson [47] list several types of fallacies: ad hominin, ad verecundiam, hasty conclusions, suppressed evidence, red herring, provincialism, ambiguity, and contextual. I suspect that when these occur, it is done consciously by the arguer knowing that the listener wants to believe the fallacy, or done in a "fast-thinking" mode not understanding that the fallacy occurred.

1. Random data and the human tendency to see regularity and order where none actually exists.
2. Incomplete and unrepresentative data and one's ability to detect and correct for these biases.
3. Humans' eagerness to interpret ambiguous and inconsistent data in light of our preferred expectations.

All this, and what was also said previously, is consistent with the work of Nobel laureate Daniel Kahneman and Amos Tversky's theory of "judgment under uncertainty" [49]. Their basic theory is that data acquisition and analysis may be so complicated and time-consuming that the human mind develops heuristics (i.e., rules of thumb) to quickly come to judgments and decisions. Certainly, this was necessary in our hominin ancestral past, where avoiding predation and securing food at times needed to be quick decisions. Their contention, and quite frankly much of what I previously presented, is that this has persisted. The vast majority of time, this works out reasonably well. However, it can lead to poor decisions or untrue beliefs. Such fallacies include the belief in the "law of small numbers," judgments of "representativeness," "availability," and "anchoring," among others. As the issues that any one person faces become more complex, the likelihood that one of these heuristics will lead to error increases. That is, a person may persist in "fast thinking" (with the social umwelt that they are familiar with), instead of switching to "slow thinking" [42], which is truly critical thinking and reasoning. Therefore, strict logical rules in an illative form of an argument may not be "heard" by the patient in the manner intended. In this type of situation, the physician should try to "slow down" the patient's thinking and try to "correct" the fallacious thinking in a manner that is not threatening to the patient social group's norms.

Again, my purpose here is not to endorse any of these particular theories but once again use it as an illustrative example of how the evolutionary path that our primate and hominin ancestors traveled have affected our rational abilities. However, there is a consistent theme that there is more to human choice that rational, material self-interest.

3.3.7 *Shibboleth Behavior*

Although not an essential feature of human reasoning, humans have evolved to be "supercommunicators" to use Hoffmann's term [50]. He asserts that the human brain is a "predication machine," meaning that it logically affirms something about another. This is done through human communication. In this communication, approximately one-third is due specifically to language, while two-thirds is due in nonverbal communication. Of this, it is estimated that of the "total impact of the message," 7% is the words one uses, 38% is the characteristics of the voice one uses, and the remaining 55% is completely nonverbal. This is the result of how human brains evolved and is an inescapable part of how humans function. It is also a part of the physician's "data gathering" about a patient. *How* the patient communicates information is almost as important and *what* information they communicate.

This brings us to acknowledge the importance of shibboleths. When reviewing the definitions of shibboleth according to Merriam-Webster [51], the most relevant definition is "a custom or usage regarded as distinguishing one group from another." In other words, this is a form of communication that allows individuals to identify their preferred groups. A rather innocuous shibboleth is wearing a cap of your favorite sports team to communicate to others what your rooting interests are. One can list numerous examples of shibboleths for all manner of associations. It is important to acknowledge that shibboleths are not only objects but also behaviors and language. That is, the displaying of socially acceptable behavior for the group is a manner of expressing loyalty to that group (consistent with one of the Moral Foundations). Similarly, the words individuals choose to use may not only carry the customary meaning of the word but also have a "social" meaning that those in the group may understand and signal to that group the speaker's *bona fides* for that group.

The reason that I bring this up is that medically related equipment, paraphernalia, treatments, etc., have become shibboleths. Patients may choose certain treatments because those choices signal to their group their allegiances to that group. I have certainly noticed that some patients come to the office wearing or speaking in shibboleths. They were signaling to me what they are and are not willing to accept with respect to medical advice. Understanding these shibboleths can be used by health care practitioners to gauge the type of communication necessary to maximize the persuasion of these individuals. In addition, health care professionals are not immune to displaying shibboleths and having reactions to them.[20] It is essential that physicians and other health care professionals have the self-discipline not to allow shibboleths to affect their relationships to their patients.

3.3.8 Human Reasoning Based on Mental Models

In the last chapter, I referred to the work of Johnson-Laird [52] that even people with no formal training in logic are able to make logical deductions. It is time to discuss his work further. Johnson-Laird acknowledges that there are large differences in the ability to reason from one individual to another. He then couples this with the assertion that almost all forms of reasoning by humans, no matter the subject, are computationally intractable. This means that as the number and complexity of the premises increase, the ability to perform the correct calculations or logical processes becomes more difficult to the point of not being able to perform the logical mechanics at all, as was discussed in Chap. 2 pertaining to formal logic. Therefore, he

[20] For example, asking the patient their pronoun will signal to the patient that you support transgender individuals and are therefore a liberal. If the patient does not subscribe to this belief, effective communication may be lost. This type of situation was written about by Lala Tanmoy Das, "The Inclusivity Trap," *The Washington Post*, February 19, 2021.

proposes an alternated view: Reasoning depends on envisioning the possibilities consistent with the starting point of the reasoner, whether it is the perception of the world, a set of assertions, a memory, or some mixture of these. Then, the reasoner constructs a "mental model" of each distinct possibility and derives a conclusion from them. Counterexamples are used to refute errors caused by systemic errors in the model. Reasoning is, therefore, a simulation of the world fleshed out with our knowledge, not a formal arrangement of the logical skeleton of sentences [52].

Considering that Chap. 2 was all about reasoning, logic and argumentation, this last assertion by Johnson-Laird is quite the broadside. He avers that until approximately 30 years ago, the consensus in psychology was that humans' ability to reason depends on a tacit mental logic, consisting of formal rules of inference (much like what was discussed in Chap. 2). However, not all forms of reasoning fit into these forms (which was also discussed at some length in Chap. 2). One can obtain logically valid conclusions that are not materially true. He bases this assertion on years of studies of actual humans using brain imaging.

A mental model is when a human perceives the world, they have a vision of what things are in the scene in front of them. They then construct a similar, but less detailed, model that can then function as a simulation of this aspect of the world [52]. This theory rests on three assumptions:

1. Each mental model represents what is common to a distinct set of possibilities.
2. Mental models are iconic insofar as they can be the structure of the representation corresponding to the structure of what is represented.
3. Mental models of descriptions represent what is true at the expense of what is false [53].

This last principle of truth reduces the load that these mental models place on working memory (as a result of human brain evolution); however, this comes at the expense of errors in deduction. The ultimate purpose is to obtain a conclusion that is true, novel, and maintains information [52]. One of the advantages of the iconic representation mental model is that it can yield relations that were not asserted when the premises of the argument were enumerated [52].

Johnson-Laird [52] acknowledges that humans have two "systems" of reasoning corresponding to Kahneman's fast and slow thinking [42]. Because of the limitations of working memory, the "intuitive" system use of working memory limits the number of items that can be processed (as noted in the previous chapter on intuition, intuition processing is nearly all unconscious). The second system is the slow thinking system with the use of a deliberate and recursive process of reasoning. This is the process of argumentation—constructing and appraising the illative core of an argument (as noted in the prior chapter). The consequence of this is that the more models needed to make an inference, the harder coming to an inference is—when it gets to more than three, it becomes quite difficult [52]. I would also contend that as the content becomes more abstract, the more difficult it is, especially for the nonexpert, to construct a mental model. For example, can we expect a patient to have the same mental model of the cholesterol molecule and its interaction with arteries that a physician does?

Content appears to affect all aspects of reasoning, from the interpretation of premises, the process itself and the formation of conclusions [52]. Because of the principle of truth (assumption #3 above), certain fallacies can occur, which can lead to false conclusions but still carry a high degree of confidence by the reasoner (which is referred to as a "cognitive illusion"). He asserts that people do not solve reasoning problems in a single, deterministic way. Humans, when they reason, do not make a distinction between deduction, induction and abduction (see Chap. 2 for details on these types of logic) because it exploits what is already known about the subject of the reasoning, that is, the subject of the reasoning influences how the person reasons. However, once a person has developed a strategy for a particular problem, this strategy tends to control their reasoning. Reasoning becomes more of a simulation of the world filled in with the relevant information the reasoner has about the subject than a formal manipulation of the logical skeleton of sentences. People build mental models, which represent distinct possibilities, or that unfold in time in a kinematic sequence, and we base our conclusion on them [52]. Certainly, this view is consistent with the brain circuitry related to "mental time travel" [1, 2], as previously discussed.

One can easily see how this type of model is relevant in medical persuasion. Recall our example of the medical encounter from Chap. 1. It is certainly easy to imagine as the patient is listening to the physician about treatment options, he develops a "mental image" of their future self after each treatment—that is, their future self-taking medications, their future self after an operation that was successful, their future self-suffering operative complications, etc. In addition, the patient may imagine how the choice of treatment may be viewed by their most relevant group(s) and how their future self may be received by their group after treatment. The physician uses his abilities as a human "supercommunicator" to try to convey to the patient the necessary information that the patient will use in his reasoning about his future self. This certainly fits into the "slow" thinking model of Kahneman [42]. In another scenario where decisions have to happen quickly, intuitive, fast thinking may be the most appropriate for the patient and physician.

3.4 Is this the Basis of the Patient's Comprehensive and Rationality?

I have taken pains to layout the evolutionary development of the human brain biologically, the development of humans need for being in social groups, and the cultural evolution of these groups for the purpose of understanding how humans actually reason, with the ultimate purpose of understanding their decision-making process and how they can be persuaded. I have tried to synthesize the salient features of theories, hypotheses, observations and arguments from evolutionary biologists, anthropologists, social and cognitive psychologists, neuroscientists, social scientists and philosophers. I have no doubt my synthesis is crude and I have missed much nuance, but I believe I have laid a foundation for persuasion.

I would first like to acknowledge that what I have focused on is how humans reason and what may be the biological/cultural/evolutionary factors that led to and constrained this ability. I have given passing acknowledgment that humans can acquire new knowledge (and like doing so), but I have not discussed in any meaningful way how humans store or use this knowledge. Abernathy and Hamm [54] discuss this in their book on surgical intuition. Knowledge is "stored" in long-term memory under the theory of *semantic networks* [55]. That is, within the brain, there are "nodes" with "ideas" that are connected to other idea nodes. The greater these nodes are accessed in critical thinking, the stronger the connections become. This will eventually lead to expertise. This use of knowledge is consistent with Johnson-Laird's [52, 53] theory of models and how knowledge content affects reasoning. Although the concepts of knowledge storage are important, it will not be addressed here are my goal is to understand human reasoning.

Although Johnson-Laird [52, 53] advocates the terms of mental models and humans "running a simulation" to future states, discounting the "sentence skeleton" model as the essential mechanism of human reasoning. I am going to understand this sentence skeleton as the illative core of an argument that was discussed in the prior chapter. Although the mental models theory may be how humans make decisions and judgments particularly for possible physical occurrences, I am having a hard time seeing how this theory explains reasoning for "abstract" ideas, say, a new medical theory. I am also going to say that the creation of new scientific knowledge and its appraisal is certainly more consistent with the "manifest rationality" of Johnson [47] rather than the mental models of Johnson-Laird [52, 53]. Moreover, most communications of new ideas *are* presented in an illative form, so the ability to appraise arguments, as discussed in the prior chapter, is still relevant (I will discuss this more in Chap. 6). Therefore, issues with respect to how individuals receive these arguments and the constraints they have on their abilities to do so need to be assessed with respect to persuasion. This includes how the social umwelt affects how an individual perceives the argument.

The social umwelt constrains the listener's argument appraisal in a "fast-thinking," intuitive way. The first part of the appraisal will have to do with who the arguer is. If the arguer is someone not considered part of the listener's group, an issue of *trust* becomes important, as previously mentioned. That is, if the listener does not trust the source of the argument, they will not even bother to determine if the illative (or for that matter, the mental model) is sound. Even if the listener grants the arguer the benefit of the doubt, the listener may not assess the voracity of the premises. If the premises are not true, then the conclusion is not true. Last, even if the listener grants that the premises are true and the conclusion sound, acceptance of the conclusion may be at odds with membership in their group. As evolution has made the listener (as well as ever other human) inclined to maintain membership in their most important salient priority (even if the consequences are not as mortal as in our evolutionary past), the listener may still reject a sound conclusion to maintain group membership. This, obviously, has great ramifications for persuasion.

Despite what has been said, I do not mean to imply that humans are held hostage to the world views of their predominate culture in which they live. Humans do have the ability with their critical thinking and reasoning to come to conclusions other than what their culture may demand. In fact, some cultures, say academic societies, have this as part of their social umwelt. However, depending on the culture, this may come at great costs. The ability to set aside the group imperative is a matter of education and intellectual self-discipline. This also requires recognition of the group dynamics that the listener finds themselves in. This is not inconsequential, as there may be a certain amount of coercion in the group toward the individual with beliefs outside the generally recognized norms. Therefore, "argument," in the broad sense, may play out more as a "power dynamic" within the group as well as between groups, rather than a logical search of the truth. Philosophically, it is curious that practical and actionable knowledge can be gained with the individual accepting the knowledge but not understanding the foundations of its production. In fact, this is how most knowledge is actually obtained. We read something or are told something by some trusted source and that then gets incorporated into our corpus of knowledge. We rarely analyze how this information was generated in the first place.

Humans have the capability of revising the way that they think as well as the content of their thought and knowledge. With considered self-reflection, an individual is capable of recognizing that his or her social and cultural beliefs require revision. Similarly, with new knowledge, an individual may reflect on their fast-thinking, intuition and slow-thinking, reasoning processes. Figure 3.5 provides a schematic of how a listener processes an argument. The flow follows from the listener's comprehension of the arguer's communication (both verbal and nonverbal), this being filtered through their social umwelt, then whether it goes into the fast-thinking mode versus the slow-thinking mode (blue arrows). If the process goes through the fast-thinking mode, the listener can either accept the results of that intuition or they may decide that it is not an optimal assessment and requires a slow-thinking approach (green arrow). Continuing following the blue arrows, eventually the listener comes to a judgment about whether to accept the communication as new knowledge. If this is substantially different than the listener's corpus of knowledge, the listener may decide that their social umwelt or processes of fast and slow thinking need to be revised (orange arrows). In other words, people can learn.

Physicians are not immune to their own version of the social umwelt. Physicians have their own groups with their own social and cultural norms. Physicians, by virtue of their profession, are part of the *Medicine* cultural group which has a long cultural history. Physicians are a product of an educational process that instills not only factual knowledge but also a method of thinking (as exemplified by the clinical vignette discussed in Chap. 1). This then leads to their own social umwelt. The process goes even further in that physicians further group themselves by specialty: there are adult internists, pediatricians, surgeons, psychiatrists, obstetrician-gynecologists, etc. All of these specialties have additional training with further indoctrination into their own cultures. These groups further consolidate their cultural differences between themselves and lay groups, as well as between themselves. It is a matter of accepted wisdom that surgeons and internists think differently. That they may look upon each other's judgments with a modicum of suspicion. It is common to refer to the "surgical" literature and "medical" literature as a way of either engendering or undermining trust. Therefore, as with the remainder of humans, physicians need to be conscious of their own social umwelt.

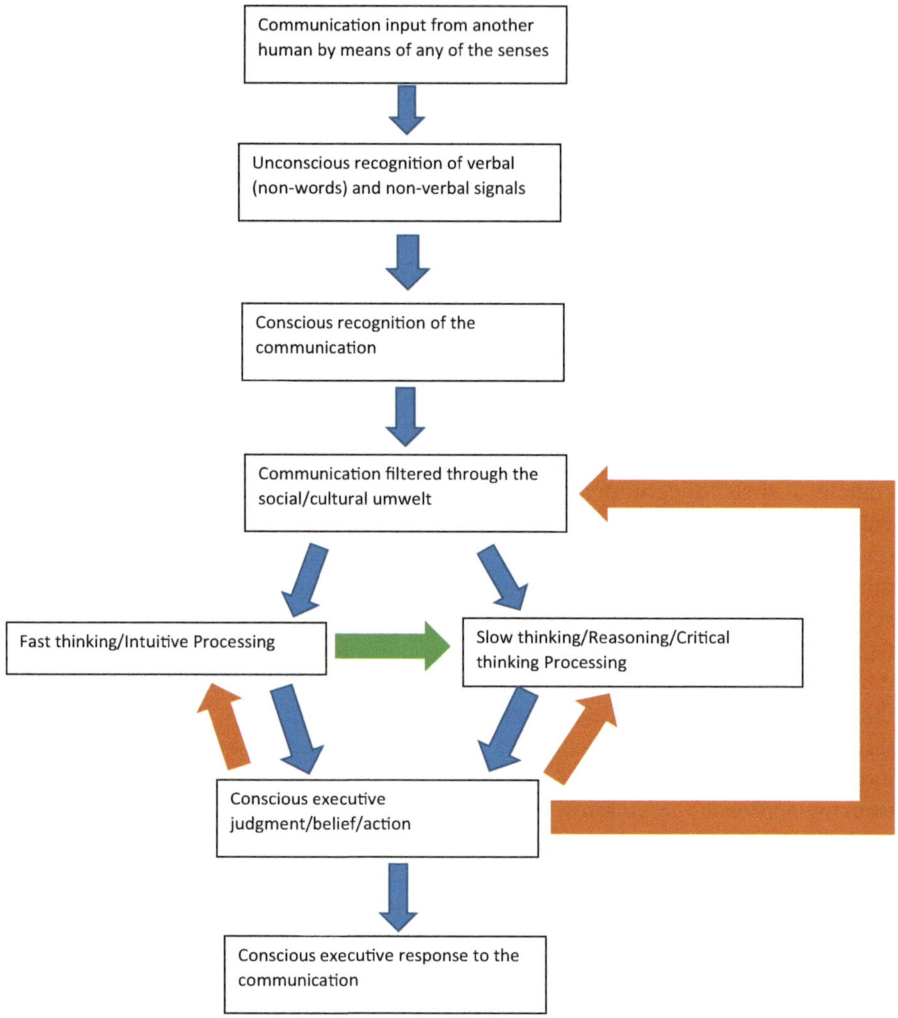

Fig. 3.5 A schematic representation of how a communication from another individual is processed into conscious understanding and executive judgment as to the truth of the communication and any need for response. The blue arrows show the flow of information. The green arrow shows that the individual recognizes the need to process the information in a "slow-thinking/reasoning/critical thinking" mode rather than relying on the "fast-thinking/intuitive" mode. The orange arrows show that the individual may recognize the need to revise their social umwelt, fast-thinking or slow-thinking modes based on their judgment of the value of the communication input

3.5 Final Thoughts

What I have provided is almost all descriptive in nature. I have given no "rules" to follow to insure that one's judgments are correct. Some philosophers, in contrast, believe that the tasks of philosophy should be normative. That is, it should provide us with guidance as to *how* to think from the standpoint of reliable mechanisms of critical thinking, as discussed in Chap. 2. They view the actual way humans think as a job for cognitive psychologists. Although it may be a failure of our educational systems that more humans are not equipped with the skills for critical thinking, from the standpoint of persuasion, we have to assume that they may not be. However, when in Chap. 6 I address issues related to the production of new medical knowledge, I will address normative standards to determine of the knowledge created is "reliable enough" for use in clinical decision-making.

It also seems obvious that the vast majority of thinking is not critical thinking because it does not have to be. Kahneman's "fast thinking" [42] probably suffices for the great majority of our decisions because those decisions simply are not that critical [44]. In other words, there is a certain amount of efficiency in thinking like this [44]. One may not put a great deal of thought into how one combs one's hair in the morning or which route to take into work. Fast thinking here is both quick and efficient. In fact, Kahneman's fast thinking, I suspect, is greatly influenced by the social umwelt of the person, which, again, for the vast majority of everyday decisions, is just fine. Much of how the world is perceived and the responses to it are already ingrained. It does require a great deal of effort to reason beyond this. This effort is probably only expended by most people for only very important questions.

Knowledge may actually be very disruptive to an individual. The value of self-ignorance is that somethings about ourselves we are better off not knowing. This preserves our sense of self and may yield a stable view of ourselves in the world [44]. When the issues are relatively trivial, there is probably no harm in this. However, if they are important, great misfortune can be the result. I have seen many patients over the years who ignored medical evaluation because they simply "did not think anything was wrong" or "did not want to know" only to lead to tragic consequences. Sometimes what you don't know can hurt you. The real issue may not be that we should be critically thinking about everything that the world throws our way but have the ability to recognize those issues that are worth critically thinking about. Medical decisions are certainly one of those issues.

In this chapter, I have not provided any guidance for assessing *how well* humans think. That is, I have not attempted to develop normative rules to ensure that some conclusions from their thinking are correct. This is a much larger task for philosophers, cognitive psychologists and neuroscientists and is not the main purpose of this book. Quite frankly, I am not sure a consensus, certainly not one imposed by others outside the trusted group, can be reached on what the rules should be. I also have provided no normative rules for when to accept an assertion that new knowledge has just been created. However, from the standpoint of new medical knowledge, I will attempt to address that issue later in the book.

3.6 Summary and Synthesis

What I have hoped to have shown is that evolution has produced a human mind that is both capable of rationality with dispassionate reasoning *and* constrained by a social imperative to remain consistent with their group. People have a wide range of abilities to “overcome” their fast-thinking social umwelt to reason outside the constraints of their social group. From the standpoint of the arguer, understanding both the social umwelt of the listener, as well as the listener’s readiness to set aside his social constraints, if necessary, is important. For example, in the vignette presented in Chap. 1, if the patient had particular religious beliefs related to medication or surgery, this may have affected their receptiveness to arguments pertaining to treatment. The physician would have to take these constraints into account when discussing treatment options. This will be the subject of the next chapter.

References

1. Hoffmann M. Assembly of the executive mind: evolutionary insights and a paradigm for brain health. Cambridge: The Cambridge University Press; 2019.
2. Hoffmann M. Brain beat: scientific foundations and evolutionary perspectives of brain health. New York: Page Publishing, Inc.; 2015.
3. Hassin RR, Uleman JS, Bargh JA. The new unconscious. Oxford: The Oxford University Press; 2005.
4. Buzsaki G. How the brain ‘constructs’ the outside world. Sci Am. 2022.
5. Dawkins R. The selfish gene. 4th ed. Oxford: The Oxford University Press; 2016.
6. Williams BA, Kay RF, Kirk EC. New perspectives on anthropoid origins. Proc Natl Acad Sci U S A. 2010;107:4797–804.
7. Wong K. How scientists discovered the staggering complexity of human evolution. Sci Am. 2020.
8. Smithsonian National Museum of Natural History. What does it mean to be human? https://humanorigins.si.edu/evidence/human-evolution-interactive-timeline. Last accessed 28 Jun 2022.
9. Pontzer H. Overview of hominin evolution. Nat Educ Knowl. 2012;3(10):8.
10. Handwerk B. An evolutionary timeline of *Homo sapiens*. Smithsonian Mag. 2021;
11. Arbib M. From mirror neurons to complex imitation in the evolution of language and tool use. Annu Rev Anthropol. 2011;40:257–73.
12. Wilkins AS, Wrangham RW, Fitch WT. The “domestication syndrome” in mammals: a unified explanation based on neural crest cell behavior and genetics. Genetics. 2014;197:795–808.
13. Wrangham RW. The goodness paradox: how evolution made us both more and less violent. London: Profile Books, Ltd.; 2019.
14. Wrangham RW. Hypotheses for evolution of reduced reactive aggression in the context of human self-domestication. Front Psychol. 2019;10:1914.
15. Darwin C. The variation in animals and plants under domestication. London: John Murray; 1868.
16. Pober BR. Williams-Beuren syndrome. N Engl J Med. 2010;362:239–52.
17. Zanella M, Vitriola A, Andriko A, et al. Dosage analysis of the 7q11.23 the Williams region identifies BAZ1B as a major human gene patterning the modern human face and underlying self-domestication. Sci Adv. 2019;5:eaaw7908.
18. Shilton D, Breski M, Dor D, Jablonka E. Human social evolution: self-domestication or self-control? Front Psychol. 2020;11:134.
19. Hare B. Survival of the friendliest: Homo sapiens evolved via selection for prosociality. Annu Rev Psychol. 2017;68:155–68.
20. Dunbar RIM, Shultz S. Why are there so many explanations for primate brain evolution? Philos Trans R Soc B. 2017;372:20160244.

21. Dunbar RIM. The social hypothesis and human evolution. The Oxford Research Encyclopedia of Psychology. 2016; https://doi.org/10.1093/acrefore/9780190236557.013.44. Last accessed 27 Jun 2022
22. Moll H, Tomasella M. Cooperation and human cognition: the Vygotskian intelligence hypothesis. Philos Trans R Soc B. 2007;362:639–48.
23. Shorter JM. Other minds. In: Edwards P, editor. The encyclopedia of philosophy, vol. 6. New York: MacMillan Publishing Co., Inc. and The Free Press; 1967. p. 7–13.
24. Culture. Merriam-Webster Dictionary. https://merriam-webster.com. Last accessed 30 Jun 2022.
25. Cultural Evolution Society. Cultural evolution is the change of culture over time. https://culturalevolutionsociety.org. Last accessed 30 Jun 2022.
26. Rosaldo RI. Foreword: defining culture. In: Baldwin JR, Faulkner SL, Hecht ML, Lindsley SL, editors. Redefining culture: perspectives across the disciplines. Mahwah, NJ: Lawrence Erlbaum Associates, Inc., Publishers; 2006. p. xv–xiii.
27. Toren C. Human ontogenesis as historical processes: an anthropological perspective. In: Lewens T, Hannan E, editors. Why we disagree about human nature. Oxford: Oxford University Press.
28. Henrich J. The secrets of our success. Princeton, NJ: Princeton University Press; 2015.
29. Lewens T. Human nature, human culture: the case of cultural evolution. Interface Focus. 2017;7:20170018.
30. Brown DE. Human universals, human nature and human culture. Daedalus. 2004;133:47–54.
31. Jung CG. The archetypes and the collective unconscious. Princeton, NJ: Princeton University Press; 1969. (1st published 1959).
32. von Uexkull J, Beer T, Bethe A. Vorschlage zu einer objectivierenden Nomenklatur in der Physiologie des Nervensystems. Biol Centralbaltt. 1899;19:517–21.
33. Clifton JDW, Baker JD, Park CL, et al. Primal world beliefs. Psychol Assess. 2019;31:82–99.
34. The 26 Primal World Beliefs. https://myprimals.com. Last accessed 4 Jul 2022.
35. Graham J, Haidt J, Koleva S, et al. Moral Foundation Theory: the pragmatic validity of moral pluralism. Adv Exp Soc Psychol. 2013;47:55–130.
36. Moral Foundation Theory. https://moralfoundations.org. Last accessed 16 Jul 2022.
37. Kahan DM, Braman D, Gastil J, et al. Culture and identity protective cognition: explaining the white-male effect in risk perception. J Empirical Legal Stud. 2017;4:465–505.
38. Kahan DM. Ideology, motivated reasoning, and cognitive reflection. Judgment Decis Making. 2013;8:407–24.
39. Baumeister RF, Leary MR. The need to belong: desire for interpersonal attachments as a fundamental human motivation. Psychol Bull. 1995;117:497–529.
40. Mackie DM, Quellar S. The impact of group membership in persuasion: revisiting "who says what to whom with what effect?". In: Terry DJ, Hogg MA, editors. Attitudes, behavior, and social context: the role of norms and group membership. Mahwah, NJ: Lawrence Erlbaum Associates, Publishers; 2000. p. 135–55.
41. Kahan DM, Peters E, Dawson EC, Slovic P. Motivated numeracy and enlightened self-government. Behav Public Policy. 2013;1:54–86.
42. Kahneman D. Thinking fast and slow. New York: Farrar, Straus, & Giroux; 2011.
43. Milovic-Prelec D, Prelec D. Self-deception as self-signaling: a model and experimental evidence. Philos Trans R Soc B. 2010;365:227–40.
44. Cassam Q. Self-knowledge for humans. Oxford: Oxford University Press; 2014.
45. Nesbitt R, Ross L. Human inference: strategies and shortcomings of social judgment. Englewood Cliffs, NJ: Prentice-Hall; 1980.
46. Harman G. Change in view: principles of reasoning. Cambridge, MA: Bradford Books; 1986.
47. Johnson RH. Manifest rationality: a pragmatic theory of argument. New York: Routledge; 2012.
48. Gilovich T. How we know what isn't so: the fallibility of human reason in everyday life. New York: The Free Press; 1991.
49. Kahneman D, Slovic P, Tversky A. Judgment under uncertainty: heuristics and biases. Cambridge: Cambridge University Press; 1982.

50. Hoffmann M. The neurobiology of human supercommunication: insights for medicine and business. World J Neurosci. 2021;11:287–306.
51. Shibboleth. Merriam-Webster Dictionary. https://merriam-webster.com. Last accessed 13 Jul 2022.
52. Johnson-Laird PN. Mental models and human reasoning. Proc Natl Acad Sci U S A. 2010;107(43):18243–50.
53. Johnson-Laird PN. How we reason. New York: Oxford University Press; 2006.
54. Abernathy CM, Hamm RM. Surgical intuition: what it is and how to get it. Philadelphia: Hanley & Belfus, Inc.; 1995.
55. Collins AM, Loftus EF. A spreading-activation theory of semantic processing. Psychol Rev. 1975;82:407–8.

Chapter 4
Persuasion in Medicine: How Medical Arguments Are Accepted

4.1 Introduction

Social influence is the process by which one human individual or group affects a change in attitude or behavior in another conspecific individual or group [1]. Social influence has probably been as an universal feature of human interaction as an inheritance from our primate ancestors as a result of the survival advantage of living in a group.[1] Persuasion is an important mechanism of human social influence for group cohesion. This chapter will review theories related to human persuasion (I will be addressing only human persuasion), the neuroscience of persuasion, various types of persuasive techniques, and how these techniques have fared in health-related communication. This will lead to an analysis of the discourse between the patient, as the listener, and the physician, as the arguer, within the context of the medical encounter. I will also discuss separately the discourse among medical professionals with respect to patient-related decisions and how that may differ from the discourse held with the patient.

However, first, let us start with definitions of persuasion. The topic of persuasion has been of great academic interest for philosophers, psychologists, communications/marketing professionals, and neuroscientists. As a basis for their studies, they provide definitions of persuasion:

> The active attempt by an individual, group or social entity to change a person's beliefs, attitudes, or behaviors by conveying information, feelings, or reasoning (Cacioppo, Cacioppo and Petty, psychologists/neuroscientists) [1].

> A human communication that is designed to influence others by modifying their beliefs, values or attitudes (Simons, as quoted by Dainton, communications/marketing professional) [2].

[1]Apparently, there is evidence that other "social" creatures also engage in social influence. These include honeybees, fish, birds, rats, and chimpanzees (references listed in Cacioppo et al. [1]).

V. Velanovich, *Medical Persuasion*, https://doi.org/10.1007/978-3-031-30371-5_4

> Any message that is intended to shape, reinforce or change the responses of another (Miller, psychologist) [3].
>
> The act or process or an instance of persuading[2] (Merriam-Webster Dictionary) [4].
>
> Is to bring another out of his bad sense into your good sense (Emerson, philosopher) [5].

Although each is slightly different and nuanced, depending on the academic viewpoint of one making the definition, they all share a common theme—namely, one individual or group is attempting to get another individual or group to accept the information and/or beliefs, with preferably subsequent behavioral changes, in a direction that the persuading individual or group would like.

4.1.1 Aristotle as a Foundational Understanding of Persuasion

The study and analysis of persuasion has a long history. In Western civilization,[3] this traditionally is thought to have begun with Aristotle's *Rhetoric* [6]. Although my intention is not to give a thorough examination of Aristotle on rhetoric (there have been numerous treatises on this by others more qualified than me, e.g., see Ref. [6]), it still will be instructive to provide a brief overview to place the subsequent discussion in context. For Aristotle, the skill of rhetoric was possessed by an individual in the activity of public speaking, especially in a public arena pertaining to public works. Such a skilled individual would have "the ability to see what is persuasive in every case" [6]. The methods the orator, as this was a spoken activity, would use would be that of *logos, pathos,* and *ethos*:

Logos—the logic of the argument. In modern terminology, cognitive elaboration or, rather, argumentation, i.e., the logical structure of the argument (i.e., illative core) with the validity of the conclusion proven.

Pathos—the emotional appeal of an argument. Modern terminology, affective appeal, i.e., the speech leads the audience to feel a certain emotion or passion that impacts the judgment they are going to make.

Ethos—factors related to the source of the persuasive message, that is, the character of the speaker. Modern terminology, perceived similarity of the listener to the message source or an authority (expert) recognized by the listener(s), i.e., whenever the speech is held in such a way as to render the speaker worthy of credence, especially in the absence of other evidence [6].

If we return to our prior discussions in Chaps. 2 and 3, we can note similarities. *Logos* at a minimum is the illative core of an argument. If there are any exchanges

---

[2] Merriam-Webster defines "persuade" as "to move by argument, entreaty, or expostulation to a belief, position, or course of action" (Persuade. Merriam-Webster Dictionary. https://merriam-webster.com, last accessed July 27, 2022).

[3] Although I am sure that persuasion-like social influence has received attention in the intellectual traditions of other civilizations, I will not be addressing those.

between the orator and the audience, it then becomes a dialectic and a version of manifest rationality. *Pathos*, as an appeal to emotion, can be elicited in oration based on the audience's Moral Foundation or Primal Beliefs proclivities. Finally, *ethos* is related to trust in the orator based on the audience's social umwelt or cultural identity.

For Aristotle, the "art" of rhetoric requires that the orator must know the reasons why some things are persuasive and some are not, must have a "complete" analysis of what is possibly persuasive and not random use of scatter persuasive factors, must provide the persuasive oration themselves, and needs to actually address the thing at issue [6]. That is, the orator must have developed a plan for persuasion, not just string together impromptu thoughts. Failing any one of these, for Aristotle, means that the orator failed as a persuader because they did not place themselves in the best possible position to persuade, whether or not the audience was actually persuaded. A proper, well-conceived attempt was more important, at least intellectually, than the success of the attempt. It certainly seems that Aristotle identified the essential components of persuasion, at least in a public, oral tradition. At the time, written persuasion was not as important as only a relatively few people could read. All that follows seems to be mere elaborations of this framework.

Let us now look at the clinical vignette from Chap. 1, specifically, Fig. 1.1 pertaining to the flow of the medical encounter and the decision-making foundations. There was quite a bit of persuasion that had to happen before and during the encounter. I will categorize only two types that I will address in this chapter: Persuasion of the patient by the physician with respect to the patient's diagnosis and treatment options and persuasion of the physician by other health care professionals with respect to the knowledge that the physician should use in their medical decision-making.

4.2 The Modern Study of Persuasion

4.2.1 Persuasion in Popular Culture

Persuasion and the techniques of persuasiveness are topics of intense interest for anyone having to communicate with the public. Business people want to persuade customers to buy their product, politicians want people to vote for them, parents want to influence their children, employers want to persuade their employees to increase productivity, and so on. During the course of any day, any one person will probably be the object of and the instigator of several persuasive attempts. There is probably no aspect of human interaction that does not include persuasion at some time or another. This came to the popular mind in earnest with the publication of Dale Carnegie's *How to Make Friends and Influence People* in 1936 [7], which was subsequently turned into courses for the education of the public on these techniques, especially those in business.

There is now a plethora of books and courses to teach supposedly effective persuasion techniques primarily, but not exclusively, to business people and administrators, as well as others who feel the need to improve these skills [8].[4] Robert Cialdini's *Influence: The Psychology of Persuasion* [9] first published in 1984 has become a very influential (pun intended) book on persuasion in popular culture. He asserts that his "Six Principles of Persuasion" work on humans via their "near-automated" responses. In fact, if one understands the biological, social and cultural evolution of the human brain/mind, it is easy to make such an assertion. Responding to the social communications of other humans is embedded into our brain, as was demonstrated in the section on the evolution of the human brain in Chap. 3, and the following section on persuasion neuroscience will show why. His six principles are: (1) Reciprocation—that is, give a favor, get a favor (in fact, this is one of the "human universals" as identified by Brown cited in the previous chapter); (2) Consistency—once we have made a choice or taken a stand, we will encounter personal and interpersonal pressures to behave consistently to that commitment. (This is consistent with the assertions of the Moral Foundation Theory, again noted in Chap. 3). Moreover, this can be used for manipulation—once one has someone's self-image where one wants it, that individual will most likely comply naturally with a whole range of one's requests; (3) Social proof—people use the actions of others to determine what their own proper behavior should be (this is consistent with our social brain defaulting to behaviors and beliefs for the promotion of group cohesion, possibly through the mirror neuron system allowing for imitation, as described in Chap. 3); (4) Liking—we are more likely to comply with the requests from people we like (consistent with both our notions of human universals and the theory of self-domestication—"survival of the friendliest"—describe in Chap. 3); (5) Authority—we tend to be more likely persuaded by authority figures (consistent with our social brain, self-domestication, Primal Beliefs, and Moral Foundation theory. Although we will identify later in this chapter, there are individuals who are reactant to authority and the implorings from such authorities will simply lead to a "boomerang" effect against the request); and finally (6) Scarcity—it is easy enough to feel properly warned against scarcity pressures, but it is substantially more difficult to act on that warning. In reviewing these six principles, it is easy to see how they are simply a consequence of our evolution, and those that understand that can communicate in a persuasive way.

There are other books that address different aspects of persuasiveness. Cialdini followed *Influence: The Psychology of Persuasion* [9] with *Pre-Suasion: A Revolutionary Way to Influence and Persuade* in 2016 [10]. Jason Harris published *The Soulful Art of Persuasion: The 11 Habits That Will Make Anyone a Master Influencer* in [11]. Of note, 4 of the 11 "habits" are truly personal characteristics and not habits in the sense of consistent behaviors but that is beside the point. These are: originality, generosity, empathy and "soulfulness." A major factor in his view is

[4] The list of publications that I will mention should not be construed in any way as an endorsement of the contents of these books by myself.

reciprocity. One should always be looking to do something for someone else. Again, the importance of reciprocity as a human universal cannot be over-emphasized. Carmine Gallo's *Five Stars: The Communication Secrets to Get from Good to Great* [12] and Kindra Hall's *Stories That Stick: How Storytelling Can Captivate Customers, Influence Audiences, and Transform Your Business* [13] both emphasize the role of the compelling narrative (i.e., stories) in persuasion. As noted in Chap. 3, the way the human brain and mind evolved the consequences of which is that humans have a natural preference for understanding the world as a sequence of events in a narrative. Such brain abilities as "theory of mind" and "mental time-travel" make humans predisposed to understanding stories as influential pedagogical tools in our cultures. Storytelling is a human universal. It is not random that the patient is encouraged to describe their symptoms in story form in the history of present illness. It is how are minds are defaulted to understand.

I do not mention these books as any type of endorsement and there are many, many more such books and courses. I use these only as examples of the overarching importance that persuasion of others has taken in our modern world, especially the world of business. However, it is also worth emphasizing that even in these popular "how-to's" of persuasion, how easy it is to see the embedded functions and preferences of the human social brain as the foundation for why these techniques can be effective. Having established working definitions of persuasion and its general importance, I move on to the more academic study of persuasion.

4.2.2 Modern Academic Study of Persuasion

As mentioned, persuasion has been a subject of study by many academic disciplines, especially philosophers, psychologists, communications/marketing professionals, and neuroscientists. Although not intended to be a comprehensive review of the extant theories of persuasion, a brief overview will provide the foundation for the subsequent discussions.

The communications professor Marianne Dainton [2] provides an informative review, especially from the perspective of the fields of communications and marketing, which obviously is concerned with cultivating attitudes and beliefs, with subsequent behavior changes pertaining to merchandise and people. She starts by saying:

> Persuasion involves (1) a goal and the intent of achieving that goal in part of the message of the sender, with (2) communication as a means to achieve that goal, and (3) the message recipient must have a free will[5] [2].

[5] This requirement of "free will" I find curious and Dainton does not explain it further. I suspect was she means by this may the legal sense of "sound mind." That is, the person has the cognitive capacity of the individual to understand the message and have the ability to accept or reject the message. However, in the greater sense, given that much of the human mind is "programmed" to receive some messages and not others, humans may not have as much free will was we would like to believe. This discussion, of course, is far beyond the scope of this book.

In this view, the "sender of the message" (whom I have previously named the "arguer") must have a goal. That is, they want something from the "recipient of the message" (whom I have named the "listener"). For the sake of consistency in terminology, I will continue to use the terms "arguer" and "listener," understanding fully that the persuasion technique used may not be an argument in the sense of argumentation as described in Chap. 2.

However, the bigger issue is what does the arguer want? Although I will expand on this later in the chapter, I will now identify two "goals" of persuasion: (1) To get someone to do something that the arguer wants them to do. For example, a manufacturer wants a customer to buy a product, a politician wants a voter to vote for them, a physician wants a patient to follow their recommendations, etc. (2) To change someone's beliefs or attitudes and/or accept new knowledge or a proposal. For example, a scientist presenting a new theory at a conference, a government official presenting a new construction proposal to a legislative body or the public, a religious leader presenting a theological doctrine to their congregation, a physician presenting the information that led to a diagnosis to the patient, etc. Dainton [2] quotes Simons from 1976 defining an "attitude" as "a relatively enduring predisposition to respond favorably or unfavorably toward something." I will only address the latter type of persuasion when I discuss persuasion in the medical context; although I am completely aware that there are medical practitioners and medical facilities that use persuasion in the first sense as a way to increase the number of customers and their revenue.[6] The theories described below, however, are applicable to either type of persuasion.

Social Judgment Theory

This theory was first proposed by Sherif and Hovland in 1961 [2, 14]. The essence of this theory is "knowing a person's attitudes on a subject can provide you with clues about how to persuade them." This is based on a person's "anchors" to a particular message. An anchor is a set of existing beliefs that a person holds. These anchors keep the individual in a range of "latitudes," that is, the range of what they are willing to accept or reject. There are three types of latitudes depending on the subject or topic of the message in this theory:

Latitude of acceptance—the range of what the person considers acceptable.
Latitude of rejection—the range of what is not acceptable.
Latitude of noncommitment—the range for which the individual has no opinion.

[6]The numerous billboards, television and radio ads for physicians in a variety of practices and healthcare facilities are certainly a testament to "medicine as a business" and the desire to increase revenue through increased patient utilization. As true as this is, this is not what I wish to focus on in this book but change in knowledge, beliefs and behaviors that are medically beneficial to the patient.

In social judgment theory, an individual's attitude toward any given subject depends on how much the individual's "ego is involved" in the subject. That is, how much they care about the subject. The more important the subject is to the individual, the more of their "ego" they have invested in the subject. When the subject becomes so important that it then becomes entwined with the individual's sense of self, this is then referred to as "ego-involved." It seems to me that this theory is consistent with the motivated cognition theory discussed in Chap. 3, and one can especially see how the person's social umwelt, as discussed in Chap. 3, can associate ego-involvement with cultural identity.

The level of ego-involvement has some consequences. The more ego involvement there is, the larger the latitude of rejection. That is, the greater the range of what is considered unacceptable. To put a finer point on it, when one feels very strongly about a topic, only their specific belief items (facts, reasons, ideas, etc.) within that topic are acceptable, and any items outside this relatively narrow range are deemed false or unimportant in order to maintain their ego.

This theory also predicts other effects. The "contrast effect" occurs when a message is perceived as farther away from the person's anchor than it truly is. With this, the listener subconsciously exaggerates the difference between the message's position and the listener's position. The "assimilation effect" is when a message received falls within the listener's latitude of acceptance; then, the listener subconsciously minimizes the difference between the message and their position. Last, the "boomerang effect" is when a message causes the person to change their mind in the opposite direction of the desired effect of the arguer. That is, the listener will be more likely to oppose the arguer's conclusion. What these effects truly say is that when a listener has strong anchors (whatever they may be) to a position, with well-defined and committed attitudes, persuasion is difficult. The listeners with wide "noncommitment" latitudes for a topic are the ones most likely to be persuaded about that topic. That is, when the listener has no strong preformed attitudes, their attitude is more likely to be shaped by persuasion.

The most significant aspect of this theory is the concept of latitudes of acceptability. It would seem that this would be consistent with what was previously discussed in Chap. 3 about the social umwelt, cognitive motivation, cultural and social identity, the Moral Foundation Theory and Primal Beliefs. Understanding these aspects of the listener can either help the arguer shape the message (or, more specifically, the illative core of the argument), try to make an emotional appeal, appeal to an authority acceptable to the listener, or decide that the attempt at persuasion would be fruitless.

Elaboration Likelihood Model

This model comes from the work of Petty and Cacioppo published in 1986 [2, 15]. This theory views persuasion as a cognitive event, with the "targets of persuasion" (i.e., the listener) using mental processes of motivation and reasoning to accept or reject a persuasive attempt. In this theory, there are two "routes" to persuasion—the "peripheral" and the "central" routes.

The central route to persuasion requires a high level of cognitive engagement by both the arguer and the listener. It is reminiscent of Aristotle's *logos.* If the arguer can achieve persuasion with this route, it is assumed that long-term attitude change in the listener can be achieved [15]. This route does require the arguer to create an illative core of an argument with a wealth of information logically constructed into a conclusion, which is the knowledge, belief or attitude that they want the listener to have. Long-term change is possible if the listener is highly motivated to mentally process all the information presented and be able to cognitively process the information [2]. That is, the listener must have both the intellectual capacity and capabilities to understand and appraise the premises of the argument as well as the logical structure of the argument. In this setting, strong arguments can create a positive cognitive response and positively align the listener's beliefs with that of the arguer. Neutral arguments may receive a noncommittal response; that is, the listener may either suspend judgment on the arguer's conclusion or simply ignore it and not change their own beliefs or attitudes. Weak arguments may receive a negative response and possibly induce a boomerang effect, as noted by Sherif and Hovland [14], where the listener not only rejects the arguer's conclusion but believes exactly the opposite of it. It seems to me that this central route is what a typical physician hopes to achieve in counseling a patient, as we noted in the clinical vignette presented in Chap. 1. That is, provide the patient with accurate, truthful information about their condition and why a particular (or set of particular) option(s) would be appropriate for the patient; and, moreover, have the patient cognitively engaged in the process, such as to produce a dialect, in the sense of Johnson's manifest rationality as noted in Chap. 2, to have a long-term change in the patient's attitude toward their health issues.

The peripheral route of persuasion relies on the listener's "emotional involvement" in the message [2]. In some ways, it is what Aristotle identified as *pathos*. This is a route that is easier for some listeners to understand, as the message is much simpler. This is one for listeners who may not have the cognitive capacity to understand arguments of the central route type. The arguer uses "cues" that the listener will respond to, such as an appeal to authority, appeal to the listener's known commitments, contrasting effects of how the appeal is made with the actual difficulty of what is requested, an appeal to how well the arguer is liked by the listener, reciprocation to a prior favor the arguer has done for the listener, appealing to the scarcity of what is being discussed in the message, and social proof of the attractiveness of what is the topic of the message (some of these points were also in Cialdini's six principles of influence, noted above). As with the central route, there are positive, neutral and negative peripheral messages. Because the peripheral route does not require the listener to "internalize" the argument, it is also less likely to produce long-term change. In my practice of 35 years, I have seen this type of persuasion used by family members to persuade a patient to either accept or reject a recommended treatment, usually done with emotional appeals, often with how the outcome of the treatment may affect other family members. Although I have seen and heard other physicians do the same, this appears to me against the "shared decision-making model" (more on this later in the chapter) for which ethical physicians should strive.

Cognitive Dissonance Theory

This theory was first proposed by Festinger in 1957 [16]. The basic foundation of this theory is that influence is often an intrapersonal event occurring when one's attitudes are incongruent with one's behavior, thereby leading to a tension within the individual which can only be resolved with a change in attitudes, beliefs or behaviors [2]. This seems consistent with the issues revolving around self-deception discussed in Chap. 3. In this theory, individuals use "schemata" as a "cognitive structure" when faced with new information to be able to link the new information with information that is already familiar[7] [2, 16]. Therefore, when new information is at odds with previously established beliefs, the individual will feel an "imbalance" or "dissonance." That is, the individual realizes that there is a discordance that needs to be resolved.

In this theory, there are three possible relationships between the individual's beliefs and their behaviors:

Irrelevance—there are no relationships between their beliefs and behaviors.
Consonance—their beliefs and behaviors are congruent, that is, they act in a manner consistent with their beliefs.
Dissonance—their beliefs and behaviors are contradictory; that is, they believe one thing but act in another [2, 16].

These relationships certainly have a similarity with "self-deception", as previously discussed in Chap. 3.

The "magnitude" of this dissonance is the "level of discomfort" felt by the individual and is dependent on three features of the individual [2, 16]. One is the level of importance of the mismatch at issue. Some things are just not that important to worry about, while others are extremely important. The second is the "dissonance ratio," which is the proportion of incongruent beliefs held in relation to the number of congruent beliefs held. That is, a certain issue may entail many behaviors required from the individual; some of these behaviors will be consistent with the individual's beliefs, while others are not. Last, the individual's ability to "rationalize" or justify the behavior. That is, the individual recognizes the dissonance but convinces themselves that this particular behavior at this particular time is justified. Individuals will then "selectively perceive" various stimuli from their environment to minimize the dissonance [2, 16]. This is done through "selective exposure"—only exposing oneself to congruent information; "selective attention"—only paying attention to congruent information, when being exposed to both congruent and dissonant information; and "selective interpretation"—that is, interpreting especially ambiguous information in a way that makes the information as congruent as possible. This appears consistent with motivated cognition as

[7] This reminds me of what I call my "Lego Theory" of education. Each bit of knowledge is similar to a Lego brick. The more bricks you have put down, the more brick prongs are exposed for even more bricks to go into the structure. That is, the more you know about a topic, the easier it is to know more about that topic. However, obviously, this discussion is beyond the scope of this book.

described in Chap. 3, or what Gilovich describes as "beliefs as property" and the need to protect one's property [17].

From the standpoint of the patient–physician interaction, the explanation from the physician to the patient must be such that the amount of dissonance that the patient experiences is as little as possible to maximize the persuasive effect of the explanation. If we return to the clinical vignette, if the risk of needing a blood transfusion was significant, a practicing Jehovah's witness would refuse such treatment. The physician will then either respect this dissonance or advise a treatment less likely to require transfusion, rather than insist on giving the patient a blood transfusion.

Narrative Paradigm

This theory proposes that "narratives," that is, stories, are an effective persuasion tool because humans are fundamentally storytelling creatures such that the most persuasive messages come in the form of a narrative rather than a rational argument [2, 18, 19]. I previously mentioned two books for business people emphasizing the need to tell stories for persuasive effects [12, 13].

In this theory, a narrative convinces the listener(s) of "good reasons" for a belief or behavior. However, it is done through hearing the consequences of the behavior within the story rather as a dictum to be followed, much in the way a fable or fairy tale contains a moral or practical message. For any given individual, their values, emotions and aesthetic preferences shape their beliefs and actions [2, 19]. Of course, emotions are a product of human evolutionary journeys. Values and "aesthetic preferences" are shaped by social interactions, culture, education, and, perhaps, primal beliefs and moral foundations, as discussed in Chap. 3. Persuasive narratives, in this theory, use symbolic words and actions that ascribe meaning in the narration for the listener [2, 18, 19]. These, it seems to me, to be a form of shibboleths that those in the in-group for which the narration is directed can readily recognize. In this sense, there is a "narrative rationality," that is, a logical method of reasoning for the listener by which they can determine how believable the story is [2, 19]. A persuasive story will demonstrate "good reasons" for the decisions made, making the story coherent, faithful to the listener's values, and congruent with their experiences. "Good reasons" are based on an individual's culture, character, history, values and experiences [2, 18, 19]. For Fisher [18, 19], most ideas cannot be proven conclusively; therefore, a narrative creates a "common understanding" for the listener with the arguer. One can see that in difficult to understand or abstract logical arguments, there may not be a "common understanding"; therefore, even when there is a preponderance of evidence, which may not be in the direct experience of the listener, the listener may reject an expert's advice. Krause and Rucker [20] performed experiments showing that when facts are "embedded" in a story, they can be more persuasive than simply stating the facts, even with evidence. This is a result of the emotional appeal of a story, especially for those who may otherwise find it difficult to understand the factual premises of an argument.

It seems consistent with what is known about the human brain and mind that storytelling has such an impact. As previously discussed, the human brain/mind evolved in such a way that narratives are a very understandable form of communication [21, 22], and very likely, storytelling increased cooperation among humans [23]. Storytelling is a human universal, and it certainly seems that its persuasive effects are embedded in the human mind. It requires a great deal of education and "retraining" the mind to think in formalized logical form (the formal, symbolic logic presented in Chap. 2 can attest to that!) and to consciously choose not to default into narratives. This is one of the reasons that Gilovich gives for so many people having fallacious beliefs [17].

Physicians and other healthcare professionals, despite their long training in "scientific" medicine, in casual moments revert to storytelling. It has certainly been my experience in nearly four decades in medicine as a student, trainee and practicing surgeon that physicians like to discuss individual cases as stories. The "case report" is nothing if not a narrative of the "character arc" (to use a term for the change in a character over the course of a story [24]) of the patient's illness, treatment and ultimate outcome. Physicians will then try to map out a particular patient's illness course with the extant information on their disease, but this does not take away from the interest of the case report as a story for medical professionals. Patients, particularly when the scientific information is difficult to understand, like to hear the stories of other patients' experiences to help in their own decision-making. One only has to note the dozens, if not hundreds, of "support groups" for almost any disease process to accept this premise. Last, and this certainly has been my experience having been interviewed by members of the media, journalists like to have an individual patient's story as an example of a larger medical topic. This creates an "emotional connection" with the audience in what would otherwise be a dry analysis of scientific data (for medical scientists, a single patients experience is "anecdotal" and not necessarily representative of the spectrum of disease, while statistically analyzed data, and the larger the data set the better, is more convincing. More on this in Chap. 6).

As with other theories that I have presented, I am not endorsing any one or all of these but just to provide examples of how persuasion has been studied by psychologists and communication professionals. I am struck, nevertheless, by how much of these theories dovetail almost seamlessly with what we know of the biological, social and cultural evolution of the human mind and brain.

4.3 General Types of Persuasion Methods

Having discussed popular and academic theories of persuasion, I would like to provide a short inventory of the types of persuasion techniques. Some may take umbrage with this list, but the purpose is to define precisely what I will address in this book.

4.3.1 Coercion

The Merriam-Webster Dictionary defines coercion as "the act, process, or power of coercing," with coerce defined as "(1) To compel to an act or choice; (2) To achieve by force or threat; (3) To restrain or dominate by force" [25]. These types of persuasion can broadly be classified into four categories:

Physical—threat or act to physical injure or kill and individual.
Emotional/mental—threat or act to cause emotional or mental anguish.
Social—threat to act to harm an individual's social standing.
Financial—threat to act to harm an individual's financial security.

Specifically, when it focuses on an individual's cognitive state, Carruthers has a specific definition:

> Coercive persuasion attempts to force people to change beliefs, ideas, attitudes or behaviors using psychological pressure, undue influence, threat, anxiety, intimidation and/or stress [26].

It should go without saying that this form of persuasion is unethical, immoral and, in many jurisdictions, illegal. Sadly, this does not make it rare. Coercion has been identified as a potential issue in intensive care medicine [27], consent [28] and psychiatric care [29]. Coercion is also an issue when family members and the patient disagree on a treatment plan [30]. I certainly have witnessed family members pressuring patients to either accept or reject treatments in a manner I thought was coercive. This is a situation that physicians must recognize, as their obligation is to the patient and uphold their shared decision-making.

Having said this, this type of persuasion is not the focus of this book, and I will not discuss it further as a valid means of persuasion.

4.3.2 Emotional (Affective)

This type of persuasion is consistent with Artistotle's *pathos*, that is, an appeal to the emotions of the listener(s). This can be done in a variety of ways and is also consistent with the "peripheral" route of persuasion, as explained in the Elaboration Likelihood Model, as well as recognized in Cognitive Dissonance Theory and the Narrative Paradigm (storytelling). These types of emotional appeals are also consistent with the social umwelt, Moral Foundation Theory, Primal Beliefs theory, motivated cognition theory, cultural identity, and self-deception, all previously discussed. These appeals can be overt elicitations of positive and/or negative emotions or more subtle shibboleths to elicit such emotions. Examples of this type of persuasion are all around us, from product advertising, to newspaper opinion pieces, to political speeches, and, yes, even in medicine. I certainly have seen healthcare professionals as well as family members give emotional appeals to a patient to accept or reject a particular treatment. These appeals do not reach the level of coercion and are certainly more common but are not the strictly logical dialectic argumentation of the risks, benefits, and potential outcomes of the treatment decision.

As with coercion, the physician's role is to maintain patient autonomy in the shared decision-making model [31, 32]. Although there is no doubt that in some circumstances of serious medical conditions, emotions will be involved in the counseling process, and the physician should acknowledge these emotions, care should be taken by the physician to ensure that "emotional decisions" are an adjunct to rational decisions, not the main driver of the decision. I will not focus on this form of persuasion in this book as a valid means of persuasion for the physician, although it may be for the patient and their family.

4.3.3 Appeal to Authority

Another form of persuasion is the "appeal to authority." That is, "*X* is a (insert whatever qualifying characteristic here), so you should do as they say." This is consistent with Aristotle's *ethos*, the character and qualifications of the speaker. It is also consistent with the "authority" Moral Foundation, as well as certain aspects of human evolution. Certainly, in the past, physicians' standing as experts in medicine has made them authority figures. Not only is this true for the general public's perception of physicians (although this reputation has developed some tarnish in recent years) but also for other healthcare professionals. Physicians refer to other physicians patients with particular problems because they are considered "experts" in that condition.[8] Nevertheless, the authority should have a better reason for a recommendation that "just because I said so." Therefore, although an appeal to authority may be a good starting point, if the authority is recognized in the field and has a record of sound advice. Nevertheless, they should not be relied upon exclusive of other input. I will not focus on this form of persuasion further in this book, although neuroscientists have identified certain regions of the brain that are activated by persuasion attempts by "experts," more on this in the next section.

4.3.4 Argumentation (Cognitive)

This will be the main focus of this book. This is Aristotle's *logos*, that is, the logical construction of the argument presented by the speaker. The logical construction of an argument is discussed in detail in Chap. 2, and I will not reiterate it here. However, I would like to discuss the issue of "bootstrapping" in persuasion.

[8] I often ask medical students and residents "What makes an expert?" The usual responses I receive are along the lines of "training and education," "experience," "publications," and the like. It is at this point that I say that "You become an expert when your colleagues recognize you as an expert." That is, the title of "expert" is one that is granted to an individual by others in the field, not by self-proclamations.

Bootstrapping is when an individual uses information delivered by a particular source to conclude that the source is reliable, without external confirmation of the source [33]. In Kolodny's article on rationality [34], he discusses bootstrapping issues as great length. To change the example used by Melchoir [35] to make it medically relevant:

A physician believes that a patient has a temperature by looking at the thermometer that just came out of the patient's mouth.
The thermometer shows that the patient has a temperature.
The physician repeats the observations of temperatures in other patients.
The physician concludes that the thermometer is reliable.

In this scenario, because the physician repeatedly uses the thermometer to obtain temperatures, they believe that the thermometer is reliable. There is a clear fallacy here in that the thermometer may be systematically in error because there is no independent "gold-standard" confirmation of its accuracy. Melchoir [35] further reduces this problem to our own senses—that is, we have no independent confirmation that what we perceive by our senses is, in fact, an accurate representation of the world. Although I do not intend to discuss the reliability of our senses to perceive the world—I have taken this as a given for the purposes of this book[9]—I want by analogy to discuss how a listener may determine if a particular source of information is reliable, in this case, a physician.

The listener can have four beliefs about a proposition: (1) they can believe the proposition; (2) they can reject the proposition; (3) they can suspend judgment about the proposition; or (4) they can be "unaware" of the proposition. Once they have received the proposition from the arguer, they are no longer unaware and must make some time of judgment about the proposition. If the listener believes that the arguer is reliable, then they accept the proposition; if the listener believes that the arguer is unreliable, they either reject or suspend judgment of the proposition. The determination of the reliability of the arguer is a key feature of judging the proposition [35]. If the listener determines the reliability of the source, say a physician, by simply listening to the physician without any other independent confirmation, then this is bootstrapping. However, in most instances of a physician–patient interaction, this is not the case. The patient will have information, perhaps from their referring physician or the fact that the physician has privileges at a given hospital, that provides *some* independent confirmation of the physician's reliability. However, this may still not engender trust in the physician's recommendation for a variety of reasons to be discussed later in this chapter.

In constructing arguments, the physician must be aware of their audience, as advised by Aristotle centuries ago. In the typical clinical encounter, as exemplified by the clinical vignette of Chap. 1, the physician's audience is primarily the patient and, if present, their family members or other significant individuals in

[9] This was Melchoir's primary thesis, and it is quite enlightening, although beyond the scope of this book.

their lives. The physician's argument must be constructed so that the patient and other participants in the decision understand the argument in such a way as to not produce reactance (more on this later). A dialectic should ensue to achieve some level of "manifest rationality," as espoused by Johnson [36] (please see Chap. 2 for details).

The second audience that the physician has are other healthcare professionals. They must also be aware of how these individuals receive the argument. As mentioned previously, because of the method of education and training that healthcare professionals have, they also have a professional umwelt that needs to be borne in mind. There are essentially two types of arguments that I am going to address: the creation of new medical knowledge (which will be addressed in Chap. 6) and how that medical knowledge should be applied to the practice of medicine (in Chap. 7).

4.4 The Neuroscience of Persuasion

Having now discussed the theories of persuasion and their types, I will proceed with a review of what is known about the neuroscience of persuasion and how this is a result of how the human brain has evolved.

I give a brief review of the evolution of the human brain/mind in Chap. 3. Let us recap the seminal developments that will later become incorporated into the "persuasion network" [37] (more on this below):

The human brain enlarged to reach its present cortical size approximately 200,000 years ago.

The human cerebellum enlarged to reach its present size approximately 28,000 years ago.

The human neuropil expanded to increase the interconnectivity of the various regions of the human brain.

The frontoparietal circuitry (neuropil) increased to allow for working memory.

A new prefrontal granular cortex developed, allowing for the ability to learn.

A ventral prefrontal cortex developed, allowing for better auditory and visual input.

A dorsal prefrontal cortex developed to allow for the ability to sequence actions.

A dorsomedial prefrontal cortex developed to allow for choosing and evaluating future actions based on previous experience and increased conspecific sociality.

A polar prefrontal cortex developed to allow for analogical reasoning, making inferences, adapting to novelty, and segregation internal from external thoughts.

A superior temporal gyrus developed to allow for conspecific gaze and facial recognition.

Enlargement of the partial lobes allowed for increased sensory input, visuospatial working memory, number, time and space computation, cross-modal sensory proficiency leading to language, metaphor interpretation, symbolism conceptualization, abstract thinking, and prospective memory function.

Increased corticocerebellar interconnectivity improved cognitive and working memory efficiency.

The prefrontal cortex becomes the center for executive functioning of the brain.

Figure 4.1 shows these regions of the brain in addition to other regions in the persuasion network.

With the advent of functional magnetic resonance imaging (fMRI), an explosion of studies on brain function is emerging. Neuroscientists interested in the neural correlates of persuasion soon started using this tool to assess which areas of the brain were involved in the persuasion process. These studies focused on the neural correlates involved in behavior change and the perceived effectiveness of the persuasion attempt [1]. More than one region of the brain is involved with persuasion, these will be enumerated and elucidated below.

In these studies, persuasive appeals that are more personally relevant produce greater motivation to engage in idiosyncratic issue-relevant thinking. When this happens, the rostral medial prefrontal cortex, precuneus and posterior cingulate are activated [1]. Highly tailored persuasive messages were more self-relevant and evoked more personal and episodic memories. When these messages were "more convincing," as acknowledged by the subjects, the lateral prefrontal cortex was activated, with "strongly convincing" messages showing more connectivity between the left inferior frontal gyrus, amygdala and insula [1]. However, these neural correlates of persuasion have varied from study to study, so the results as yet cannot be generalized.

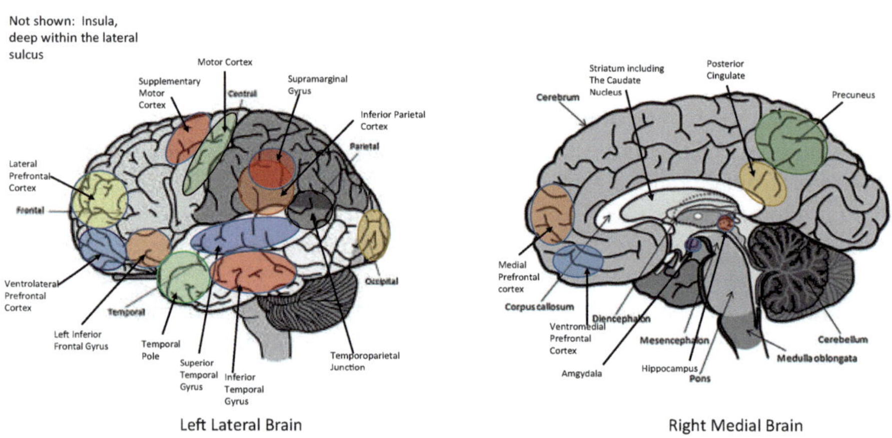

Fig. 4.1 Anatomic illustration of brain regions involved in the persuasion network

Activity in the medial prefrontal cortex during a persuasive message predicted subject-reported change in use of the product advertised [1]. Moreover, regional activity with the rostral medial prefrontal cortex predicted behavior change beyond the self-reported measures of attitude or intentional change by the subject [1]. That is, when this portion of the brain is activated by a persuasive advertisement, subjects' attitudes and behaviors change more than what they think they will. Other areas associated with behavioral change include the posterior superior temporal sulcus, temporoparietal junction, temporal pole, hippocampus, supplementary motor cortex, inferior parietal cortex, occipital cortex, motor cortex and insula [1]. Such behavior change can result from encoding information into one's own self-concept and planning to execute the relevant behaviors [37]. Falk et al. [37], using fMRI and text-based persuasive messages, demonstrated increased activity in the posterior superior temporal sulcus bilaterally, the temporal poles bilaterally, and the dorsomedial prefrontal cortex. This also occurred with video-based messages. Moreover, they referred to this as the "persuasion network", and activity in this network has been associated with social cognition and mentalizing [37], which was previously noted as an important milestone in human brain evolutionary function.

The processes underlying behavioral change reside in the medial prefrontal cortex, which is related to the sense of self [1]. This is the area associated with self-reported intentions, self-efficacy, and the ability to relate to messages, which predict behavior change upon activation of the medial prefrontal cortex. This area is involved with various kinds of self-referential thinking and information processing. Specifically, the anterior zone of the medial prefrontal cortex is associated with persuasion and behavior change but is also associated with affect, decision-making, social cognition, and episodic memory [38].

Individuals who are recognized as an "expert" in a particular area have additional effects on persuasion. Klucharev et al. [39] used fMRI to assess the brain activity of subjects exposed to both "expert" and "nonexpert" messages. Expert messages were associated with activity in the left prefrontal and temporal cortices, which are also associated with semantic elaboration. Experts also enhanced subsequent memory effects in the medial temporal lobes in the hippocampus and parahippocampal gyrus, which are involved in memory function. Expert messages also affected attitudes toward the topic of the message by activating the caudate nucleus, which is involved in trustful behavior, reward processing and learning. This activity in the caudate nucleus results in a "re-evaluation" of the object in terms of its perceived value, which is also mediated through the dorsal striatum [39].

Experts are an important "source variable," that is, the person who is actually presenting the message to the listener [40]. It appears that persuasiveness generally increases with the communicator's expertise (or rather, *recognized* expertise). This is due to recognized expertise being a source of credibility and trustworthiness

(Aristotle's *ethos*, as well as what was previously said about trust in the arguer) [40]. To have a lasting persuasive effect, attitude change must be accompanied by successful memory formation [41]. Hence, the need to involve those areas of the brain that process long-term memories.

Similar neural correlates were found when the persuasive attempts were related to changing social norms. Yomogida et al. [42] used fMRI to study areas of brain activation in participants exposed to messages about social norms. In general, in most modern societies, norms change through interpersonal communication and persuasive messages found in the media. What these investigators found was that the temporal poles, temporoparietal junction, and medial prefrontal cortex were activated. Interestingly, when the persuasion attempt was to direct away from the accepted norm, the left middle temporal and supramarginal gyri were activated. The left supramarginal gyrus activity represented a participant's attitude toward social norms and tracked the persuasion-induced attitude changes. Because there is a strong bias, presumably from how the human brain evolved, to conform to social norms for group cohesion [43], an individual's attitude to change away from these norms requires deep logical reasoning and/or reappraisal, consistent with the middle temporal gyrus's role in cognitive appraisal [44], logical reasoning regarding deontic rules [45], and conceptual/language processes essential for logical reasoning [46, 47]. The left supramarginal gyrus is recruited when persuasion decreases agreement with the norms [42]. The left middle temporal gyrus and left supramarginal gyrus cooperate in changing attitudes by the interconnectivity of the perisylvain pathway [48], which is related to the evolution of verbal communication [49]. Yomogida et al. [42] make the following proposal: the dorsolateral prefrontal cortex and dorsomedial prefrontal cortex provide the common basis for attitude change. The temporal pole, temporoparietal junction, and dorsomedial prefrontal cortex process the social information inherent to issues related to norms. The left middle temporal lobe handles the extra reasoning/reappraisal necessary if the proposed direction of the change is away from the accepted norms, while the left supramarginal gyrus represents attitudes toward these norms and tracks persuasion-induced changes in attitudes. These areas are also used in other belief changes (as noted in the previously cited work).

Although there is a great deal of work in progress pertaining to the neural correlates of persuasion, several keys points are fairly well established. The first is that the neural persuasion network is complex, involving several regions of the brain (Fig. 4.1, Table 4.1). Next, these regions of the brain are also the regions that are involved in highly social self-referential activities, such as language, social cognition, and moral and intellectual judgment (Table 4.1). This makes complete sense when one reflects on human brain evolution. Our survival imperatives were to stay within the group; persuasion is merely a form of social influence that is part of the social fabric of the group. These neurophysiological studies are consistent with the psychological and communications theories of persuasion previously cited, in that areas of the brain that are activated correlate well with the psychological mechanisms of these theories. Therefore, much of what makes a message persuasive is already embedded in the human brain.

Table 4.1 Brain regions involved in persuasion and their associated functions

Brain region	Function in addition to persuasion
Right dorsolateral prefrontal cortex Ventromedial prefrontal cortex Insula	Norm compliance and adaption
Dorsomedial prefrontal cortex Posterior cingulate cortex Temporo-parietal junction Ventromedial prefrontal cortex Striatum	Moral judgement
Dorsomedial prefrontal cortex Posterior superior temporal sulcus Temporal poles	Social cognition
Ventromedial prefrontal cortex Striatum Insula	Social equity
Medial prefrontal cortex Precuneus Posterior cingulate	Self-referential processing
Dorsomedial prefrontal cortex Ventromedial prefrontal cortex Inferior frontal gyrus Right dorsolateral prefrontal cortex	Attitude change through persuasion
Left medial temporal gyrus	Cognitive reappraisal
Left supramarginal gyrus	Decrease agreement with norms
Dorsal anterior cingulate Dorsal medial prefrontal cortex Insula Amygdala	Conflict-related activity
Striatum	Reward-related activity, social interaction
Lateral prefrontal cortex Parietal cortices	Deliberative reasoning
Limbic system	Emotional processing
Medial temporal lobe Left ventrolateral prefrontal cortex	Memory encoding
Medial prefrontal cortex	Affective processes of valuation, reward and fear
Anterior zone of the medial prefrontal cortex	Affect, decision-making, social cognition, episodic memory
Posterior superior temporal sulcus Temporo-parietal junction Temporal poles Hippocampus Motor cortex Supplementary motor cortex Inferior parietal cortex Occipital cortex Insula	Behavior change
Caudate nucleus	Trustful behavior, reward processing and learning
Supramarginal gyrus	Spoken and written language, emotional responses

4.5 Factors Involved in Persuasion

The purpose of the previous sections expositions of the theories and the neural correlates of persuasion was to provide a foundation for discussing factors that may be involved in persuading some people. Of course, humans vary greatly in their characteristics, and there is no way that any particular factor will always be true for any one particular person. However, the general premise of this book is that human brain/mind biological, social and cultural evolution have embedded a reasoning framework that prioritizes social group cohesion and that it requires focused cognitive reasoning and no small amount of moral courage by the individual to make choices that would be against their social norms. In fact, the psychological/communications theories of persuasion as well as the neural correlates of persuasion are consistent with this view.

One of the primary factors related to persuasion is the listener's cognitive abilities to understand the message or argument, thereby being able to appraise the argument in a dispassionate manner to achieve manifest rationality. This may not always be the case, however. People have varying levels of intelligence, education, and experiences so that some will be better able to comprehend arguments or messages of varying complexity and the information content within these arguments. Therefore, one of the first assessments for an arguer is to assess just how much that the listener can understand. This was one of Aristotle's first requirements for an orator. Again, for clarity, although I will be addressing persuasion from the standpoint of trying to logically persuade someone of new knowledge or a recommendation for a decision, even in this scenario, there is more to persuasion than just the illative core of the argument.

4.5.1 The Social Union

I spent some time in the last chapter developing the concept of the social umwelt. In this conception, just as the biological umwelt of animals depends the animal's senses and that which the animal cannot register with their senses is not part of their world, the social umwelt is the person's "cultural and social senses." In this sense, there are some cultural elements that will not be accepted by the listener. In this setting, the arguer needs to couch their presentation in a way that will not threaten the cultural identity of the listener. This may lead to resistance to any messaging attempts, as noted in Chap. 3. Clearly, there may be at times some aspects of the listener's attitude that the arguer may find repugnant. An overt challenge may be appropriate in some circumstances; however, in the setting of the physician–patient relationship, it will require self-discipline on the part of the physician not to engage the listener in a contest pertaining to which values are more nobler and simply focus on the issues that are relevant for the medical benefit of the patient.

4.5.2 Emotionality

The intensity of the emotion used in the message or argument can affect the effectiveness of the persuasive attempt. Emotion can be expressed in both written and oral arguments but more acutely felt with verbal messages. The intent to persuade other people spontaneously increases the emotionality of the individual's appeals via the words that the arguer uses [50]. One of the consequences of using emotion in an appeal is that it tends to enhance memory, and there is an association between memory and persuasion [50] (see the above section on the activation of memory in persuasive appeals [39]). Both positive and negative emotions can enhance persuasion under specific circumstances [51]. On the other hand, escalating the emotional appeal when the circumstances are not right for it may backfire on the arguer [50], the so-called boomerang effect that more than one persuasion theory has warned.

It is not surprising that emotional appeals can be persuasive. The human mind is programmed to send and receive emotions as a form of communication (see Chap. 3). Social-functional approaches to emotion propose that emotions facilitate and direct social interactions between individuals [52]. Furthermore, outward displays of emotions evolved largely to influence others [53], that is, as a form of persuasion. Specifically, Andrade and Ho [54] demonstrated that anger can have a significant impact and change the behavior of others. Certainly, one would be hard pressed to find an individual who did not become angry or was subject to angry rhetoric when milder forms of persuasion have failed.[10]

Part of the reason some feel that injecting emotionality into their persuasion technique is that it has worked in the past. The "Persuasion-Knowledge Model" asserts that people accumulate experiences with persuading others over a lifetime, which can lead to learned associations that can be triggered when the person intends to persuade [55]. Friestad and Wright [55] found a causal relationship between participants' intent to persuade and the emotionality of their language, even when emotionality threatened to backfire. Therefore, they specifically aver that more emotional audiences may be more open to emotional appeals while warning that more "cognitive" (by which, I think the authors mean, more logically intellectual) may not be persuaded by such emotional appeals [55].

From the standpoint of the physician trying to persuade a patient, expressions of empathic emotions can build trust. I had a former mentor who would say, "Patients don't care how much you know, until they know how much you care." However, this display, although trust-building, should not be the main persuasion tool—a logically constructed argument of how the patient's diagnosis was determined, followed by another pertaining to treatment options should be. The physician must understand

[10] Stories of the "hot-headed" boss, or, in my field of surgery, the "demanding" (to use a euphemism) surgeon are legendary. Later, when asked why they threw the tantrum that they did, the usual response is that the receiver of the tirade did not "understand" the urgency of the situation, a point they were trying to make clear.

that family members may use emotional appeals, but as long as this does not escalate into coercion, this should be allow to play out among the family.

4.5.3 Mimicry

Mimicry in persuasion is when one individual takes on a few of the overt bodily and linguistic characteristics of another individual to elicit a favorable response to the persuasion message. This has been termed the "chameleon effect' [56]. Characteristics mimicked are such things as posture, physical mannerisms, modes of speech, etc. Those who successfully mimic another person were, in general, better liked by that person [56]. This extends into the business of consumerism. Participants who were mimicked in a sales interaction were more likely to choose those goods and rate these goods higher than those who were not [57]. They also showed more positive attitudes toward the product being presented to them by the mimicker [57]. Importantly, the participants who were mimicked were not aware that they were being influenced by the mimicry [57]. In other words, the persuader can achieve a successful persuasion attempt with the appearance of trying to persuade by mimicry.

Although it is worthwhile for the physician to understand how mimicry can affect the persuasive interaction between the physician and the patient, the use of mimicry just to "get the patient to agree to a treatment" does not strike me as ethical on a routine basis. Perhaps there are times where mimicry can be used to enhance the physician's likability in the patient's eyes or perhaps build trust, but it should not be used as a form of manipulation.

4.5.4 Voice Modulation

Most people have probably heard or said the phrase, "It's not what you said, it's how you said it!" This could pertain to the actual words used (i.e., language) or pertain to the way the voice was used. The field of "paralinguistics" studies "paralanguage," which is the acoustic property of speech, such as volume, pitch, timber, cadence, etc. [58]. Paralanguage adds a layer of additional communication than simply the words used. It is common to hear someone say of an interaction "I do not like your tone," for example. Obviously, this applies when the arguer is actually speaking to the listener—although certainly written communication can have a "voice" and a "tone," it does not produce actual sound that speaking does. It is also abundantly clear that from an evolutionary standpoint, the human brain is quite attuned to the sound of another human voice.

Studies on how paralinguistics can influence persuasion are based on "acoustic cues" provided by the arguer while speaking in the form of volume, pitch, speech rate, etc. These acoustic cues can enhance persuasion by making the speaker seem more confident in their message without undermining their perceived sincerity. That is, the speaker's confident vocal demeanor persuades others by serving as a signal that they strongly endorse the conclusion of their argument [58]. In the patient–physician interaction, such confidence can be comforting to the patient. Therefore, paralinguistics can uniquely persuade when linguistics alone cannot.

Part of the reason this may be so is that when someone knows that someone else is trying to persuade them, they are placed "on guard" [59]. They then try to "inoculate" themselves against the persuasive message [60] because they feel that those who are trying to persuade them might have "devious" motives [59]. Because paralinguistics evades detection, these techniques may be more successful; however, if there are linguistic cues that allow for the persuasion attempt to be detected, then the persuasion advantage of paralinguistics is nullified [58]. However, Van Zant and Berger's studies [58] suggest that changes in voice volume and volume variability appear to make the speaker more confident in their message and, therefore, an implied reliability in the message.

Certainly, there is no doubt that the paralinguistic features of our voice when we speak will affect how particular individuals will hear the message. These are features of how our brains developed language ability. Although I am not aware of any specific study evaluating this in the physician–patient relationship, I have had patients report to me that they found so-and-so doctor inspiring "confidence" just by the way that they talked. I will admit that I have nothing but anecdotal evidence in this regard, the acoustic cues that are heard as "confidence," "mastery," or "expert" cues will be persuasive to many patients, in conjunction with the neural activation of those brain centers influenced by expertise (Fig. 4.1) [39].

4.5.5 Body Language

Another aspect of nonverbal communication in persuasion is body language [61]. There is no question that in our primate evolution that much communication developed through physical demonstration.[11] Oullier and Basso [62] aver that "in real social life, the signals sent by the body and the physical presence of others influence the way we act and decide," and it is "not always about inferences of someone's else's state of mind." That is, we "read" someone's body language, which may send a more convincing message than the words they are saying. These authors, who are from the cognitive psychology and economic fields of study, refer to this as "embodied economics," which they define as "how information provided by bodily signals, the physical presence and displacement of others (or its imaginations) influence the way we make economic decisions." Specifically, it is about how "movement, posture, sensitivity to mimicry, and every kind of information the body conveys." In

[11] Our primate brethren still communicate predominantly with physical gestures and with "paralinguistic" verbalizations. It is very probable that we received such abilities from our common primate ancestors.

reality, although these authors are studying this from an economic point of view, this is truly about how body language can persuade.

Oullier and Basso [62] integrate the importance of the body in human perception of the world with other aspects of cognition. For example, they seem to adhere to Changuex's "neuronal habitus" model [63] in which the nerve synapses change as a result of learned concepts. They further link bodily activity with the concept of "embedded cognition," use of metaphors, "frames" and "prototypes"[12] [64]. In particular, embodied cognition is the cognitive dynamics of how our bodies interact with the physical and social world. Moreover, the way people move conveys information to predict their intentions and goals [62]. They further reviewed studies showing how individuals will "link" or coordinate their movements when information is exchanged.

What all this means for the physician is that their body language, as well as the patient's and the families, will communicate information about the message and how message is received. Such things as posture, eye gaze, head nods, being in a seated position, etc., all convey a message to the patient about the physician's interest in the patient. Arms or legs crossed, shaking heads, and tense posture all convey information about how the patient is receiving the argument presented by the physician. Physicians need awareness of these bodily cues when trying to persuade a patient.

4.5.6 Resistance to Persuasion (Reactance)

Reactance was first described in 1966 by Brehm [65]. The concept centers around an individual's motivation to regain freedom after it has been lost or is threatened [66]. Reactance is an amalgam of anger and "negative cognitions" that is preceded by a perceived threat to freedom [67]. It is clear that much advice that comes from physicians to patients is asking them to behaviorally restrict their freedom for the sake of their health. It is also clear that many will not heed this advice. Understanding reactance will help understand this resistance to change behavior to improve health.

There are many ways reactance manifests. Those who are reactant to advise will generally follow one of four strategies: avoidance, contesting, biased processing, and empowerment [68]. The motivations for this resistance are a threat to freedom, reluctance to change, and concerns for deception. The avoidance strategy can be used for all three types of motivations; the contesting strategy is generally used for the concerns for deception motivation (deception motivation is a trust issue, which is related to believing the premises of an argument); and the empowerment and biased processing strategies used for the reluctance to change motivation [68].

People who are reactant are opposed to being influenced [68]. Highly reactant individuals are characterized by a resistance to rules and regulations, have a high

[12] This appears to be an echo of the Jungian archetypes discussed in the last chapter.

desire for personal autonomy, are highly defensive, have a low concern for social norms, are more prone to risky behaviors, and experience more threats to their freedoms[13] [67]. A person's experience of reactance strongly depends on their goals and values when the threat occurs [66]. Those who express "motivated resistance" simply do not want to be persuaded. Some individuals may be "trait reactant," that is, it is part of their character, having the strong need for independence, autonomy, confrontational/rebellious behavior, and a tendency to resist authority in general [69]. These individuals are armed with resistance strategies to reduce attitudinal and behavioral change and maintain their current attitudes and behaviors [68]. Those with "outcome resistance" simply do not change their attitudes in response to a persuasive attempt—that is, they have not been persuaded but do not necessarily feel threatened.

These strategies are put into practice in different ways. In the avoidance strategy, the person simply avoids persuasion attempts through a physical process (e.g., not showing up to an appointment, walking out the room, etc.), a mechanical process (e.g., turning the channel on the television or radio, not clicking on an internet site), or cognitive process (e.g., simply ignoring the message despite hearing it) [68]. Avoidance may be a way to avoid cognitive dissonance (as described earlier in the chapter); that is, they wish to avoid messages that conflict with their beliefs [68].

The contesting strategy is more adversarial. These individuals will contest the content of the message, the source of the message, or the persuasive strategies used in the message. That is, they do not believe the premises of the argument are true; they do not trust the arguer; and/or they think the argument is logically flawed or whatever other persuasive method used is used incorrectly [68]. With the contesting strategy, the individual actually thinks about the content of the message or argument (as opposed to the avoidance strategy with which the individual purposefully does not want to think about the content of the message) to create a counterargument to refute it.[14] It also appears that when the individual is "forewarned" of a persuasion attempt, he may be more prone to contest [68] (this appears to be the boomerang effect previously discussed). Interestingly, when the attempt is constructed as a narrative, there appears to be less counterarguing [68] (consistent with the power of storytelling to influence because the persuasion attempt is hidden in the story). Another method of contesting is "source degradation," that is, dismissing the credibility, expertise or trustworthiness of the source. One such method is "defensive stereotyping", in which a negative stereotype of the message sender is brought to mind. Ultimately, contesting strategies are used because individuals develop beliefs about how persuasion agents try to influence them, and the use of such persuasion

[13] This is certainly consistent with the "white, male effect" previously discussed in Chap. 3.

[14] If this leads to a goodwill, honest exchange of viewpoints such that the arguer is willing to revise his premises according to valid criticisms of the listener and the listener would be willing to accept a revised conclusion based on his criticisms, this is actually the manifest rationality of Johnson. However, here, we are discussing the individual who has no intention of being persuaded but is simply being contradictory.

knowledge may be automatic and unconscious [70] (consistent with what was said about the neural habitus in the prior section).

In biased processing, the message either fits the extant attitudes or beliefs of the individual, or if not, the message simply becomes less relevant [68]. They do this by weighing attributes and reducing the impact of the message by distorting the information received that is inconsistent with a particular attitude or behavior, and by optimism bias which allows for dismissing the relevance of the message for them (e.g., "I know smoking causes cancer but I have a great immune system so it won't cause cancer in me.").

The empowerment strategy is self-affirming. That is, the individual "empowers" or "strengthens" their sense of self and their beliefs in their own attitudes to reduce their vulnerability to external influence. They do this by attitude bolstering and social validation, which reinforce a particular attitude, and self-assertion, which increases their self-confidence [68]. With attitude bolstering, they do not refute or challenge the argument; they believe that their beliefs and attitudes are better. With social validation, they see that other people who are important to them believe the same, so their beliefs are also valid (consistent with the evolution of group cohesion and the moral foundation of loyalty). With self-assertion, the individual reminds themselves that their attitudes and behaviors are important despite the argument presented [68].

The last reactance concept I would like to discuss is "vicarious reactance," defined as a person experiencing feelings of reactance to a threat to another individual's or group's freedom even if the threat does not directly affect their own freedom of choice [66]. This comes in two forms: (1) as a consequence of people cognitively taking the role of the restricted person and asking themselves what the restricted person might experience, (2) people experience reactance themselves while observing a threat to another person's freedom. People from "collectivistic" cultures tend to experience more vicarious reactance than those from more "individualistic" cultures. With respect to the medical encounter, this may be a reaction of a family member predisposed to reactance to authority seeing their loved one's freedoms threatened.

I have spent some time on reactance as it is a key feature as to why some individuals will not be persuaded. Breaking through this reactant barrier may be exceptionally difficult if the physician cannot couch their argument in a way that threatens the perceived freedoms of the patient.

4.5.7 Ambiguity of Words or Phrases

Words and phrases frequently have more than one meaning or an imprecise meaning; or, rather, they can be construed to have more than one meaning. As was mentioned in Chap. 2, ambiguity can either be lexical (having to when a word has more than one meaning) or structural (when a phrase can be interpreted in more than one way). The listener of such an ambiguous message will tend to hear what is consistent with their underlying beliefs and biases [17]. In my estimation, it is also consistent with their social umwelt, that is, they have always attached certain meanings to words and phrases and simply to not "hear" the alternative meanings. In such a situation, persuasion may have appeared to have happened, but in reality, there is a discordance between the conclusion that the listener heard and the conclusion the arguer thought they reached. Moreover, even when the message is unambiguous, there is a tendency for people to try to fit the new information into their established belief system (i.e., change the meaning of the message to fit their belief schema) or to be so critical of it as to not accept the conclusions, as in the reactant individual described in the preceding section.

For the physician, there is both an advantage and disadvantage to ambiguity. Many clinical situations are not clear-cut. The trajectory of a particular illness can take many paths. In which case, being ambiguous about the potential paths may be appropriate. This is usually couched with the patient and family that there are several possibilities, and, at this point, it is not possible to determine which. I will give an example from my practice, a patient with a newly diagnosed cancer will often ask, "How much time do I have left?" That is, what is my life expectancy? I would never give a specific answer of x number of months, but rather, show what is the survival curve is for past patients with their particular cancer at that particular stage with the treatment available at the time. I would point out that some patient unfortunately die relatively soon after diagnosis, and some die a long timc after diagnosis, and many in-between. I do not know where a particular patient will fall in that survival curve. I would also point out that this curve was based on what happened to patients in the past, and how it applies to future patients may not be exactly the same, particularly as new treatments may be forthcoming. The advantage, in my opinion, of this ambiguity is that it is both an honest appraisal of our lack of predictive knowledge and does not rob the patient of hope.

The disadvantage is that one believes that one has come to some type of agreement with the patient, but, in fact, the patient believes they have agreed to something else. This will result in poor patient compliance. This is one of the reasons why it is recommended that the patient repeat what was said to them by the physician, and vice versa for that matter, so that one ensures that the message sent was the message understood.

4.5.8 Memories in Persuasion

In the neuroscience of persuasion section, it was previously noted that those regions of the brain that are involved in memory are also activated during a persuasion attempt. The importance of memory, especially working memory, in human reasoning and understanding was discussed in Chap. 3. The human mind evolved to understand the world as a narrative sequence. As such, memories are used to predict future events based on past experiences. For Kahneman and Tversky [71], these then become the "anchors" that an individual may use when trying to make a judgment in uncertain conditions. Memories are also critical in the "mental models" theory of reasoning, as put forth by Johnson-Laird [72], also discussed in Chap. 3. Therefore, what an individual holds in their memory will affect their ability to be persuaded by any one particular means.

4.5.9 Self-Persuasion

Self-persuasion is a technique by which individuals can increase the self-relevance of an argument [73]. This can be considered the opposite of the reactance described above. It is not surprising that people are generally more persuaded by arguments that they themselves construct rather than arguments that are presented to them by others [74]. This is opposed to "direct persuasion," which are those arguments presented by others [74]. This is because in self-persuasion, people assume that the motivation for the persuasion comes from within themselves [74]. This would also eliminate the concern for deceptive motives of other people trying to influence the person, which is a motivation for reactance[15] [68]. Self-generated arguments are also tailored to match each individual's values and attitudes [75], so issues with cognitive dissonance, motivated cognition, and conflict with their social umwelt will presumably not occur. In addition, self-persuasion seems to have a larger effect when the person believes that a majority of other people hold the same attitudes and beliefs [76]. This is consistent with the finding that conformity tends to increase when people identify with the group communicating the attitude or social norm [77]. Of course, this is consistent with the evolutionary imperative of group cohesion, human universals, and moral foundation theory.

Self-persuading norms are a combination of self-persuading techniques and social descriptive norms [73]. In their experiments, Berquist and Ejelov [73] found that self-persuading norms strengthen social influence by 17–25% by having individuals provide reasons consistent with their values. These norms tend to be more effective in regulating behavior when there is some argument in favor of the norm. Therefore, when an individual can produce a self-constructed argument in favor of the social norm, they are more likely to adhere to that norm. This speaks again to both the need to maintain group cohesion and the social umwelt.

Some of this may have to do with the culture from which the individual comes. Li et al. [78] found that self-persuasion is more effective with people from "individualistic" cultures (i.e., those cultures where individuals' freedoms are tantamount), while direct persuasion (i.e., messaging from others) is more effective in "collectivistic" cultures (i.e., cultures where the group welfare is tantamount). This clearly harkens back to the discussion of the importance of cultural identity discussed in Chap. 3. This clearly has implications for persuasion in the physician–patient relationship.

[15] However, it may not eliminate the actual occurrence of self-deception (see Chap. 3).

The value here for the physician is in understanding whether their patient would be better persuaded by encouraging a self-persuasion approach or a direct persuasion approach. This will require some knowledge of the patient's cultural orientation (individualistic vs. collectivistic). Failure to take this into consideration may risk reactance from the patient. It is important that the physician does not try to impose their cultural orientation, as it may also lead to reactance.

4.5.10 Storytelling as an Instrument of Persuasion

I have previously noted the importance of storytelling (i.e., the narrative paradigm) as a means of persuasion [12, 13, 18–24]. I will not reiterate what was previously said here. However, from the standpoint of patient–physician communication, there may be times where the patient may better understand their situation as a story rather than numerical probabilities. Bullock et al. [79] confirmed experimentally that a narrative has its persuasive power because of its ease of understanding for most people. What I mean here is that the physician can take the best case scenario, worst case scenario, and probable in-between scenarios of the patient's potential course of their illness and present them as a story to the patient and the family, with the relative likelihoods for each scenario. Although I usually begin such counseling with "I am not God, I don't know what is exactly going to happen to you, me or anybody else," I have frequently found this method effective so that the patient and family can elicit images, perhaps conjure memories of others in different health crises, and engender emotions so that the patient and family will be able to create the mental models or future event sequencing to all for better decision-making.

4.6 Persuasion as Manifest Rationality

In Chap. 2, I spent some time developing the concepts of rationality, reasoning and argumentation (I also spent time on intuition, but that will be brought up again in Chap. 7). I discussed the different types of persuasion and linked the ability to persuade and be persuaded to the way our brain and mind evolved biologically, socially and culturally, as reviewed in Chap. 3. In discussing persuasion as it pertains to medical decision making for the patient, I have rejected those forms of persuasion whose goals are simply to "get someone to do something that I want them to do." Rather, the type of persuasion that I view as ethical in medicine is to create an argument in such a fashion, understanding the patient's cognitive abilities and social restraints, so that the patient accepts the conclusion to, in fact, be in their best interests. This, I believe, is done under the broad framework of manifest rationality as described by Johnson [36]. Namely, that the physician will present the illative core of their argument in a manner both understandable and non-socially threatening to the patient, the patient (and/or family) will ask questions (i.e., criticisms of the argument for clarifications), and a mutually acceptable conclusion will be reached.

In the Elaboration Likelihood Model of persuasion as put forth by Petty and Cacioppo [2, 15], there are two routes of persuasion, the peripheral and central routes. The peripheral route tends to use emotional appeals, and although they may have short-term effectiveness, the effects tend to wane in the long term. The central route requires active engagement by the listener. It requires the arguer to present a coherent, understandable argument and the listener to critically appraise the argument. This route is most likely to lead to long-term changes in attitudes and beliefs. There are probably few issues that will engage an individual more than their health, so it is very likely that the physician will have the focused attention of the patient. This, I believe, is the argument constructed by the physician to get to a diagnosis and the argument constructed by the physician presented in a counseling session for appropriate treatment options (see Fig. 1.1). This is the route of persuasion I will be discussing now.

Going back to our clinical vignette from Chap. 1 as well as the foundations of the different aspects of the clinical encounter, the physician has taken in information from the patient and pertinent objective testing to come to a diagnosis (I will explore why obtaining specific information through the patient encounter and objective testing can lead to a diagnosis in Chap. 7, but, for now, let us assume the diagnosis is correct). With respect to obtaining information from the patient, the physician has to have trust that what the patient is telling the physician about their symptoms is, in fact, true. In the explanation to the patient, the physician will start off by reiterating the patient's symptoms and any pertinent physical examination findings. They then will say that these findings can be found in a certain number of disease processes, the differential diagnosis, each of which has a prior probability of being present before any testing is done. To determine which is most likely, the physician will order one or more tests. When the results return, the posterior probabilities of the possible differential diagnoses will be assessed. This is a typical Bayesian approach to diagnosis [80], although quite frankly, it is usually done qualitatively in the physician's mind rather than a rigorous quantitative assessment. If no one diagnosis reaches a level of satisfactory confidence, then additional testing is performed until such confidence is reached. The one diagnosis with the posterior probability high enough that the physician judges should be treated will be presented to the patient. This is the general structure of the illative core of the diagnosis (the "Illative Core of the Argument" in Fig. 4.2).

How does the patient then appraise this argument? The first thing that the patient needs to do is determine the truth of the premises. The patient is, of course, aware of this symptom, so they should be able to trust that this premise is true. The patient experiences the physical examination as the physician conducts it, although they may not be able to interpret the findings the way that the physician can.

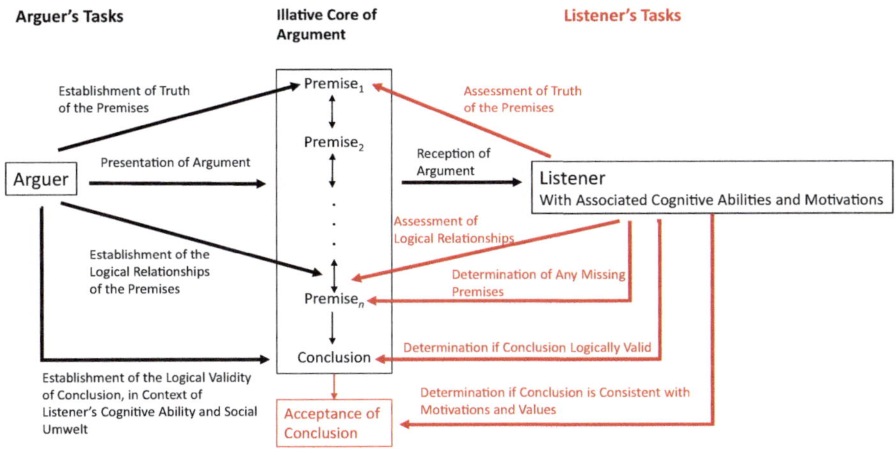

Fig. 4.2 Flow of the argument from the arguer to the listener, with the tasks required of the arguer to persuade the listener and the tasks required of the listener to accept the conclusions of the argument

Therefore, the patient must trust the physician's interpretation.[16] Similar to the objective findings of the test, unless the patient "does their own research" into how to interpret the tests they have just undergone, they rely on the physician's interpretation. Even if the patient does find information about the tests (through the internet or otherwise), they still have to trust these sources as well. Therefore, much of the assessment of the truth of the premises has to do with trust in the physician and how the validity of the tests were determined, that is, the scientific medical "establishment" (for the physician, the testing validity comes under "Techniques of Evidential Foundation Appraisal" column in Fig. 1.1—more on this in Chaps. 6 and 7). If the patient has a satisfactorily high level of trust in the physician and the scientific medical establishment, then they will accept the truth of the premises (or, at least, true enough). However, if the patient lacks this trust, by virtue of their social umwelt, trait reactant character, or any other reason, they will not accept the truth of the premises. If this is the case, the conclusion lacks relevance to the patient and will be rejected. In addition, even if the patient accepts the truth of the presented premises, they must make the further determination of any other relevant premises that were not used in the construction of the argument. For example, maybe the patient feels that other test needs to be done to further increase or decrease the reliability of the conclusion (Fig. 4.2, "Listener's Tasks" column). So, going back to Fig. 3.5, this occurs through the boxes of the "communication filter," the "slow thinking processing," and conscious executive

[16] It is certainly not an unusual experience for a physician to have a patient either diminish or exaggerate their symptoms for a variety of reasons. In my practice, this is where having family members present to confirm or refute what the patient is saying can be quite helpful.

judgement" with the associated feedback loops. That is, Fig. 4.2 is a subset task of person-to-person communication.

If the patient accepts the truth of the premises, they must now determine that the premises are logically related in such a way that the conclusion (i.e., the diagnosis) is acceptable. In Chap. 2, I explored the different forms of logic. I came to the conclusion then that formal, deductive logical methods are, at best, too cumbersome, or, at worst, inappropriate for this task. Informal and/or inductive methods would be more appropriate. In a more formal way, each premise is related to the next dependent on the relationship to the diagnosis. The more closely it is linked, the more relevant the premise becomes. In the clinical vignette pertaining to GERD, the symptoms of heartburn are very closely linked to GERD, as gastric acid is a known cause of the symptoms (the "Physician's Metacognition: Theoretical Framework" column of Fig. 1.1, more on causation in Chap. 5). The objective finding of a $pH < 4$ within the esophagus for a time exceeding the threshold of being pathologic, especially if the patient feels heartburn symptoms at the same time that the pH is <4, is a strong indicator that the premises are linked. The patient will not necessarily know these logical relationships prior to their encounter with the physician, but if the physician is able to explain the relationships in a matter understandable to the patient, then the patient can assess the logical relationships.

It is at this point that the patient must accept or reject the conclusion. If the patient is a "rational agent" or *Homo philosophicus*, to use Cassam's term,[17] they will accept the conclusion. However, as I have tried to emphasize in this chapter, the "persuasiveness" of an argument is related to, but not exactly the same, the structural validity and propositional soundness of an argument. There are other aspects of what people believe and what they want to believe. Assuming that we have a "good faith" effort on both the physician and patient to come to an agreement on the conclusion, a dialectic leading to manifest rationality will ensue. Now the example I gave is that of an elective encounter where the stakes, although high, do not require an immediate decision. The necessary degree of confidence in a decision is correlated with the stakes of the decision, given the time constraints that the decision needs to be made. For example, after an acute trauma, where the patient is bleeding significantly, decisions have to be made in an emergent manner. The time of the clinical encounter to definitive treatment is necessarily shortened, with less time for a dialect to occur. However, in most situations, the patient will be able to ask questions (i.e., provide criticism of the argument, in the sense of trying to give the physician an opportunity to strengthen the argument). Once the patient believes that the conclusion is logically sound, they then have to determine that the conclusion is consistent with their values and beliefs. A similar process would go on for decisions about treatments.

[17] Please see the discussion pertaining to *Homo philosophicus* in Chap. 3.

However, despite this, patients may not accept conclusions that they would agree are valid yet fail to satisfy other conditions that are mandatory for that particular patient to accept the conclusion and change their attitude and behavior.

4.7 Effects of Patient Beliefs and Motivations on Persuasion

4.7.1 Health Care Communication

Similar to what was previously shown with respect to the neuroscience of the brain regions used in persuasion, Huskey et al. [81] showed that the same brain regions are involved in health care communication. When a message is "tailored" to an individual, the message aligns the source, the message, the receiver and the context [81]. It appears that interventions that modify attitudes, norms and self-efficacy are effective in promoting health behavior change [82]. This may be related to beliefs concerning the appeal and consequences of behavior (attitudes), other people's approval and performance of the behavior (social norms), and one's ability to execute the relevant responses (self-efficacy) [82]. These changing attitudes go through two phases: (1) "Deliberate phase," where one considers the desirability and feasibility of the goal and culminates in the decision or intention to act, and (2) the "implementation phase," in which there is a translation of the intentions into action involving a set of processes that have to do with action preparation [82]. What does this mean for communication between the physician and the patient?

4.7.2 Patient Motivations

Yates [83] defined a "decision" as "a course of action that is intended to produce a satisfying state of affairs." Although this might be a satisfying definition when the decision is to take a certain action or not, some decisions are not action-oriented, such as decisions about beliefs and attitudes. A perhaps more inclusive definition would be *a conclusion pertaining to an individual's state of mind or course of action.* Regardless of the definition, in the setting of the clinical encounter that I am discussing, the decision that the patient must make is whether to accept the diagnosis rendered by the physician and then decide on a treatment plan.

The patient will have a constellation of motivations for both. The patient's primary motivation when seeking health care is "to get better," that is, return to a prior state of good health. Certainly, there are medical encounters that are preventative in nature; that is, the patient is in satisfactory health and wishes to maintain it. However, for my present discussion, I am using the clinical vignette from Chap. 1, where the patient consults with a physician due to troublesome symptoms—in the case of the vignette, heartburn from GERD. This particular patient's treatment options as presented by the physician include lifestyle modifications, medications or surgery.

Beyond returning to a state of good health, the patient may have a number of other considerations when making a decision. These include health-related decisions, financially related decisions, personal and/or family-related decisions, and socially related decisions (Table 4.2). A patient's particular circumstance will determine the relative importance of each of these factors. Note that from the standpoint of the physician's argument for the diagnosis and treatment options, none of these factors were considered in the premises in their argument. These must have to be identified by the patient and/or family in order for the physician to then revise their argument to reach a mutually agreeable conclusion (Fig. 4.2).

The health-related motivations listed in Table 4.2 are relatively self-explanatory and do not require exposition. When disease is potentially fatal, prolonging survival is a motivation. Beyond that, relief of symptoms, improvement of quality of life, avoidance of treatment-related adverse events or complications, and avoidance of medications are important motivations for some patients. During the course of my 30-year career, I have heard all of these as motivation to seek medical care. In addition, for most physicians, this is, in fact, what they consider their task to be. However, there are other motivations that patients have that physicians generally do not consider (but, perhaps, traditional healers do, which will be explored in Chap. 8).

Unfortunately, financial strain can be a major driver of healthcare decisions for some patients. Nguyen et al. [84] demonstrated that financial strain of medical care involved trade-offs between household needs and an individual's medical needs, a search for alternative remedies as affordable substitutes when standard care is a financial burden, and, sadly, a reluctance to discuss financial strain in a clinical setting with their healthcare provider. In another study of decisions pertaining to non-facial skin growth, Li et al. [85] noted that in some patients, the financial impact of the procedure affected the decision to remove the skin growth. Beyond actually paying for the treatment, if the treatment affects the patient's ability for employment, this may be a factor in the decision, particularly if their health insurance is based on their work. I have heard all of these considerations, as I am sure many other physicians have.

The patient's family may play a role (Table 4.2). Family members may have their own considerations when assisting a patient in a medical decision. Dijkman et al. [86] determined that there were five broad categories of factors that influenced

Table 4.2 Patient's possible motivations that are potentially persuadable in a medical encounter

Health-related	Financially-related	Personal/family-related	Socially-related
Survival/longevity Quality of life Symptomatic improvement Adverse events/ complications Medication dependency	Insurance costs Out-of-pocket costs Loss of income Employment restrictions	Loss of independence Change in status within family Family dynamics Family coercion Family obligations Effects of costs on family Travel Personal goals Change of sense of self	Social umwelt Group coercion Shibboleth behaviors

family involvement. These included (1) patient characteristics, (2) family characteristics, (3) family system characteristics, (4) physician's role, and (5) cultural influences. One can easily see in these categories some of the effects of the social umwelt. Sometimes, family-doctor conflicts can occur, especially if the patient is incapacitated and critically ill [87]. Beyond these circumstances, other factors related to the patient's sense of self, such as loss of independence, feelings of their own status within the family (e.g., they are "breadwinner"), family obligations (e.g., they are the caregiver for another family member), guilt over burdening the family, and their own personal goals in life (e.g., witnessing an important family event), can all be factors (i.e., premises in their own argument of self-persuasion) in their decision.

Last, social and cultural considerations can also affect decisions (Table 4.2). With some decisions, a patient's social and cultural group's attitudes and beliefs can be an important factor. We have discussed previously about risk-taking in white males and blood transfusions among Jehovah's Witnesses. We have certainly seen Covid patients refuse to acknowledge that they have the disease and refuse certain types of treatments or preventative measures. These decisions act as shibboleths to confirm the loyalty of the individual to their cultural/social group and maintain group cohesions. Tariman et al. [88] showed that in cancer treatment decisions in older adults, the patient's beliefs and values, ethnicity (which is a surrogate for culture), decision control preferences, health-care related experiences, patient perceptions of the decision-making process, and personal factors (such as I described) all can become premises in a self-constructed argument of self-persuasion.

However, patient involvement in shared decision-making may not be ideal. Buljac-Samardzic et al. [89], in a study of patients with chronic illness, found that patient engagement was dependent on (1) enabled involvement—the extent to which patients are facilitated and empowered to participate, (2) relationship-driven involvement—the relationship between the patient and healthcare professional, (3) disease-impact driven involvement—the severity of the disease, and (4) cognitive-driven involvement—knowledge and information. All of these issues have been discussed in how people are persuaded. Therefore, there is consistency in the persuasion model presented from the rationality-logic-argumentation to the evolution of the human brain/mind to persuasion theories.

From a purely economic standpoint, a "rational agent" may not be as complex as what we described. We have developed a formula for the costs of the treatment of GERD for quality-adjusted life expectancy[18] [90]. This takes into account patient survival, improvement in quality of life, and all the costs associated with the treatment. In this particular analysis, the Nissen fundoplication was the most cost-effective for the patient, yielding 2.99 quality-adjusted life years per $1000 cost to

[18] We also analyzed the value propositions for the other stakeholders: the surgeon, the hospital and the private insurance company [90]. One of the most significant findings is that each will have a different metric when analyzing the value of a treatment. Therefore, it cannot be surprising that there are conflicts among the stakeholders—they each value something different. This will be discussed further in Chap. 7.

the patient. There is a growing field of "Bayesian persuasion" in economics in which the probability of accepting a persuasive attempt is changed by information produced by the persuading agent, that is, prior probability of acceptance → information (argument) given → posterior probability [91, 92]. As interesting as this is, as with formal, symbolic logic, its practicality in a medical encounter setting is not feasible.

In summary, in the setting of the clinical encounter (Fig. 1.1), the physician's goal is to persuade by achieving cognitive agreement with the patient for the conclusions pertaining to the diagnosis and treatment options. Evidence from human evolution, anthropology, social psychology and neuroscience has demonstrated that much of how one is persuaded is embedded in the brain's neural pathways. Therefore, the arguer cannot assume that the listener will be persuaded by the same argument that the arguer is. For the medical encounter to end in a truly rational decision, respecting the autonomy of the patient, not only premises related to the scientific data accumulated by the physician but also the patient-specific motivational factors have to be part of the argument to achieve manifest rationality. This requires understanding of how persuasion is carried out but, more importantly, the cognitive, emotional, social and cultural milieu (i.e., social umwelt) of the patient (Table 4.2 and Fig. 4.2). Although others may attempt to persuade the patient via more emotional or coercive routes, the physician should shun these approaches and try to redirect the patient and family to a route of manifest rationality.

4.8 Persuasion of Other Medical Professionals

Thus far, in this chapter, as well as the preceding chapters, my focus has been on the patient's rationality, social umwelt, and motivations for their capacity to be persuaded by an argument put forth by the physician in the clinical setting. However, what was said about the patient also applies to other healthcare professionals.[19] They are the products of the same evolutionary history, and the same "persuasion network" exists in them. The only substantial difference is education and training. As mentioned previously, this education and training also creates their own professional umwelt; that is, they expect information to be presented in a certain way, and they will have the same issues pertaining to accepting the conclusions as the patient's, albeit, just different constraints. They will have a theoretical framework into which pertinent information must be placed (more on this in Chap. 6).

[19] What I mean by "healthcare professionals" is not only physicians but also nurses, dietitians, psychologists, physical and occupational therapists, etc., trained in the paradigm of Western medicine. Practitioners of other medical traditions, i.e., non-Western medicine, or of alternative medicine will have separate theories and social umwelt, which will affect their capacity for persuasion.

Like with the patient, although unlike the pure sciences, healthcare professionals must make diagnoses and treatment decisions, often under sometimes severe time constraints and substantial uncertainty, then implement these decisions. Therefore, the level of confidence of the information in the theoretical framework is pertinent to the clinical problem at hand. In other words, they do not have the luxury of always being absolutely certain of their conclusions (the above discussion of ambiguity in persuasion is relevant here). Therefore, in medicine, the practitioner does not have to prove that something is absolutely true, all they need is to prove that it is "true enough"—either as a probability or reliability—to act. An "act" in this sense is a decision to either do one thing, something else, or nothing at all.[20] For not to act is an action. There are consequences of not acting when one needs to and adverse consequences of acting when one does not have to. This will be discussed more in Chaps. 6 and 7.

4.9 Summary

What I have hoped to have demonstrated is the ability to persuade and be persuaded in embedded in the human brain and mind through the "persuasion network" [37], which is a consequence of human biological, social, and cultural evolution. It is not an insignificant association that many of the regions of the brain are involved in both the persuasion network and functions related to sociality, cognition and judgment. It is also, in my opinion, not coincidental that theories and practices related to persuasion activate these regions, although perhaps the individuals proposing such theories and practices may not have been aware of this.

Although there are different methods that can be used in persuasion, the most ethical for physicians is constructing an argument that will lead to the most likely and beneficial conclusion, most often using informal or inductive logical methods (although in some instances, deductive logic or intuition would be appropriate, see Chap. 2). Premises in this argument can be challenged by the patient as well as the patient inserting missing premises that are important to the patient. This is the dialect process of rationality proposed by Johnson [36]. This will give the physician (the arguer) and opportunity to revise their argument to lead to a mutually agreeable conclusion, i.e., manifest rationality. We will see in Chap. 6 how the peer-review process does the same with respect to medical and scientific studies submitted to journals for publication.

[20] I had a mentor in my training, who, when he was confident that the natural history of the condition was such that the afflication would resolved itself, would say, "Don't just do something, *stand there*!"

References

1. Cacioppo JT, Cacioppo S, Petty RE. The neuroscience of persuasion: a review with an emphasis on issues and opportunities. Soc Neurosci. 2018;13:129–72.
2. Dainton M. Explaining theories of persuasion. In: Dainton M, Zettey ED, editors. Applying communication theory for personal life: a practical introduction. 2nd ed. Thousand Oaks, CA: Sage Publications; 2010. p. 103–31.
3. Miller GR. On being persuaded: some basic distinctions. In: Roloff ME, Miller GR, editors. Persuasion: new directions in theory and research. Beverly Hills, CA: Sage Publications; 1980. p. 11–27.
4. Persuasion. Merriam-Webster Dictionary. https://merriam-webster.com. Last accessed 27 Jul 2022.
5. Emerson RW. Letters and social aims, vol. 4. Cambridge, MA: Riverside Press; 1880.
6. Rapp C. Aristotle's rhetoric. In: Zalta EN, editor. The Stanford encyclopedia of philosophy. Stanford, CA: Stanford University; 2022. https://plato.stanford.edu/archives/spr2022/entries/aristotle-rhetoric. Last accessed 19 Jul 2022.
7. Carnegie D. How to win friends and influence people. New York: Simon & Schuster; 1936.
8. Harrell E. Persuasion—and resistance. Harvard Business Review, Nov–Dec 2019.
9. Cialdini R. Influence: the psychology of persuasion. New York: William Morrow and Company; 1984.
10. Cialdini R. Pre-suasion: a revolutionary way to influence and persuade. New York: Simon & Schuster; 2016.
11. Harris J. The soulful art of persuasion: the 11 habits that will make anyone a master influencer. New York: Crown Publishing Group; 2019.
12. Gallo C. Five stars: the communication secrets to get from good to great. New York: St. Martin's Press; 2018.
13. Hall K. Stories that stick: how storytelling can captivate customers, influence audiences, and transform your business. New York: Harper Collins Leadership; 2019.
14. Sherif M, Hovland CI. Social judgment: assimilation and contrast effects in communication and attitude change. New Haven, CT: Yale University Press; 1961.
15. Petty RE, Cacioppo JT. The elaboration likelihood model of persuasion. Adv Exp Soc Psychol. 1986;19:123–205.
16. Festinger L. A theory of cognitive dissonance. Evanston, IL: Row, Peterson; 1957.
17. Gilovich T. How we know what isn't so: the fallibility of human reason in everyday life. New York: The Free Press; 1991.
18. Fisher WR. The narrative paradigm: in the beginning. J Commun. 1984;34:74–89.
19. Fisher WR. Human communication as narration: toward a philosophy of reason, value and action. Columbia, SC: University of South Carolina Press; 1987.
20. Krause RJ, Rucker DD. Strategic storytelling: when narratives help or hurt the persuasive power of facts. Personal Soc Psychol Bull. 2020;46:216–27.
21. Boyd B. On the origins of stories: evolution, cognition, and fiction. Cambridge, MA: Harvard University Press; 2009.
22. Dunbar RIM. How conversations around campfires came to be. Proc Natl Acad Sci U S A. 2014;111:14013–4.
23. Smith D, Schlaepfer P, Major K, et al. Cooperation and the evolution of hunter-gathered storytelling. Nat Commun. 2017;8:1853.
24. Bell JS. Write great fiction: plot & structure. Cincinnati, OH: Writer's Digest Books; 2004.
25. Coerce. Merriam-Webster Dictionary. https://merriam-webster.com. Last accessed 31 Jul 2022.
26. Carruthers M. Prevent coercive persuasion and mind control. https://systemiccoaching.com/coercion.htm. Last accessed 31 Jul 2022.
27. Jobges S, Mouton Dorey C, Porz R, et al. What does coercion in intensive care mean for patients and their relatives? A thematic qualitative study. BMC Med Ethics. 2022;23:9.

28. Wendler D, Wertheimer A. Why is coerced consent worse than no consent and deceived consent? J Med Philos. 2017;42:114–31.
29. Chieze M, Clavien C, Kaiser S, Hurst S. Coercive measures in psychiatry: a review of ethical arguments. Front Psych. 2021;12:790886.
30. Sedig L. What's the role of autonomy in patient- and family-centered care when patients and family members don't agree. AMA J Ethics. 2016;18:12–7.
31. Alston CZ, Berger C, Brownlee G, et al. Shared decision-making strategies for best care: patient decision aids. Discussion paper. Washington, DC: Institute of Medicine; 2014. http://nam.edu/wp-content/uploads/2015/06/SDMforBestCare. Last accessed 31 Jul 2022.
32. Deniz S, Akbolat M, Cimen M, Unal O. The mediating role of shared decision-making in the effect of the patient–physician relationship on compliance with treatment. J Patient Exp. 2021;8:1–5.
33. Weisberg J. The bootstrapping problem. Philosophy. Compass. 2012;7:597–610.
34. Kolodny N. Why be rational? Mind. 2005;114:509–64.
35. Melchoir G. The persuasiveness puzzle about bootstrapping. Ratio. 2020;33:27–36.
36. Johnson RH. Manifest rationality: a pragmatic theory of argument. New York: Routledge; 2012.
37. Falk EB, Ramesson L, Berkman ET, et al. The neural correlates of persuasion: a common network across cultures and media. J Cogn Neurosci. 2010;22:2447–59.
38. de la Vega A, Chang LJ, Banich MT, et al. Large-scale meta-analysis of human medial prefrontal cortex reveals tripartite functional organization. J Cogn Neurosci. 2016;36:6553–62.
39. Klucharev V, Smidts A, Fernandez G. Brain mechanisms of persuasion: how 'expert power' modulates memory and attitudes. Scan. 2008;3:353–66.
40. Cialdini RB, Goldstein NJ. Social influence: compliance and conformity. Annu Rev Pscyhol. 2004;55:591–621.
41. Bless H, Strack F, Walther E. Memory as a target of social influence? Memory distortions as a function of social influence and meta-cognitive knowledge. In: Forgas JP, Williams KD, editors. Social influence: direct and indirect processes. Philadelphia: Psychology Press; 2001. p. 167–83.
42. Yomogida Y, Matsumoto M, Aoki R, et al. The neural basis of changing social norms through persuasion. Sci Rep. 2017;7:16295.
43. Panchanathan K, Boyd R. Indirect reciprocity can stabilize cooperation without second-order free rider problem. Nature. 2004;432:499–502.
44. Buhle JT, Silvers JA, Wager TD, et al. Cognitive reappraisal of emotion: a meta-analysis of human neuroimaging studies. Cereb Cortex. 2014;24:2981–90.
45. Fiddick L, Spampinato MV, Grafman J. Social contracts and precautions activate different neurological systems: an fMRI investigation of deontic reasoning. NeuroImage. 2005;28:778–86.
46. Vigneau M, Beaucousin V, Herve PY, et al. Meta-analyzing left hemisphere language areas: phonology, semantics, and sentence processing. NeuroImage. 2006;30:1414–32.
47. Wei T, Liang X, He Y, et al. Predicting conceptual processing capacity from spontaneous neuronal activity of the left middle temporal gyrus. J Neurosci. 2012;11:481–9.
48. Catani M, Jones DK, Ffytche DH. Perisylvian language networks of the human brain. Ann Neurol. 2005;57:8–16.
49. Rilling JK, Glasser MF, Preuss TM, et al. The evolution of the arcuate fasciculus revealed with comparative DTI. Nat Neurosci. 2008;11:426–8.
50. Rocklage MD, Rucker DD, Nordgren LF. Persuasion, emotion, and language: the intent to persuade transforms language via emotionality. Psychol Sci. 2018;29:749–60.
51. Wegener DT, Petty RE. Mood management across affective states: the hedonic contingency hypothesis. J Pers Soc Psychol. 1994;66:1034–48.
52. Keltner D, Haidt J. Social functions of emotions at four levels of analysis. Cogn Emotion. 1999;13:505–21.
53. Frijda NH, Mesquita B. The social roles and functions of emotions. In: Kitayama S, Markus HR, editors. Emotion and culture: empirical studies of mutual influence. Washington, DC: American Psychological Association; 1994. p. 51–87.

54. Andrade EB, Ho TH. Gaming emotions in social interactions. J Consum Res. 2009;36:539–52.
55. Friestad M, Wright P. The persuasion knowledge model: how people cope with persuasion attempts. J Consum Res. 1994;21:1–31.
56. Chartrand TL, Bargh JA. The chameleon effect: the perception-behavior link and social interaction. J Pers Soc Psychol. 1999;76:893–910.
57. Tanner RJ, Ferraro R, Chartrand TL, et al. Of chameleons and consumption: the impact of mimickry on choice and preferences. J Consum Res. 2008;34:754–66.
58. Van Zant AB, Berger J. How the voice persuades. J Pers Soc Psychol. 2019; https://doi.org/10.1037/pspi0000193. Epub ahead of print.
59. Kirmani A, Zhu R. Vigilant against manipulation: the effect of regulatory focus on the use of persuasion knowledge. J Mark Res. 2007;44:688–701.
60. Kirmani A, Campbell MC. Goal seeker and persuasion sentry: how consumer targets respond to interpersonal marketing persuasion. J Consum Res. 2004;31:573–82.
61. Pease A, Pease B. The definitive book of body language. New York: Bantam Dell; 2006.
62. Oullier O, Basso F. Embodied economics: how bodily information shapes the social coordination dynamics of decision-making. Philos Trans R Soc B. 2010;365:291–301.
63. Changeux JP. Croyance, Raison et Deraison. Paris: Odile Jacob; 2006.
64. Lakoff G, Johnson M. Metaphors we live by. Chicago: University of Chicago Press; 1980.
65. Brehm JW. A theory of psychological reactance. New York: Academic; 1966.
66. Steindl C, Jonas E, Sittenthaler S, et al. Understanding psychological reactance: new developments and findings. Z Psychol. 2015;223:205–14.
67. Reyonlds-Tylus T. Psychological reactance and persuasive health communication: a review of the literature. Front Commun. 2019;4:56.
68. Franzen ML, Smit EG, Verlegh PWJ. Strategies and motives to persuasion: an integrative framework. Front Psychol. 2015;6:1201.
69. Quick BL, Scott AM, Ledbetter AM. A close examination of trait reactance and issue involvement as moderators of psychological reactance theory. J Health Commun. 2011;16:660–79.
70. Laran J, Dalton AN, Andrade EB. The curious case of behavioral backlash: why brands produce priming effects and slogans produce reverse priming effects. J Consum Res. 2011;37:999–1014.
71. Kahneman D, Slovic P, Tversky A. Judgment under uncertainty: heuristics and biases. Cambridge: Cambridge University Press; 1982.
72. Johnson-Laird PN. Mental models and human reasoning. Proc Natl Acad Sci. 2010;107(43):18243–50.
73. Berquist M, Ejelov E. Self-persuading norms: adding self-persuasion techniques strengthens the influence of descriptive social norms. Soc Influ. 2022;17:1–16.
74. Aaronson E. The power of self-persuasion. Am Psychol. 1999;54:875–84.
75. Baldwin AS, Rothman AJ, Vander Way MW, Christensen AS. Examining causal components as a mediating process underlying self-generated health arguments for exercise and smoking cessation. Health Psychol. 2013;32:1209–17.
76. Gordijn ED, Postmes T, de Vries NK. Devil's advocate or advocate of oneself: effects of numerical support on pro- and counterfactual self-persuasion. Person Soc Psychol Bull. 2001;27:385–407.
77. Fielding KS, Terry DJ, Masser B, Hogg MA. Integrating social identity and theory of planned behavior to explain decisions to engage in sustainable agriculture practices. Br J Soc Psychol. 2008;47:23–48.
78. Li S, Halen C, Baaren R, Muller B. Self-persuasion increases healthy eating intention depending on cultural background. Int J Environ Res Public Health. 2020;17(10):3405.
79. Bullock OM, Shulman HC, Huskey R. Narratives are persuasive because they are easier to understand: examining processing fluency as a mechanism of narrative persuasion. Front Commun. 2021;6:719615.

80. Velanovich V. Bayesian analysis in the diagnostic process. Am J Med Qual. 1994;9:158–61.
81. Huskey R, Turner BO, Weber R. Individual differences in brain responses: new opportunities for tailoring health communication campaigns. Front Hum Neurosci. 2020;14:565973.
82. Sheeran P, Maki A, Montanaro E, et al. The impact of changing attitudes, norms, and self-efficacy on health-related intentions and behaviors: a meta-analysis. Health Psychol. 2016;30:1178–88.
83. Yates JF. Judgment and decision-making. Englewood, NJ: Prentice-Hall Inc.; 1990.
84. Nguyen OK, Higashi RT, Makam AN, et al. The influence of financial strain on health decision-making. J Gen Intern Med. 2018;33:406–8.
85. Li DG, Xia FD, Rana J, et al. Factors influencing patient decisions regarding treatments for skin growths: a cross-sectional study. Dermatol Res Pract. 2018;2018:3941347.
86. Dijkman BL, Lattik ML, Van der Wal-Huisman H, et al. Factors influencing family involvement in treatment decision-making for older patients with cancer: a scoping review. J Geriatr Oncol. 2022;13:391–7.
87. Spijkers AS, Akkermans A, Smets EMA, et al. How doctors manage conflicts with families of critically ill patients during conversations about end-of-life decisions in neonatal, pediatric, and adult intensive care. Intensive Care Med. 2022;48:910–22.
88. Tariman JD, Berry DL, Cochrane B, et al. Physician, patient and contextual factors affecting treatment decisions in older adults with cancer: a literature review. Oncol Nurs Forum. 2012;39:E70–83.
89. Buljac-Samardzic M, Clark MA, van Excel N, Job A, van Wijngaarden JDH. Patients as team members: factors affecting involvement in treatment decisions from the perspective of patients with a chronic condition. Health Expect. 2022;25:138–48.
90. Zheng QV, Velanovich V. Modeling stakeholder valuation: a example using the surgical treatments of gastroesophageal reflux disease. Cureus. 2021;13(11):e19559.
91. Kamenica E, Gentzkow M. Bayesian persuasion. Am Econ Rev. 2011;101:2590–616.
92. Bergemann D, Morris S. Information design, Bayesian persuasion and Bayes correlated equilibrium. Am Econ Rev. 2016;106:586–91.

field. The [illegible]
are explicit and dem[illegible]
even a [illegible]
cannot [illegible]

[illegible]

Chapter 5
Causation Attribution in Clinical Medicine

5.1 Introduction

The previous chapters have laid the foundation for this and the succeeding chapters by establishing how humans are persuaded to accept new knowledge. The next two chapters will address how medical knowledge is generated and what evidence is necessary to persuade mostly other health care professionals but even lay people as well, that this new knowledge should be accepted as true (or, rather, true enough upon which to act). The prior chapter discussed several techniques of persuasion. Due to both efficacy and ethical reasons, I have chosen to focus on the method of argumentation of manifest rationality, that is, both the arguer and listener have come to a mutually agreeable conclusion based on a dialectic exchange.

One of the features of this exchange may require an explanation. An explanation, although having some characteristics of an argument, is not an argument in that a new conclusion is not reached. Rather, it is an exposition of a sequence of already established facts for the enlightenment of others, as in how the physician explained the GERD to the patient in the clinical vignette in Chap. 1. One of the features of an effective explanation, when needed, is attribution of a cause or causes. This is true for both lay people and health care professionals. This chapter establishes the features of causal attribution from a common experience, everyday perspective, philosophical perspective, and medical perspective. I will argue that for both medical professionals and their patients, the most important property of causal attribution is in reliable predictability and identification of action points (i.e., therapeutic targets); and, because of this, accepting that there are multiple concepts of causation that can support these aims is the most practical approach.

V. Velanovich, *Medical Persuasion*, https://doi.org/10.1007/978-3-031-30371-5_5

5.2 Causal Attribution in the Common Experience

People going about their everyday business will routinely identify causes for the events in their lives:

The tire went flat because it ran over a nail.
My football team won because of a last second field goal.
I don't have anything for dinner because I forgot to go shopping.
I cleaned by room because my mother told me to do it.
I have heartburn because I have acid reflux.

In these examples, the word "because" identifies a causal connection. In fact, the word origin of the word "because" comes from middle English "by cause" [1]. These everyday phrases could be more formally reworded as follows:

The cause of the tire going flat is that it was punctured by a nail.
The cause of my football team winning is that the kicker made a field goal in the last second.
The cause of me having nothing for dinner is that I failed to go shopping.
The cause of me cleaning my room is that my mother insisted that I do so.
The cause of my heartburn symptoms is that I have acid reflux.

If one were having a conversation with the individuals making these statements, one would have no trouble understanding that the person speaking was trying to convey causal attribution in these particular events.

Once again, let us start with definitions. The Merriam-Webster dictionary defines "cause" as follows:

(a) A reason for an action or condition.
(b) Something that brings about an effect or a result.
(c) A person or thing that is the occasion of an action or state.
(d) Sufficient reason [2].

Similarly, for "because", the Merriam-Webster dictionary gives the following definition:

(a) For this reason.
(b) The fact that [3].

Therefore, when most people, who are not philosophers, think of a cause, they have the notion that, whether it was an inanimate object to living being, there was something that induced a change in something else, whether it was a physical change, change of action, a change of mind, or change of outcome.[1] Cause or causation has

[1] In the examples given above, one can identify many "intermediate" causes. For example, with the tire and the nail, the nail was on the road because it fell off of a truck, the nail caused the tire to go flat because it punctured the tire allowing air to leak out, etc. However, these intermediate causes still follow the same basic pattern.

many synonyms, a few examples are explanation, motivation, origin, purpose, source, account, beginning, consideration, creator, determinant, foundation, genesis, inducement, maker, producer, among others [4]. As one can see, most of these synonyms, also well as part of the definitions, have more to do with human actions, rather than phenomena in the universe. In science, it is common to hear terms such as force, power, influence, catalysis, among other more specific words, to identify causal attribution. I have presented these definitions and synonyms because in both everyday life and in science, cause, causation and causality are imprecise terms that can lead to confusion. The discussion below exemplifies that perhaps some issues with causation will have to do with semantics.

Most people will not attribute causation haphazardly; they have rules for doing so. The basic rules that are associated with causal attribution are (1) the cause must come temporally before the effect[2] and (2) the cause must have some type of influence that promotes the change of the phenomenon to the effect. This is graphically depicted in Fig. 5.1. Most people will describe causation in a mechanistic way; for example, the nail punctured the tire, allowing air to leak out, resulting in the tire going flat. They will also imply a level of determinism; for example, once the nail punctured the tire, there was no other outcome but for the tire going flat. I have chosen to call this attribution "influence" as an all-encompassing term for anything that can promote a change in any phenomenon, be it physical or mental, rather than "force", which has more of a physical nature connotation to it or "persuasion", which has more of a mental nature connotation to it.

This causation heuristic certainly works very well for most people most of the time when the causal attribution is relatively simple and straightforward. However, this can be prone to error. To provide a trite example, the kicker made the winning field goal because I was wearing my lucky jersey while I was watching the game on TV. This meets the causal attribution as illustrated in Fig. 5.1 only because of my belief that the mechanism of influence (my wearing my lucky jersey) did indeed have an effect on the outcome (the kicker making the field goal). As farcical as this example sounds (and, for the record, I don't believe in lucky jerseys), Gilovich provides numerous such examples, especially in health-related beliefs that people actually do believe [5].

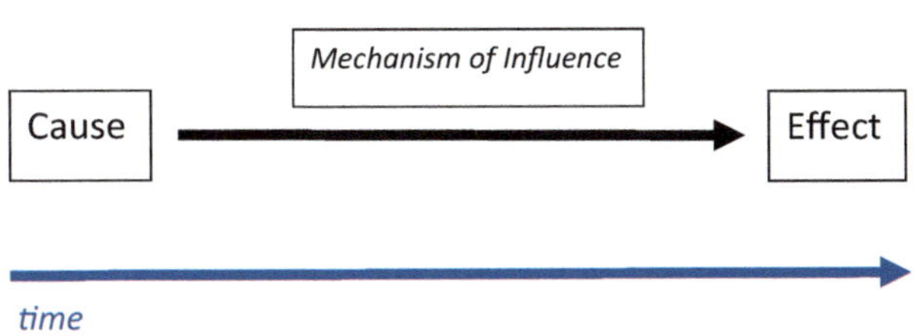

Fig. 5.1 The common understanding of a causal connection

[2] There are aspects in the theories of quantum mechanics that allow for some causes to occur after their effects, but that is not in the purview of this book.

Therefore, part of causal attribution has to include normative standards to distinguish reliable (as opposed to true, more on this later in the chapter) causes from spurious or coincidental temporally juxtaposed phenomena. Philosophers and scientists (as well as lawyers and judges) have been pondering this issue for centuries. The next section reviews some of this thinking.

5.3 Philosophical Approaches to Causation

Let me start by saying that this is a very big topic and I have no intention of giving it a comprehensive review. In the philosophical literature, there is still quite some controversy, and I refer the interested reader to the excellent review by Broadbent [6] or the numerous entries in the *Stanford Encyclopedia of Philosophy*, as well as the many books on the issue. Nevertheless, a review of a few of the basic philosophical issues is pedagogical.

Not surprisingly, Aristotle had something to say about causation. He defined four types of causes:

1. The efficient cause—that by which change is wrought.
2. The formal cause—the end purpose for which the change is wrought.
3. The material cause—that in which a change is wrought.
4. The final cause—that into which something is changed [7].

Taylor [7] gives the example of a marble statue: The sculptor chisels (the efficient cause) the marble (the material cause) for the purpose of producing a statue (the formal cause); hence, the statue is created (the final cause). This has led to the "traditional" (or, rather, commonsense view) that a cause is that which produces something and, in terms of what is produced, its effects, so to speak, can be explained [7]. Alternatively, perhaps as a more general statement, "in the process of change, a quality disappears and another quality comes into existence, the sources of this process are causes" [8]. Even in Ozen's [8] description just quoted, one a suspect a certain amount of bootstrapping[3] as "source" can be a synonym of "cause." However, this only speaks to the difficulty in being able to give a precise, all-encompassing definition of causation.

David Hume in his *A Treatise on Human Nature* questioned the traditional view, and philosophers ever since have been trying to answer his challenge [9]. In summary, which may perhaps be inadequate, Hume identified two essential characteristics that motivate humans to recognize a cause-effect relationship. First, there is a contiguity of cause and effect in space (i.e., the cause and effect are close enough together in space that it can appear that the cause has plausibly influenced the effect). Second, there is a succession in time from cause to effect (i.e., the cause comes before the effect, but close enough in time that they can appear to be related). In fact, this is

[3] Please recall from the prior chapter that "bootstrapping" is the process of confirming the reliability of a measuring device by repeatedly using it to make measurements. In this sense, I am using it here; it is using the synonym of the word to define the word.

exactly the understanding of cause and effect that most people have, as illustrated in Fig. 5.1. However, for Hume, since the "force" that supposedly caused the change cannot be observed, there is no "objective" evidence of its existence. Hence, Hume deemed this relationship to be a human construct to explain the events witnessed and *not* a logical necessity. Immanuel Kant in *Critique of Pure Reason* [10] took this further in that the connection that we make between objects is not given by the objects themselves but an action of the human observer. That is, it is to say, it is the human that decides that a succession of events that are observed is a causal relationship. (Perhaps some animals also have such a concept as cause, as observed by their behavior. Sadly, this is unknowable.) It is the regularity of the relationship that is observed that makes us declare such a sequence of successive events a causal relationship.

Of course, this view does lead to difficulties. It is clear that not all events that occur in succession regularly are causal. The most cited example is that day always follows night, but, of course, night is not the cause of day. Another issue is that of nonrecurrent events. For example, if, as some evidence suggests,[4] an asteroid impacting the Earth caused the extinction of the nonavian dinosaurs, this is certainly a nonrepeatable event. This was a one-time event; therefore, something other than its "regularity" has to be invoked to support the claim of causation. Next, there are times when the cause is present, but the effect does not occur. For example, although it is now generally accepted that smoking causes lung cancer, there are numerous examples (as my smoking patients tell me) of individuals who smoked their whole lives and never developed lung cancer. On the other end, a cause may have numerous effects. Continuing with the smoking example, smoking causes not only lung cancer but also emphysema, head and neck cancers, coronary artery disease, and peripheral vascular disease, among other ailments. The last issue that I will identify (there are certainly others) is that of multiple causes for the same event. For example, there are certainly numerous causes for an automobile accident—reckless driving, drunk driving, mechanical failures, weather conditions, etc.—so that the presence of one (or a few) will suffice to produce the effect.

Many of these issues were recognized by John Stuart Mill [11]. Mill identified that an effect could have multiple causes. Moreover, he developed his "law of causation," which states that for every event, there is a "natural law" that describes the event's occurrence, ala Newton's laws of motion. For Mill, the cause of the event is the entirety of the phenomena sufficient and necessary for the occurrence of the event coupled with the law governing those types of events. If one only knew the law and all the data needed to solve the law's equation(s), then the event would be completely predictable. This is the essence of "determinism"—the eventuality of the event is determined by the law governing the event and the conditions required to produce it. This gives its ultimate form in Laplace's demon.[5]

---

[4] I understand that this may not be the sole factor in the extinction of the dinosaurs. However, for my purposes as an example of a nonrepeating causation event, it will serve.

[5] Laplace in the nineteenth century conjured an omniscient being that had knowledge of all the natural laws for every extant phenomenon and all the pertinent data for each of these laws and, therefore, was able to predict with absolute certainty all future phenomena.

There are many ways to describe causation, including deterministic or probabilistic relationships, as a mechanism or process, or what happens after an intervention [12]. I will review what I feel are the most pertinent ones related to medicine.

5.3.1 Deterministic Causation

Causal determinism is the idea that are natural laws governing the occurrences of phenomena [8]. This can be summarized formally deductively as

General law
and
Pertinent data

Therefore, invariable outcome.

Carnap [13] defined this type of causal relationship as a conditional statement, which is a logical relationship. That is, the event is a particular instance of a general law that is universal with respect to time and space. This is best exemplified by the laws of classical physics, such as Newton's laws of motion. What I have identified as the "pertinent data" are the conditions required for the outcome to be determined. In the laws of motion, these are things such as mass, velocity, gravity, etc. This conception is very practical—we can predict tides, the movement of bodies, engineer a plethora of structures and machines, etc. Clearly, this concept is "good enough" for many practical endeavors and should not be underestimated.

More difficulty occurs when the laws are not known. Then, we have a regularity that has been observed in nature, such that "an observed factual relation between X and Y, such that Y always follows X or goes together" [8]. This is considered the "empiricist's" view [8]; that is, this observation is an empirical fact. The rationalist's view is that there is a "necessary connection" between the conditions, that is, X and Y *necessarily* go together [7, 8], such as Carnap avers [13]. That is, there exists some mandatory influence of the cause over the phenomenon in question. In the context of a general law, it is the law that is the necessary component linking X and Y. When such laws are not known, there is effort to determine if the conditions (i.e., pertinent data) are necessary, sufficient or both [7]. A necessary condition must be present for the phenomenon to occur, but its presence does not ensure that it will occur. While a sufficient condition may be enough for the phenomenon to occur, it is not necessary for its occurrence. Much of the deterministic effort is in identifying such conditions.

Nevertheless, the problems of multiple causes and multiple effects still exist. One answer to this comes from Mackie [14] with his INUS conditions: a cause is an *i*nsufficient but *n*onredundant (or *n*ecessary) part of an *u*nnecessary but *s*ufficient condition. This is part of a greater "causal sequence", which is the conjunction of necessity-in-the-circumstances and is associated with causal priority. Formally, X is necessary in the circumstances for and causally prior to Y provided that if X were kept out of the world in the circumstances referred to and the world ran on from there, Y would not occur [14]. Broadbent [6] describes this more formally, as *c* is a cause of *e* if and only if *c* is a necessary but insufficient part of an unnecessary but sufficient condition for *e*. This also has the flavor of counterfactual causation to be discussed below.

Even with this, there may be continued difficulties. Let us take the example of our clinical vignette and ask the question: Does this patient's acid reflux the cause of their heartburn symptoms? An abbreviated causal sequence could be as follows: The stomach produces hydrochloric acid; due to an incompetent lower esophageal sphincter, the acid is allowed to reflux into the esophagus. While in the esophagus, it inflames the esophageal mucosa. This inflammation produces a noxious stimulus that stimulates the nerve receptors in the esophagus to send a signal to the brain that a noxious event is occurring. The brain then recognizes this signal as a burning in the chest, which the patient's consciousness interprets as "heartburn." Are the INUS conditions met for acid? Is the presence of acid insufficient to cause heartburn? The answer is yes, because several other conditions must be present for the acid to be eventually interpreted by the patient's consciousness as heartburn.[6] Is it nonredundant (or necessary)? The answer here is more complex. Certainly, in the present causal sequence, it is. However, many patients suffer from "functional heartburn" [15], such that they consciously perceive heartburn, but there is no acid in their esophagus. Therefore, although acid being a nonredundant component of a causal sequence may be true for an individual patient, it is not true for the entire population of patients suffering from heartburn. To continue, is it unnecessary? The answer is the opposite of the above: It would be necessary for this particular causal sequence in this particular patient but not for the entire population. Last, is the entire causal sequence sufficient? The answer here is an unequivocal yes. Nevertheless, the conclusion of this exercise does produce an example of the inadequacy of the INUS conditions.

Therefore, in conclusion, although a deterministic approach can produce something of causal understanding in some circumstances, it is not applicable to all situations. Although we would like to identify phenomena that have causal "influence," "power," "efficacy," or however else one would like to describe it, it is nevertheless that we cannot pinpoint what that influence is. It also appears that in our search for this influence, we create names for it, for example, "gravity" in physics. In fact, humans have done this for everyday phenomena as well. For example, humans have created the word "strength" as a way to identify the influence of some entity. It is common to say that a particular individual is "strong" by observing their abilities. We cannot "see" strength as a force, as Hume suggests, only the effects of what we have chosen to identify as strength. Scientists have created and, no doubt, will continue to create such words.

[6] Certainly, many individuals have "silent reflux." That is, they clearly have a pathologic amount of acid refluxing into the esophagus but have no symptoms whatsoever.

5.3.2 *Counterfactual Causation Theory*

The essence of counterfactual theory is that if the cause did not happen, the effect would not have happened [16]. Formally, *c* causes *e* if and only if there is a causal chain running from *c* to *e* whose links consist of a chain of counterfactual dependence [6]. Here, what is meant by "counterfactual dependence" is that phenomenon *c* must be present; otherwise, phenomenon *e* would not have occurred. Again, in application to our clinical vignette, there certainly appears to be difficulties. In this particular patient, they certainly would not have heartburn if they did not have acid reflux (in fact, this is the rationale for anti-acid treatment). However, this counterfactual is not true for the entire population of patients suffering from heartburn. Nevertheless, counterfactual causation is very important in medical reasoning. Illari and Russo [17] have suggested that counterfactual reasoning is the underlying logic for all medical interventions—specifically, if the treatment was not administered, the cure would not have been achieved.

5.3.3 *Probabilistic Causation*

This has received much attention, and, certainly, from the medical knowledge standpoint, this is central to understanding medical causation. The foundational concept in probabilistic causation is that the occurrences of some phenomena are stochastic. That is, even in similar circumstances, sometimes the phenomenon occurs and at other times it does not, such as the lung cancer example given above. Moreover, this is a result of either the intrinsic property of the phenomenon or that we still do not know all of the factors involved in the causal sequence that would make it deterministic.

The underlying premise is that stochastic processes follow "statistical laws" in the manner that deterministic processes follow natural laws [18]. Suppes [19] defined a "probabilistic cause" as

> There is an event B, occurring at time t′, that is a *prima facie* cause of A, occurring at time t, if and only if $t' < t$, and the probability of B at time t′ is greater than 0, $P(B_{t'}) > 0$; and the probability of A occurring at time t given that B occurred at time t′ is greater than the probability of A occurring at t given the B did not occur at t′, $P(A_t|B_{t'}) > P(A_t)$.

Giere [20] further expands on this concept to include populations, such as C being a positive causal factor of E in a population U (or, more generally, in a stochastic system S) if and only if the probability of E given the presence of C in the population U is greater than the probability of E given that C is not present in the population U (although unsaid, it must be for a given time). More formally, $P_c(E) > P_{notC}(E)$.

To return to our clinical vignette example, let us say that this patient also had obesity, in addition to the other conditions. Is the obesity a cause of his heartburn? According to the above view, the patient's probability of having heartburn should be higher if they were obese than if they were not. However, this is an impossible task because it is impossible to measure such probabilities at the present point in time. The physician can ask the patient if there was a time that they were of normal weight, and, if there was, did he have heartburn then? If not, then it certainly supports the assertion that the obesity *may have played some role* in his symptomatology, but that is the best we can do. On the other hand, the relationship between obesity and GERD has been extensively studied, and it is generally accepted that obesity increases the likelihood of the presence of GERD [21]. Therefore, point estimates exist for the increased likelihood of the presence of GERD with the presence of obesity; yet, how this applies to any one individual patient is still a quandary (more on this in Chap. 7).

A greater question is whether we use probabilistic causation because we simply do not know enough about the causal sequence. For example, for a given occurrence of a phenomenon, Z, we know that the probability of its occurrence at time t_z is $P(Z_{tz})$. If, through research, we find that the occurrence of A at t_a increases the probability of Z occurring such that

$P(Z_{tz}|A_{ta}) > P(Z_{tz})$, given that t_a comes before t_z, such that $t_a \rightarrow t_z$ in temporal sequence.

However, what if, through additional research, we discover the existence of the phenomenon, B, such that the occurrence of B at t_b, which occurs between t_a and t_z, such that $t_a \rightarrow t_b \rightarrow t_z$, which improves the probability of the occurrence of Z, such that

$$P\left(Z_{tz}|\left(B_{tb}|A_{ta}\right)\right) > P\left(Z_{tz}|A_{ta}\right) > P\left(Z_{tz}\right).$$

In fact, this is nearly the whole enterprise of medical research (more on this Chap. 6). It may eventually be possible to obtain the occurrence of some phenomenon X at t_x with intermediary occurrences from A to X, such that

$$P\left(Z_{tz}|\left(X_{tx}|\left(W_{tw} \ldots|A_{ta}\right)\right)\right) = 1.$$

Therefore, this is now a deterministic rather than a stochastic system. It is not beyond the pale to think that such a phenomenon cannot be seen at one time to be a chance occurrence to be a deterministic occurrence. For example, many genetic diseases, once the genetic component is determined to be present, are now thought of as completely deterministic occurrences [22].

Nevertheless, until the day when research can finally convert a heretofore recognized stochastic system into a deterministic system, we are left with probabilistic causation. Additionally, there may be some biological systems that are inherently stochastic so that we will never achieve deterministic causation. In addition to the above, other causal probabilistic methods include Bayesian analysis/networks, contingency tables, and structural and multilevel models [17], such as multiple logistic regression. In fact, the above descriptions from Suppes and Giere are somewhat elementary. Most modern approaches to probabilistic causation have great concern for bias, and there are study designs and statistical techniques available to reduce the amount of bias in these assessments of causation attribution. More on these in Chap. 6.

5.3.4 *Causation as Agency (Interventionalism)*

The concept of agency in causation is based on the notion that individuals are agents who make decisions and do things to bring about goals that we have decided upon [6]. This does harken back to Aristotle's forms of causation. In this account, there is no point is trying to identify causes of natural phenomena as these are mere constructs of the human mind (make sure this is a correct statement). I am not prepared to argue this point of whether or not there are "real" causes in nature; however, from the standpoint of medical causal attribution, our purpose in identifying a cause is both for prediction and to be able to intervene (more on this below).

5.3.5 *The Pluralism of Causation*

Some philosophers now assert that causality is a hopelessly ambiguous term in science, as in everyday life, and those who try to reduce causation to a single concept are naïve and do not take into account how scientists are actually motivated [23]. That is, philosophers have tried to create theories that would account for all manner of causation (see the discussions above); such an effort is reminiscent of physicists trying to unify four the theories of force into one. In addition to the causality concepts listed above, Ben-Menachem [23] listed other concepts as well: stability, locality, symmetry, conservation laws, and least action principles. She further avers that causality is truly a "cluster concept." Illari and Russo, in apparent agreement, describe causality as a "pluralistic mosaic" [17]. My intention is not to analyze each of these concepts, as that would be outside the scope of this book. However, the notion of a plurality of causes is very appealing in medical causation attribution, as this is very practical for the practicing physician and their patients. Certainly, my experience of how physicians attribute causation, either for an individual patient or a population of patients, confirms that several types of causal attribution concepts are used, more on this in Chaps. 6 and 7.

5.3.6 *Causation as a Constraint*

Ben-Menachem [23] argues that rather than seeing causation as a phenomenon causing another phenomenon to occur, it is better to see causation as a constraint forcing a state of being from its present state to another. To understand this better, expounding on stability would be helpful. For Ben-Menachem, *stability* implies a property of a state to which it will return after a perturbation. For example, after a rock is thrown into a pond with smooth water, the ripples will dissipate until the water is smooth again. All living organisms strive for stability through their homeostatic mechanisms; for example, one's heart rate will return to its normal rate after exercise has increased it. In this way, stability dictates how much a system can change as a result of certain interactions [23]. When a causal constraint occurs, it does not allow the system to remain or return to its present, normal state. Such a way of thinking about causation can be applied to all "hierarchies" of phenomena—from subatomic to galaxies.

5.3.7 Summary and a Practical View

One can easily see that the "issue" of causation is not settled among philosophers. Some, such as Bertrand Russell, have suggested dispensing with the idea altogether [6]. For example, Bertrand Russell asserts that physics, as a science, rarely, if ever speaks of a "cause." I am not going to argue any of these points, because I doubt I would achieve a better solution than what have already been proposed. However, although the concept of causality may not be necessary in theoretical physics,[7] causal notions are useful in "higher-level" sciences (i.e., sciences that are not reduced to physics) and "everyday" observations [24]. As one can see for the types of causality listed, as well as GERD examples to illustrate them, causality as a concept does not have a succinct, universally applicable theory. Specifically, in medicine, we have the quandary of trying to determine a cause for one particular patient's ailments as well as trying to assess the cause of a disease in a population. These are two completely different tasks. As I asserted at the beginning of the book, my approach is practical. Therefore, it certainly seems to me that a search for a universal concept of causation is both impractical and unnecessary for the concept to be useful. I will accept the pluralistic view with the intent that whichever concept provides the most understandable explanation of the phenomenon in question and can provide points of prediction and intervention is what will be used. As a foretelling, these causative concepts will be overwhelmingly deterministic, probabilistic, and counterfactual. I will use the term "causal attribution" to denote that these are the observations and connections that medical professionals have accepted as causal, with the caveat that they might be wrong or incomplete. However, I am not overly concerned about these potential errors as I am more interested with how this attribution actual occurs and how it is used.

[7] Although not discussed here as it is not the purpose of this book, some philosophers have proposed that the terms "causation," "causality," and "cause" be dispensed with, especially in physics. The proposal was initially forwarded by Bertrand Russell.

5.4 Causation Attribution in Medicine: The Inter-Level and Inter-Field Nature of Medical and Biological Theories

5.4.1 Inter-Level Nature of Medical Theories

Schaffner [18], whom I will also refer to in Chap. 6, starts by identifying the issues in explanation in biology and medicine as prediction, causation, historicity, teleology, organization, and autonomy. New hypotheses and theories attempt account for data (i.e., observations); that is, provide some type of explanation for them. In the context of causation, Schaffner approaches this as "a how well it could be used as explanation" purpose. One of these explanatory models is the "deductive-nomological" model, which is essentially determinism. The other is the "statistical relevance" model, which is essentially probabilistic causation. In the statistical relevance model, statistical generalizations, which are treated as natural laws, with event occurrence (i.e., the conclusion) probablistically following after some set of premises, which is a type of inductive logic (see Chap. 2). When used to explain the causative connection of A to B, a property C_i "explains" because it is *statistically relevant* due to B and A having similar properties. Philosophers have identified problems with these models, as they have, quite frankly, with nearly all models. Nevertheless, these are good starting points in understanding biomedical theory.

These types of causal generalizations are generally framed as interlevel explanations (i.e., from molecular to organ system to organisms, etc.) and interfield (i.e., physics, chemistry, biology, population ecology, etc.) [25]. Understanding biomedical theories in this way is quite useful. Certainly, in medicine, explanations for medical phenomena extend from the atomic to the broad Earthly environment.

The temporal sequence in a biological explanation or theory is a causal sequence, and in the interlevel causal sequence, one level of causation (e.g., the cellular level) is reinterpreted into another level (e.g., the organ level). This is very common in medical causal attribution. This is different from the deductive model, as premises in these arguments are not laws but a set of causal sentences of varying degrees of generality, the "perspective sequence," which is what happens going from one level to another. Moreover, Schaffner [18] states that the causal interlevel sequence does not go in reverse, that is, from the organism level to the biochemical level. Quite frankly, I am not sure about this, as certainly there are examples of organism behavior which affect physiology and molecular secretion, e.g., grooming leads to oxytocin release as described in Chap. 2, and poor eating habits associated with diabetes.

To continue with Schaffner's account [18], the explanation proceeds by identifying the system under investigation with the relevant theoretical system, thereby exhibiting the explanandum (i.e., what is to be explained) as the causal consequence of the system's behavior. Much of this has to do with the interlevel nature of the theory. Many explanations in biology and medicine are understood in the "overlap" range between levels, where few hidden mechanisms can account for a wide range of phenomena by exhibiting complex causal pathways leading to the phenomena.

An example of the overlap range would be that of high blood cholesterol levels (molecular level) and creation of plaques in the coronary arteries (organ level). Understanding the causal sequences in these overlap areas between levels leads to most biological explanations being causal and mechanistic. Certainly, the physician from our clinical vignette in Chap. 1 had such an explanation.

For Schaffner [18], there are three components to causation:

1. Logical—an explication of what type of conditional (e.g., necessary, sufficient, etc.) is used to distinguish causal from noncausal sequences. That is, "necessity-in-the-circumstances."
2. Epistemological—evaluate the generation and evaluation of causal notions.
3. Metaphysical—a process of metaphysics as undergirding causation.

As I interpret this, the logical component has to do with the logical arrangement of the causal sequence such that the phenomena for which cause is attributed are logically sound. The epistemological component has to do with how justified we are in accepting purported causative factors as knowledge. Finally, the meta-physical component has to do with how well the causal explanation satisfies human emotion.

5.5 Medical Science and the Attribution of Cause (Integrating the Clinical Vignette)

5.5.1 Pitfalls in Causation Attribution: An Example of a Change in the Accepted Cause

I would like to start this section by recounting a disease process that had undergone a sea-change in how physicians have ascribed causal attribution. Peptic ulcer disease, known as benign ulceration of the stomach and duodenum, was a common and severe problem in the latter half of the nineteenth century and the first two-thirds or so of the twentieth century [26]. The intellectual route that established that gastric acid was the cause of peptic ulcer disease started with the famous gastric physiological studies of William Beaumont on his patient, Alexis St. Martin, who was treated for a chronic gastrocutaneous fistula after a gunshot wound in 1825, established that the stomach produces acid (which was later determined to be hydrochloric acid). Theodor Billroth revolutionized the surgical treatment of peptic ulcers with gastric resection and the gastroenterostomies that still bear his name. In 1902, Ivan Pavlov demonstrated that the vagus nerve was important in initiating gastric acid secretion during the cephalic phase of digestion, for which he won a Nobel Prize. In 1910, Karl Schwarz, a student of Billroth's, published his series of 14 patients with peptic ulcers that he treated surgically and ascribed acid as the cause, based on the observation that these ulcers only occurred in the regions of the gastrointestinal tract that were in contact with gastric acid. He coined the dictum "No acid, no ulcer," giving causal attribution to gastric acid for the development of peptic ulcer disease.

Although vagotomy was used as early as 1921 by a few surgeons, Lester Dragstedt made the connection between vagal nerve stimulation and gastric acid hypersecretion. He advocated truncal vagotomy in the treatment of peptic ulcer disease to reduce gastric acid production. The causal sequence of peptic ulcer disease appeared to be settled. Standard operations for the treatment of peptic ulcer disease, depending on its associated complication of obstruction or bleeding, including some type of vagotomy, with some type of "drainage procedure," such as pyloroplasty or antrectomy.

We see in this abbreviated recounting (as there is much detail I left out for brevity), an interlevel, interfield theory of peptic ulcer disease developed around the production of gastric acid. This theory includes interactions at the organism level (patient symptomatology), organ level, and biochemical level. It included concepts of anatomy, physiology and biochemistry. It identified a cause mechanistically, and this cause provided agency for a treatment plan. It actually worked quite well, with not only surgical but also medical treatments, directed at acid production curing these ulcers in a majority of patients. This was taught as dogma, certainly to surgical residents, for decades. Older surgeons repeated this dogma to me as if it was gospel during my surgical training in the late 1980s to early 1990s. The trouble was—at worst, this theory was wrong; at best, it was incomplete.

Not quite parallel to these concepts, other observations were being made. Although "spirochaetes" were initially identified in the stomach of human autopsies in 1938, it was not until 1983 when Robin Warran and Barry Marshall identified *Campylobacter*-like bacteria in patients suffering from dyspepsia and peptic ulcer [26] in the mucosa of the gastric antrum. To "prove" that these organisms produced gastric inflammation, Marshall self-inoculated himself with isolates of these organisms. This led to a 14-day illness, and on the tenth day, he underwent an endoscopy which both documented gastric inflammation and these bacteria in the mucosal lining of his antrum. Subsequent studies confirmed the relationship between what is now known as *Helicobacter pylori* and peptic ulcer disease and gastritis in general. Warren and Marshall received a Nobel prize for this discovery in 2005. Currently, the modern treatment for peptic ulcers includes antibiotic therapy for these bacteria [27]. In fact, the American College of Gastroenterology's guidelines review on peptic ulcer disease no longer mentions acid as a cause [27]. Looking back, it is also quite interesting that the "best" operation for peptic ulcer disease was a vagotomy with antrectomy and either a gastroduodenostomy (Billroth I) or gastrojejunostomy (Billroth II). I do not think it is coincidental that the antrum is the location where the most *H. pylori* is located and resection of the antrum was probably the most successful means of eradicating (or at least reducing the bacterial load of) *H. pylori* prior to the routine use of effective antibiotics.

The point that I am trying to make with the above story is that causal attribution is a task of humans, as Hume noted. And these humans, despite their best efforts, may be wrong. I must acknowledge that the causation attribution of peptic ulcer disease is still more complex than what I have recounted here. Gastric acid can still be a factor in general, and for diseases such as Zollinger-Ellison syndrome from a gastrinoma, it is still the primary factor. Nonsteroidal anti-inflammatory agents are also a causative factor [26, 27]. This "error" is causal attribution could be because, in fact, the role of *H. pylori* was not recognized because we did not have a way to isolate it, and it was the cause of peptic ulcer disease all along, or perhaps, the cause changed from the late nineteenth and early twentieth century to the late twentieth century. Most likely, there were several confounding variables that other medical scientists and practitioners simply either did not take into account or for which they were unaware. That is, they suffered from missing premises. Nevertheless, I do think that this illustrates Hume's observation that causation is a quality that humans attribute to a phenomenon, and establishing whether this human-attributed cause is what occurs in the universe may not be as conclusive as we would like.

Why is this? The term "causality" is ambiguous, as previously mentioned. It denotes a relationship between entities that cannot be easily captured in words and is impossible to ascertain beyond a lingering doubt [28], as the above historical account illustrates. Part of this pitfall may have to do with the problems that medical science tries to address. Illari and Russo [17] identify five scientific problems in causation:

Inference—does X cause Y?
Prediction—what will happen?
Explanation—how does X cause Y?
Control—how to control the causal sequence.
Reasoning about causality.

One can see elements of all of these in the historical account of peptic ulcer disease. Both the observations of Schwarz pertaining to ulcers only occurring where there is contact with gastric acid, and the actions of Marshall infecting himself with *H. pylori* were both attempts to answer the question of inference. Similarly, both theories attempted to address questions of prediction, or, rather, natural history, and control, with treatments directed at the presumed causative agent. Although I did not state it in the historical account, there is a vast literature for both acid and *H. pylori* to address the explanatory question. Both demonstrated reasoning about causality. However, there are problems for both theories of peptic ulcer causation. There are those who are not ready to abandon the acid causal sequence [26], and *H. pylori* certainly does not account for all ulcers of the gastroduodenal tract. This example of difficulties in causative attribution in medicine was certainly not isolated to peptic ulcer disease. Additional considerations in medical causation was felt to be needed. Russo and Williamson [29] proposed that causal claims in health science need to be supported by evidence of difference-making *and* evidence of mechanisms. This is, the cause had to affect the otherwise steady homeostatic state of the organism (consistent with the "causal constraints" view of causation discussed above), and a biological mechanism needs to be part of the causal sequence. More on this below.

5.5.2 *Identifying a Cause as a Means of Predictability*

Identifying a cause for the medical practitioner is essential as a means of predictability [30]. For the practitioner, there are two main questions when confronted with a patient with an illness. What will happen to the patient if I do nothing (i.e., let the natural history of the disease take its course)? And, if this is unacceptable, what treatment should I recommend to change the course of the disease? Both of these questions are questions of predictability. I have argued that this is the most important quality for the physician of identifying the causal sequence and making a causal attribution [30]. It is a practical matter—more on this below.

5.5.3 *Causation and the Reliability of Disease Diagnosis*

It is unequivocal that the causes of many disease processes appear to be multifactorial. Therefore, as mentioned previously, the physician is tasked with identifying a cause of a particular patient's illness, while the medical scientist is tasked with identifying a cause for a disease process generally. What follows is a general causality account of disease causation as it relates to symptom manifestation and, hence, diagnosis, from Rizzi and Andur Pedersen [31]. Singular causality, as in a specific patient, is a relation between a concrete sequence of causally linked events. General causation, as in disease etiology, includes various categories of causal relations between event types. The "reference" case serves as a source of causal inference. The "reference case" is the extensive account of (all) possible causal factors that are known or believed to be potentially able to lead to the effect; that is, a hypothetical, absolute and exhaustive representation of causes, causal connections and conjunctions that could be relevant for an effect of the given kind. The chain of events that induce a disease state are effective causal complexes, each composed of nonredundant components, which separately contribute to the effect of the complex, without the individual component being necessary or sufficient in itself to produce the effect. This is clearly consistent with Mackie's INUS components [14]. Furthermore, causes, defined as nonredundant components, can be further differentiated according to their avoidability or by the potential for eradication of the cause.

Traditionally, physicians think of diseases in humans in the following manner: (a) the disease manifestations (signs and symptoms) are due to (b) the disease itself, which is the result of (c) a certain pathogenesis, based on (d) an etiology, such that

$$\text{Etiology} \rightarrow \text{Pathogenesis} \rightarrow \text{Disease} \rightarrow \text{Manifestations}$$

which is a general causal sequence of the generation of the disease to its human symptoms and physical signs. Therefore, knowledge of a causal connection of a general kind customarily has been the result of determining causality in an array of many singular cases.[8] This is an inductive process, that is, going from the particular to the general, as previously discussed in Chap. 2. Links between causal factors are due to mutual dependance and/or reflect statements of general causality. It is by operating among the factors in an actual singular case, as well as the reference case, that the causal search is performed. A causal complex consists of some important, nonredundant factors that together refer to a singular event or a group of singular events [31].

Rizzi and Andur Pedersen go on to define a "causal field" as the sum total of features and properties that (a) must be present in all counterfactual situations and (b) gives a comprehensive, yet scientifically detailed setting so the phenomenon or event of which we are trying to find the cause(s) is adequately characterized. They define a "token" as an individual event in a sequence of events; for example, for the concept of an event type, a token is an instance of this type of event. When justifying that a token of X is a cause of token Y in a singular case, one refers to the general case, where X is an approved cause of Y, which was previously established through observations of numerous cases of this disease type.

These sequences of events as they occur in the universe are continuous processes. However, when establishing a causal explanation, humans segment the dynamic flow of continuous changes in time into a sequence of discrete events, as the above traditional causal sequence from etiology to manifestations illustrate. Therefore, these effective causal complexes are human constructions, and the construction of the connected complexes signifies a partial description of actual, complete constituents contained in the circumscribed space-time relation of the human-declared events [31]. Humans define the boundaries of a causal event, which is important in our understanding of the causal attribution of the event. Effective causal complexes are finite and purportedly used to characterize specific phenomena, but the proclamation of the phenomenon as a semantically meaningful set of components is a product of massive numeric and qualitative reduction of all the prevailing circumstances [31]. This is what is in the physician's meta-cognition of both the theoretical framework and evidence for theory (Fig. 1.1). The nonredundant components denote necessary factors of that event and reflect a rather larger group of unexpressed conditions [31]. Such unexplained conditions are the enthymemes of a logical argument. The structure of the causal complex components is accomplished according to a sense of acceptability that can be agreed upon because they serve to characterize cognitive features [31].

Categorization of phenomena is vital to humans' ability to understand the world around us and to be able to effectively interact with that world. This is a result of how the human brain and mind evolved, as discussed in Chap. 3. This ability to categorize has two important features for cognition: (1) cognitive economy—helps handle large quantities of objects in the mind, and (2) categories mirror intersections between groups, which are organized in a specific manner [32].

---

[8] Recall the example of acute appendicitis from Chap. 2. That, as well as most diseases, was the result of physicians carefully documenting disease presentations and natural histories of many patients and recognizing patterns for future aid in diagnosis.

Rizzi and Andur Pedersen [31] suggest causes (nonredundant components) can then be differentiated and classified:

1. Avoidable causes—those causes that if they did not happen, the event would not have occurred (this is truly an example of counterfactual causation)
2. Impervious causes—those causes for which there is no way to prevent them from occurring.
3. Susceptible (Responsive) causes—those causes that have potential therapeutic targets.

One can see in the classification clear practicality. In fact, this is cause as agency, as discussed above.

5.5.4 Causation and the Reliability of Therapeutic Intervention

One of the most important aspects of causal attribution is identifying targets for therapeutic intervention. This was mentioned by Rizzi and Andur Pedersen [31] in item #3 of their classification above, as well as causality as predictability [30]. This is consistent with causality as agency or interventalism. However, the reliable identification of targets is important, as the peptic ulcer disease historical account presented above attests. Many confounding variables can lead to erroneous causal attribution. This will be discussed more in Chap. 6 on the generation of new medical knowledge.

5.5.5 Extent of Deterministic in Medical Causation

Sequences of events or phenomena are thought to be causal only because we have observed that these sequences happen invariably, or at least frequently enough, together in the past and believe that they will continue to do so into the future *and* believe that the preceding phenomenon has some type of influence over the emergence of the succeeding phenomenon. If phenomena are always linked, e.g., if A occurs, B will always occur, and we therefore believe that they are causally linked. Humans will attempt to characterize the influence of A over B with words that speak to this influence, with either an existing word in the language or a novel word which may be unique to this particular relationship.

However, what if research discovered that there were intermediary phenomena between A and B, such that, for example, A → A′ → B′ → B? Do we still say that A caused B? Returning to our clinical vignette of Chap. 1, there were several "intermediate" steps in the causal sequence of gastric acid reflux into the esophagus and the patient's conscious perception of heartburn. It is clear that each step is necessary (or, necessary to a greater or lesser extent), but none by themselves are sufficient. However, the entire sequence is sufficient to cause heartburn. This is also a satisfactory explanation for heartburn symptoms, using the structure of the causal theories discussed above, as well as for targeting therapeutic interventions.

Nevertheless, as appealing as such a causal attribution is, there is abundant reason for caution.[9] There is always the issue of "true-true, but unrelated" in medical causation. This is a particular problem in assigning causation to an individual patient. Therefore, although cause and effect may not be required to be, according to Hume, "logically linked" (whatever that means, quite frankly), there must be some type of compelling factors that make them physically or, at least, practically, linked; that is, there must be some mechanism of influence. This is why medical scientists continually try to identify mechanisms of pathogenesis.

5.5.6 Probabilistic Causation in Medical Theories

The probabilistic causation concept is one of the most frequently used in medical science. Certainly, nearly all epidemiology is based on probability (or rather, frequencies, which are point estimates of probabilities), and the "gold standard" for assessment of a therapeutic intervention, the randomized controlled trial, is also based on probabilistic causation. (More on this in Chap. 6.) This has been termed by Rubin [33] the "potential outcomes approach," such that an individual who is given a certain treatment (or not) could experience a certain outcome (or not). Of course, *post hoc*, for an individual patient, the outcome occurred (posterior probability of 1), or it did not (posterior probability of 0). The *a priori* determination of probability is accomplished by assessing groups of individuals, such that the outcome difference (presence or absence of the outcome of interest) between two groups (treated and untreated) is *defined* as being causal if certain additional requirements are fulfilled [34]. Once again, we see that causation as an near-arbitrary construct of the human mind in the Humean sense to create a foundation for understanding (in a way, tell a story).

Figure 5.2 shows one such hypothetical comparison of the cure of a particular disease after treatment compared to no treatment, i.e., the natural history of the disease. In this comparison, 60% of patients with the disease were ultimately cured of the disease with the treatment, while 40% of patients with the disease were cured of the disease even though they received no treatment. For the sake of argument, let us say that this difference is statistically significant by the appropriate statistical tests. Most would say that treatment is superior to no treatment and offered the best probability of cure. In fact, the "manipulationist" view point is such that an exposure E causes outcome O if and only if changes in E are due to its manipulation being followed by changes in O [28], which appears to me as a type of counterfactual. Let us now say that patient *X* is this trial, received the treatment, and was cured.

---

[9] As I have told innumerable individuals over the years, just because it makes sense doesn't mean its true and just because it doesn't make sense doesn't mean it's false.

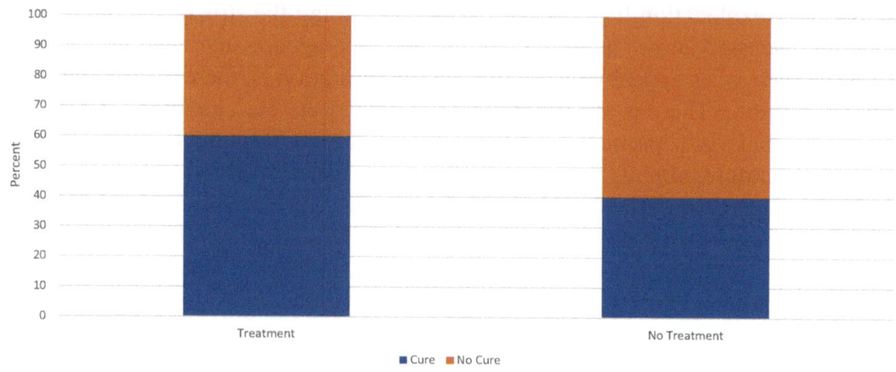

Fig. 5.2 The results of a randomized, controlled trial of treatment vs. observation

Did the treatment cause the cure in this patient? For ease of explanation, let us say that there were 100 patients in each group. Twenty more patients in the treatment group achieved a cure than those in the no treatment group. However, given the information presented, it is impossible to say whether patient *X* would have been one of the 40 patients who achieved a cure without treatment or whether they would have been one of the 20 who presumably were cured because of the treatment (as the other 40 in the treatment group may also have been cured without treatment as in the no treatment group). This is the main criticism of assessing causality in this manner as the assumption that the *observed* outcome in a group of *untreated* individuals is a solid estimate of *what would have been* observed, but was not, if the treated individuals had not been treated. This is sometimes referred to as the "missing data problem"; that is, the missing data are not knowing what would have happened to *X* if *X* had not been treated. In other words, we have a "black box" of sorts for each individual outcome [35].

These types of probabilistic causation studies can be prone to confounding. Therefore, claims of causal relations are often based on applications of statistical methods to frequency data [36]. In the following, Ward [36] explains the difficulties: The source and type of data place important constraints on the choice of statistical methods and on the warrant attributed to the causal claims based on the use of such methods, especially with making claims from nonexperimental, observational studies in which random allocations to treatments and control groups are not present. That is, these types of studies are at risk of bias. Bias can affect the attribution of probabilistic causation. To address this, some have proposed "causal criteria." However, such causal criteria may not be appropriate for either deductive or inductive inferences; nevertheless, they do have a role in inferring the best explanation. (Please recall that an explanation is not intended to be an argument.) This then led to the introduction of the randomized controlled trials, where like experiments, potential bias, known and unknown, is randomly distributed to the comparison groups. This is what made the randomized controlled trial the gold standard determining the causal effect of treatments. Unfortunately, it is not a panacea, as it may still suffer from confounding. Moreover, even if the results of an idealized randomized controlled trial are internally valid, generalization from these results to a wider population may be limited. (More on this in Chap. 6.) Another standard for assessing probabilistic causal attribution is repeating the observation/trial/experiment. However, repetitions of randomized control may not be "ideal"; in that, there may be some methodological and population differences with the first observation/trial/experiment. Real-life repetitions of randomized controlled trials are more likely to increase the likelihood of other kinds of biases, such as differential attrition, which are not controlled for by the use of a randomized controlled trial. In causal inferences, therefore, using statistical techniques are neither deductive nor inductive but are "inferences to the best explanation." Even though potentially problematic, they still have pragmatic value for the preliminary assessment of statistical association to be further studied. Moreover, for observational studies, other methods of treatment allocation are necessary to reduce potential bias and improve the reliability of probabilistic causal attribution. Cartwright [37] asserts the view that randomized controlled trials may tell us something about causal relations in the very specific circumstances of the experiment but tells us nothing about what the cause does elsewhere. This is a very important point when addressing diagnostic categories (Chap. 7).

5.5.7 Integrating Mechanism with Deterministic Causation

As previously mentioned, biomedical theories are interlevel and interfield. Phenomena at one level can influence phenomena at another level. Such causal sequences can include aspects of population ecology, physiology, anatomy, cellular and molecular biology, and biochemistry. These causal sequences can apply to disease manifestation at the individual up to the population level. They are constructed in such a manner as to imply a mechanism that is deterministic in its causal attribution. In fact, as an explanation for biomedical phenomena, they are satisfying from the standpoint of human understanding, as our minds, as previously mentioned, evolved to understand the world in this manner. I would assert that a mechanistic explanation is just another way of telling a story, which the human mind evolved to prefer.

Randeau et al. [38] studied causal attribution in cancer progenesis, which illustrates this point. To the question of: What causes cancer? They provide an answer covering many types of causation theories (i.e., a pluralist's view) in conjunction with an interlevel and interfield view of biological theories. They divide possible causal attribution into two broad categories. One is "mechanistically"—how a tumor grows and spreads within an organism. The second is "etiologically"—what are the factors that initiate and favor cancer development? With the first, the causal sequence has to do with identifying the molecular and cellular mechanisms of how a cell transforms from a benign to a malignant cell, then how this malignant cell divides to expand its numbers, with changes in the local tissue environment establishing a tumor, how the cells of this tumor "hide" from the host's immune system, and then how it eventually spreads to other regions of the body. These mechanisms, each part of a causal sequence, are generally described in molecular terms leading to cellular behavioral changes. In essence, these causal attributions tend to be deterministic in nature. The second, etiological, has to do with what promotes the molecular derangements in the cell's genetic material. These factors can be intrinsic within the organism, such as preexisting genetic anomalies that predispose the organism to develop cancer cells, or environmental, such as smoking or radiation exposure. These causal attributions tend to fall into probabilistic causation.

Within these broad categories, six characteristics are identified [38]. These are (1) multicausality—many different factors influence cancer initiation and dissemination; (2) causal variability—the factors that influence the formation and dissemination of tumors can vary from tumor type to tumor type; (3) causal necessity and/or sufficiency—some factors are necessary (or required), while others are just one of many sufficient factors; (4) causal intricacy—factors can, and often do, interact in complex ways;[10] (5) sequence-dependent causality—cancer is an evolving process, with different factors having different effects at different stages; and (6) spatially situated causality—factors can affect tumor development within the microenvironment or at a distance.

Having established these categories and characteristics, these authors then propose two explanatory schemata: the tumor cell-centric view and the tumor environment-centric view. The tumor cell-centric view focuses on somatic mutations, that is, the genetic alterations that a cell must undergo to become malignant. The tumor environment-centric view focuses on the tissue organization around and within the tumor. These authors then aver that while deterministic explanations may be sufficient to understand causation in some of these models, stochastic explanations will be required for other models. Furthermore, they state that causality in cancer is frequently "nonlinear"; that is, causality may not follow linearly transformable quantitative-dependent relationships, unlike, say, correlations and linear regressions.

This account is a fine example of interlevel and interfield biological causation attribution that rests on deterministic, probabilistic, and, most likely, counterfactual notions of causation. As the authors assert, this approach to causation can establish hierarchical causes that can be prioritized for treatment targets. In other words, there purpose in understanding cancer causation is a practical one—namely, to improve therapeutics. It also improves predictability.

[10] Clearly, William of Ockham, of Occam's razor fame, of did not do cancer research. Perhaps his razor would not have been so sharp.

5.5.8 *Integrating Mechanism and Probabilistic Causation*

In an attempt to better identify causative candidates, especially, but not exclusively, in epidemiology, Sir Austin Bradford Hill in 1965 proposed a list of "causative considerations" [39]. The basic problem is that correlations or associations between variables can be a fallible indicator of causation [40]. A "modified" version of these considerations is given in Table 5.1. Even a cursory examination of this list once again shows the interlevel, interfield nature of medical causal attribution. Of these considerations, only the first three—temporal proximity, spatial proximity, and mechanism—were determined to be required by Evans et al. [40], consistent with what Hume previously proposed. The remainder are not needed, but would add to the evidence that there may be a causative connection. Some view this as a hierarchy of evidence [41]. These authors view disease as a "causative pathway" through the often overlapping stages of etiology, pathology, and pathophysiology, as others

Table 5.1 The Modified Bradford Hill list of causal considerations for medical causation

Consideration	Necessity	Reason
Temporal proximity	Yes	The outcome must occur after or during the exposure to the active causative factor, never before
Spatial proximity	Yes	Causative factors must be able to act upon the individual and eventually the site(s) of outcome
Mechanism	Yes	A mechanism of interaction between the causative factor and the biology of the recipient must exist. However, it is not necessary to know the details of the mechanism to measure its effect
Coherence	No	Cause-and-effect interpretations should not seriously conflict with known facts of the condition and causative factor. Generally, evidence from basic science and population studies should be mutually supportive
Specificity	No	To infer a causal relationship, it helps if the effect has only one likely cause. However, in reality, outcomes often have multiple causative factors, and exposures can simultaneously cause more than one effect
Biological gradient (dose-responsiveness)	No	Greater exposure should generally lead to greater incidence of the effect, if the purported mechanism predicts such a relationship. Strongest "dose-response" evidence comes when the process is reversible, when reduced exposure reverses the effect
Experiment	No	The size of the observed effect is not likely attributable to confounding
Replicability	No	Replicability of research results, faithfully repeated and consistently observed by different persons in different places, circumstances and times, with different samples, strengthen the likelihood of a causal relationship
Similarity	No	Similar effects of observed factors in similar populations may be considered as strengthening the likelihood of causation

Adapted from Evans, et al. [40]

have [31]. For them, for an intervention to change the natural course of the disease, it must occupy the same time and space and share a "common form," the point at which the two pathways converge and interact [41]. Clearly, this fits into the interventionalist (agency) theory of causation [6]. A mechanism of interaction between the intervention and the biology of the recipient must necessarily exist, whether known or not. The problem becomes when this mechanism is unknown; we are left with the black box of probabilistic causation. This may have to do, as Howick et al. [42] point out, that until every mechanistic "link" in the causative "chain" is known, the highest common form between the intervention and disease pathway should suffice as an acceptable understanding of such a mechanistic interaction.

Although the Bradford Hill list is useful, it has endured criticism. For example, some have asserted that they are not truly "criteria" as such [43]. Hofler [43] further goes on to say that "the heuristic value of Hill's [sic] considerations converges to zero as the complexity of a causal system and the uncertainty about the true causal system increase." That is, as the system becomes more complex, the harder it is to create considerations or criteria to determine its cause. Phillips and Goodman [44] counter that this is just good scientific common sense. They aver that when we postulate causal sequences, we create "causal diagrams" that take as inputs some of the known or postulated elements of a worldly system of causes and effects and schematize them in a way that new knowledge (i.e., beyond the inputs themselves, which is an assertion that the new knowledge is not being bootstrapped, as discussed in the prior chapter) can be extracted. Moreover, uncertainty about input assumptions (e.g., assumptions that measurements are accurate and for which confounding is controlled) is almost always ignored in epidemiological results, and people (including experts) have been shown to be quite bad at quantifying the possible magnitude of error without mathematical aids [44]. They further go on and state the "Duhem-Quine problem of any study used to test a claim is simultaneously testing many ancillary hypotheses about the study methodology and thus we cannot be sure the observed results inform the causal hypothesis of interests" [44]. To restate this quandary to hopefully improve clarity—whatever methods we use to generate data is also testing the method used to generate the data; therefore, there may be some level of uncertainty about both the data and the method. That is, this has the potential to be a bootstrapping problem. The conclusion to be made is that reliance on a set of considerations or criteria does not guarantee reliable causation attribution.

5.5.9 *Cause as a Target of Intervention*

I have alluded to several times in passing that one of the essential purposes for humans of assigning causal attribution is in identifying targets for intervention. The underlying concept, as previously put forth, is that of a counterfactual. That is, if the cause can be eliminated, the disease can be eliminated. If the disease is eliminated, the human manifestations of the disease are eliminated. There is also a component of causation as agency and as mechanistic determinism. This, however, is based on the assumption that the disease, once established, is reversible. There are clearly instances where this is true, for example, eliminating acid reflux results in eliminating heartburn (if, indeed, acid reflux is the cause of the heartburn) or removing the inflamed appendix eliminates the cause of sepsis. However, both have a certain probabilistic nature as well. In that, there are "treatment failures." This produces a whole host of questions regarding causation, which I will further explore in Chap. 7. Other disease processes, such as emphysema, once established, are not reversible even if the patient quits smoking (although quitting smoking will help prevent worsening of the emphysema). However, for the time being, the essential point is that identifying causal attribution is used to identify treatment targets. Moreover, there are multiple causation notions that can be used in this endeavor, consistent with the pluralistic concept of causation.

5.6 Causation in Explanation, Argument and Persuasion

Causality is a human concept for attributing influence to "forces" that transform one state of being into another. Although the example I have used has to do with physical ailments, the same notions can be applied to mental illness and broadly to nonmedical causation, as the examples at the beginning of the chapter illustrate. Confusion over how to attribute causation probably has less to do with these forces being present in the universe but rather our performance in identifying these forces. It is painfully obvious that humans have made errors in the past about medical causation, and no doubt, much of what is accepted now in medical knowledge is wrong as well. Having said this, let us apply these causal concepts to our patient from Chap. 1 with GERD.

Please recall that the patient presented with heartburn. After an evaluation with a history and physical examination, which determined that the patients had class I obesity, the physician ordered additional testing that confirmed a sliding hiatal hernia, esophagitis, a hypotensive lower esophageal sphincter (consistent with an incompetent lower esophageal sphincter) and a pathologic level of acid reflux into the esophagus. All this is depicted in Fig. 5.3. To construct the causal sequence, the patient's stomach produces hydrochloric acid. The patient's lower esophageal sphincter is hypotensive, which may be related to the patient's hiatal hernia and, therefore, incompetent, meaning that the sphincter is not "completely shut." The patient's obesity produces an increase in his intra-abdominal pressure. The intra-abdominal pressure exceeds the esophageal sphincter pressure, thereby allowing gastric acid to enter the esophagus. The amount of gastric acid overwhelms the esophageal anti-acid defenses of the esophageal mucus lining of the esophageal mucosa, the neutralizing effects of the more alkaline saliva, and the esophageal motility clearance mechanism. This allows hydrochloric acid to remain in contact with the esophageal mucosa long enough to cause inflammation of the esophageal mucosa. This inflammation causes the nociceptors of the vagal afferent nerves and spinal afferent nerves to signal to that brain that a noxious event is occurring in the

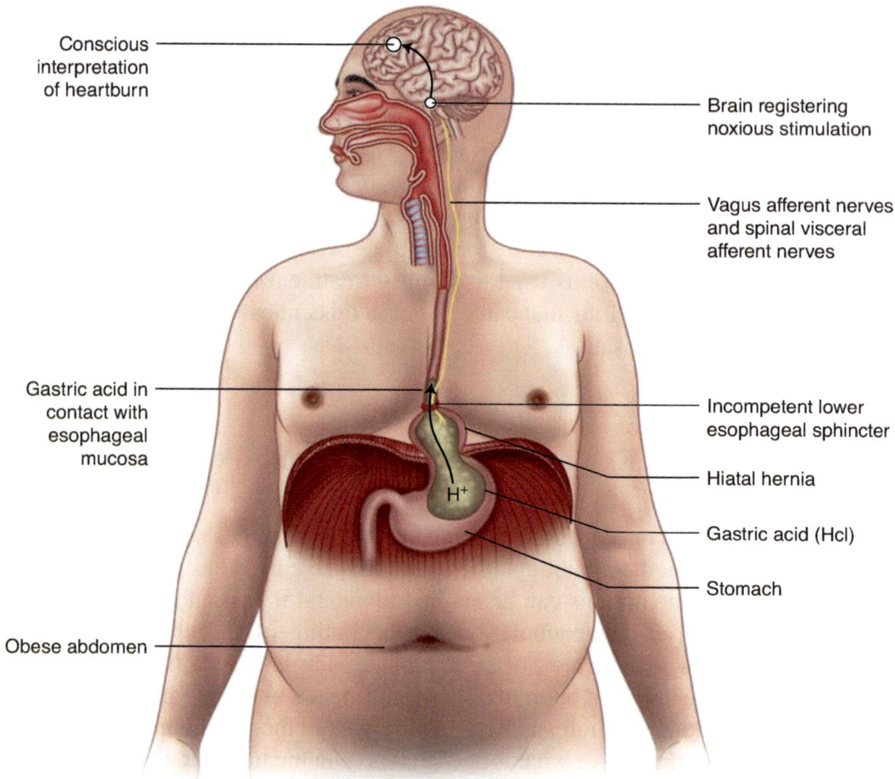

Fig. 5.3 The anatomico-physiologic causal sequence of a patient with heartburn from gastroesophageal reflux disease

esophagus. The receiving brain nucleus then signals to the frontal cortex that a noxious stimulus is being detected in the esophagus. The patient's consciousness then registers this event as heartburn [45].

Again, we can see this causal sequence using a pluralistic approach to causation. The causal sequence described in the passage above is mechanistic in nature. This type of presentation is quite satisfying and understandable to most, as the human mind evolved to temporally sequence events. Therefore, as an explanation, this causal sequence works well. Earlier in this chapter, it was noted that causal attribution was quite valuable as an effective explanation. There are clearly a few deterministic elements in this sequence. For example, to have acid reflux, the stomach must produce hydrochloric acid. However, this does not automatically entail that the patient will or will not have heartburn. This part of the causal sequence is probabilistic, as there are a certain number of individuals who will have "silent acid reflux," i.e., gastric hydrochloric acid in the esophagus, yet no heartburn symptoms, and another number of individuals who will have functional heartburn, i.e., perceived symptoms of heartburn, but no hydrochloric acid in the esophagus. Obesity and hiatal hernia are also probabilistic causative factors, as not all obese individuals or those with hiatal hernias will have reflux. Causal interactions are when two causal factors are interactive if in combination they act as a single causal factor whose effects are different from at least one of the two acting separately [46]. There is a counterfactual component as well—if the lower esophageal sphincter were competent, i.e., with normal functioning, there would be no acid reflux. Similarly, both deterministically and counterfactually, the nervous system signally the noxious stimulus to the brain, making the patient consciously aware of the heartburn all have to be intact.

Returning to Fig. 1.1, the above causal sequence fits into the physician's meta-cognition theoretical framework, which informs the physician's cognition. The patient's symptoms, physical examination findings and objective testing are explained by and causally attributable to the anatomic and physiologic alterations found in this patient, as well as the normal hydrochloric acid production. This is further linked to the physician's meta-cognition evidence for theory, and this will be further addressed in the next chapter.

5.6.1 *Medical Attribution of Causation Is About Predictability*

In 1992, when writing about causality concepts in surgery [30], I proposed that for physicians, the practical issue in causality is predictability. To that I would now add identifying targets for treatment. This fits with the physician's meta-cognition and cognition (Fig. 1.1). A more general account of predictability is given by Mulaik [47]; causal relations and functional relations are those associated with any given value of some independent variable, revealing the unique outcome associated with that independent variable. This is how multivariate analysis works, which I will explore in the next chapter. Moreover, Granger causality is a causality of predictability: if knowing all earlier values of x, our estimate of x at time t is improved by knowing all earlier values of y, then a causal relationship exists between y and x [48]. The prediction of natural history and treatment response is of paramount concern for practicing physicians.

5.6.2 *The Role of Causation in the Persuasion of Lay People and Professionals*

I started this chapter with everyday examples of causal attribution. I end it with medical causal attribution as presented to people as a form of persuasion. A selection of what is a cause is the result of a choice that reflects the interests of the person who makes the choice [49]. This is consistent with what was previously said, by Hume and others, that causation is a human-invented concept to help us understand the universe we live in. I also suggest that this choice will be influenced to a greater or lesser extent by the individual's social umwelt. Although unfortunately, causation is somewhat an ambiguous term in science, with most people, it is understood reasonably well. In this sense, causal attribution serves two purposes in persuasion—(1) as a vehicle for explanation and (2) as a premise in an argument.

Causation Used in Explanation

An explanation is a human desire for descriptive information to better understand the phenomenon in question. An explanation is not the same as a proposition, an argument, or a list of propositions; it is an *answer* [18]. For van Fraazen [50], an explanation is an answer to the question *why*? I have certainly had to answer that question innumerable times over the years. The patient in the clinical vignette in Chap. 1 required an explanation for his symptoms before they could even begin to contemplate consenting to a treatment plan. Providing such an explanation is part of the physician's cognition and meta-cognition (Fig. 1.1), as well as an obligation to the patient. All explanations in medicine rests on biomedical models; that is, medical scientists construct an account that will allow for the best fit of the data known. Not all models are explanatory. However, mechanistic models, such as the one used to explain heartburn above, appear to have explanatory value [51]. That is, according to Schaffner [18], it tells "the whole story," or, I would say, at least, what is known of the story (once again, we see the desire for storytelling). "Explanatory information" is based on the context, interests, and background knowledge given or what aspects of the ideal explanatory text will be selected [18]. Very little should be of more interest to the patient than this explanation. Similarly, an explanation will be required to persuade the patient of the best treatment options as well (Figs. 1.1, 3.5 and 4.2).

However, I will add the caveat that acceptance of medical causes as true or relevant to the individual is dependent on many things, not the least of which is their social umwelt. Some patients will listen to the explanation and choose not to be persuaded by it. Each item in the causal chain can be treated as a premise in an argument, although for the physician, it is merely a recounting of known facts. The reaction to the listener of the explanation would be similar to that of Fig. 4.2 in the persuasion chapter. I certainly have had patients over the years who simply do not accept the explanations I have provided for a number of reasons, mostly because they view these explanations as simply not applicable to them or as contrary to their core beliefs. This is where belief systems recounted in Chap. 4, such as Primal Beliefs, Moral Foundations, cultural identity and the social umwelt, may lead to such rejections.

Causation as a Premises in an Argument

In determining new medical knowledge or justifying a treatment decision, the causal sequence is invariably used in the illative core of the argument a physician puts forth to patients or colleagues. Specifically, with other healthcare professionals, the causal sequence provides the counterfactual basis for treatment decisions. The argument's basic form is:

This patient has these symptoms and these findings (by physical exam or objective testing).
I have determined that disease *x* is the cause of these symptoms and findings.
The cause of disease *x* is *y*.
Elimination of cause *y* will cure disease *x*.
Treatment *z* will eliminate cause *y*.
Therefore, treatment *z* should be administered to this patient.

Variations in this illative core are the bedrock of medical practice. In this argument, the "cause" is described mechanistically, although the scientific foundations were most likely probabilistic. The causes were accepted as actionable items because they were accepted into the physician's meta-cognition of evidence for theory, which was a result of their acceptance of how the relevant information was generated from the techniques of evidential foundational appraisal (Fig. 1.1). Although much of the accepted medical causal attribution is deterministic, even more is probabilistic. As such, it is open for interpretation, which will be addressed in Chaps. 6 and 7.

5.7 Summary

What I have hope to have shown is that causation in medical science is an ambiguous, albeit useful, term with no one clear definition and mode of assessment. There are many concepts of causation that are acceptable as modes of explanation but, more importantly from a practical standpoint, as a means of predictability and therapeutic target selection. These include deterministic, probabilistic, counterfactual and interventionalist (agency) concepts. Although my opinion is that much of the differences among philosophers are semantic in nature, there is no denying the practical value of recounting the causal sequence in persuasion for both existing knowledge and new knowledge. With respect to causation in the production of new medical knowledge, I will address that in the next chapter.

References

1. Because etymology. https://etymologeek.com. Last accessed 16 Aug 2022.
2. Cause. Merriam-Webster Dictionary. https://merriam-webser.com. Last accessed 16 Aug 2022.
3. Because. Merriam-Webster Dictionary. https://merriam-webster.com. Last accessed 16 Aug 2022.
4. Causation. https://thesaurus.com. Last accessed 16 Aug 2022.
5. Gilovich T. How we know what isn't so: the fallibility of human reason in everyday life. New York: The Free Press; 1991.

6. Broadbent A. Causation. The Internet encyclopedia of philosophy. https://iep.utm.edu/causation. Last accessed 9 Aug 2022.
7. Taylor R. Causation and determinism. In: Edwards P, editor. The encyclopedia of philosophy, vol. 2. New York: MacMillian and the Free Press; 1968.
8. Ozen U. Causality in the philosophy of science: from Hume to today. Int J Hum Soc Sci. 2011;1(11 special issue Aug):191–7.
9. Hume D. A treatise on human nature. Oxford: Oxford University Press; 2000. (first published 1739)
10. Kant I. Critique of pure reason. Dover Publications; 2003. (first published 1781)
11. Mill JS. A system of logic: ratiocinative and inductive. New York: Longman's Green and Co.; 1882. (first published 1843)
12. Beebee H, Hitchcock C, Menzies PC. The Oxford handbook of causation. Oxford: Oxford University Press; 2009.
13. Carnap R. An introduction to the philosophy of science. New York: Basic Books; 1966.
14. Mackie J. The cement of the universe. Oxford: Oxford University Press; 1974.
15. Fass R. Functional heartburn. Gastroenterol Hepatol. 2014;10:381–3.
16. Lewis D. Counterfactuals. Cambridge, MA: Harvard University Press; 1973.
17. Illari P, Russo F. Causality: philosophical theory meets scientific practice. Oxford: Oxford University Press; 2014.
18. Schaffner KF. Discovery and explanation in biology and medicine. Chicago: University of Chicago Press; 1993.
19. Suppes P. A probabilistic theory of causality. Amsterdam: North-Holland; 1970.
20. Giere R. Causal models with frequency dependence. J Philos. 1984;81:384–91.
21. Chang P, Friedenberg F. Obesity and GERD. Gastroenterol Clin N Am. 2014;43:161–73.
22. Jackson M, Marks L, May GHW, Wilson JB. The genetic basis of disease. Essays Biochem. 2018;62:643–723.
23. Ben-Menachem Y. Causation in science. Princeton, NJ: Princeton University Press; 2018.
24. Price H, Corry R. A case for causal republicanism? In: Corry R, Price H, editors. Causation, physics and the constitution of reality: Russell's republic revisited. Oxford: Oxford University Press; 2007.
25. Darden L, Maull N. Interfield theories. Philos Sci. 1977;44:43–64.
26. Gustafson J, Wellig D. "No acid, no ulcer"—100 years later: a review of the history of peptic ulcer disease. J Am Coll Surg. 2010;210:110–6.
27. Peptic Ulcer Disease. The American College of Gastroenterology. https://gi.org. Last accessed 22 Aug 2022.
28. Dammann O. Causality, mosaics and the health sciences. Theor Med Bioeth. 2016;37:161–8.
29. Russo F, Williamson J. Interpreting causality in the health sciences. Int Stud Philos Sci. 2007;21:157–70.
30. Velanovich V. Causality concepts in surgery. Theor Surg. 1992;7:197–200.
31. Rizzi DA, Pedersen SA. Causality in medicine: toward a theory and terminology. Theor Med. 1992;13:233–54.
32. Lakoff G. Women, fire and dangerous things: what causes reveal about the mind. Chicago: University of Chicago Press; 1987.
33. Rubin DB. Causal inference using potential outcomes: design, modeling, decisions. J Am Stat Assoc. 2005;100:322–31.
34. Imbens G, Rubin DB. Causal inference for statistics, social and biomedical sciences: an introduction. Cambridge, UK: Cambridge University Press; 2015.
35. Fiorentino AR, Dammann O. Evidence, disease and causation: an epidemiologic perspective on the Russo-Williamson thesis. Stud Hist Philos Biol Biomed Sci. 2015;54:1–9.
36. Ward AC. The role of causal criteria in causal inference: Bradford Hill's "aspects of association". Epidemiol Perspect Innov. 2009;6:2.

37. Cartwright N. Hunting causes and using them: approaches in philosophy and economics. Cambridge: Cambridge University Press; 2007.
38. Rondeau E, Larmonier N, Pradeau T, Bikfalvi A. Characterizing causality in cancer. eLife. 2019;8:e53755.
39. Bradford Hill A. The environment and disease: association or causation? Proc R Soc Med. 1965;58:295–300.
40. Evans DW, Lucas N, Kerry R. Time, space and form: necessary for causation in health, disease and intervention. Med Health Care Philos. 2016;19:207–13.
41. Howick J, Glasziou P, Aronson JK. The evolution of evidence hierarchies: what can Bradford Hill's 'guidelines for causation' contribute? J R Soc Med. 2009;102:186–94.
42. Howick J, Glasziou P, Aronson JK. Evidence-based mechanistic reasoning. J R Soc Med. 2010;103:186–94.
43. Hofler M. The Bradford Hill considerations on causality: a counterfactual perspective. Emerg Themes Epidemiol. 2005;2:11.
44. Phillips CV, Goodman KJ. Causal criteria and counterfactuals: nothing more (or less) than scientific common sense. Emerg Themes Epidemiol. 2006;3:5.
45. Bennett RD, Straughn DM, Velanovich V. Gastroesophageal reflux disease, hiatal hernia, and Barrett esophagus. In: Zinner MJ, Ashley SW, Hines OJ, editors. Maingot's abdominal operations. 13th ed. New York: McGraw-Hill Education; 2019. p. 393–422.
46. Eells E. Probabilistic causal interaction. Philos Sci. 1986;50:35–57.
47. Mulaik SA. Toward a synthesis of deterministic and probabilistic formulations of causal relations by the functional relation concept. Philos Sci. 1986;53:313–32.
48. Carr K. Causality, predictability and explanation. Theor Surg. 1989;4:88–90.
49. Wulff HR, Andur Pedersen S, Rosenberg R. Philosophy of medicine: an introduction. Oxford: Blackwell Scientific; 1986.
50. van Fraazen B. The scientific image. New York: Oxford University Press; 1980.
51. Carver CF. When mechanistic models explain. Synthese. 2006;153:355–76.

Chapter 6
Generation and Acceptance of New Medical Knowledge

6.1 Introduction

The previous chapters are an account of the attributes that humans have and the mechanisms humans use to determine the truths of the phenomena around them. When I use the word "truths" what I mean by this it that the truth of the given phenomenon in question is judged on a gradient from absolutely false to plausible to possible to unlikely to likely to probable to absolutely true, and descriptors (or even quantitative values) in between. This will be the basis for the following chapters, as the topics will be the acceptance of new knowledge and how this knowledge is used with respect to the science and practice of medicine (or in the case of Chap. 8, the theoretical foundations and practices of non-Western traditional and alternative medicine). Toward this end, I will discuss how new medical knowledge is created. This entails observations, as presented to the keen-eyed observer who comes upon them serendipitously or through controlled experimentation by the scientist. These observations are then communicated to the community of humans who would have some interest in them. This communication is done in some type of argument. This argument needs to be persuasive for the audience it was intended.

In the construction of arguments, premises are presumed facts that bear some type of relationship to the conclusion. A key quality of these facts, if they are to be persuasive, is that they are true, or at least believed to be true enough. Therefore, how these facts are determined to be true to justify belief in them is an crucial characteristic of these facts. These facts come from observations of the pertinent phenomena. The philosophical descriptive and normative study of this process is epistemology. As the purpose of this chapter is to describe how medical knowledge is generated and its use justified in the application of medical practice, I will address two broad categories of how this knowledge comes to be accepted: the "scientific" generation of new knowledge and the individual physician's accumulation of knowledge through experience and reflection.

V. Velanovich, *Medical Persuasion*, https://doi.org/10.1007/978-3-031-30371-5_6

As a foundation, I will discuss the broad tenets of epistemology to better understand how and why medical knowledge should be accepted.

6.2 Basic Tenets of Epistemology

Epistemology, in its broadest sense, is the philosophical study of knowledge [1]. Another way to characterize it is that epistemology seeks to understand one or another kind of "cognitive success" (or cognitive failure) [2], such that one attitude or belief is more reasonable for a person to have than another at a given time. Of course, determining what is "reasonable" is part of the normative epistemological process. Needless to say, epistemology is a big subject that is nuanced and full of controversy, for which I am only to state the most basic, relatively uncontroversial tenets.

Epistemology wants to understand the "nature of knowledge." That is, what does it mean to say that someone knows or does not know something [1]. It also wants to understand the "extent of human knowledge." That is, how much do we, or can we know [1]. Truncellito [1] describes three different kinds of knowledge: (1) Procedure knowledge—how to do something; (2) Acquaintance knowledge—to be aware of someone or something; and (3) Propositional knowledge—knowledge that purports to describe a fact or state of affairs. We can think of these as *knowledge how, knowledge of,* and *knowledge that,* respectively. In the everyday affairs of humans, all of these types of knowledge are important for getting about our daily lives.[1] In fact, because "knowing how" is fundamentally different from "knowing that," the concept of "optimality" involves the promotion of ends that are practical rather than simply alethic (i.e., solely relating to propositional truths) [2, 3]. Certainly, as my approach has been to promote the practical, this has an appeal. However, for the epistemologist, it is propositional knowledge, *knowledge that*, which is of interest. Nevertheless, knowing how is quite important in medical knowledge as many healthcare professionals in the course of their practice are performing manipulations and procedures on patients. These manipulations can be the source of knowledge, such as a physical examination, or a treatment, such as a surgical operation.

That being said, with respect to propositional knowledge, epistemic consequentialism is the school of thought that one should form beliefs about the world that are true and avoid beliefs that are false [2]. That is, the "consequence" of having a corpus of beliefs is that these should expand the breadth of true knowledge (later I will also discuss understanding and wisdom) of the universe. To do this, one can acquire knowledge that is "nonempirical" (sometimes referred to as *a priori*), which requires

[1] Certainly, for me as a practicing surgeon and an educator of future surgeons, *knowledge how* is part and parcel of my professional life, namely, how to do and how to teach operations, which combines the cognitive skills of problem solving with the manual handicraft to accomplish them. For all physicians, *knowledge of* patients and their families is nearly the greater part of medical practice.

the individual only to use their own reasoning talents, without the need for experience or observation [1]. A good example of this would be developing a new mathematical proof, for example, the proof of the existence of imaginary numbers ($i^2 = -1$, or i is defined at the square root of -1). There is no overt world experience for imaginary numbers (although they were later found to be useful); they were created by pure thought. The other type is "empirical" (sometimes referred to as *a posteriori*), which is obtained only through "sensory" experiences [1]. That is, by physically (through one of our five sensory organs) the phenomenon in question is observed or experienced. Knowledge, by this account, is a mental state—a belief. In Chaps. 2–4, we discussed the various ways humans come to believe what they do, with some of these beliefs not based on rational argumentation, more on this below. Moreover, these beliefs can be "occurrent"; that is, the individual is consciously activating and using these beliefs at the present time. Or they can be "nonoccurrent"; that is, these are beliefs that reside within the individual's mental corpus dormantly but are not being accessed or used at the present time [1]. Knowledge, therefore, is the individual's stock of "true beliefs"; that is, matching one's mind with the world [1] (assuming, of course, that there is such a thing as "objective" truth[2]).

"Truth," therefore, becomes a condition for knowledge. False beliefs cannot count as knowledge, since these beliefs have no corresponding phenomenon in the universe, past, present or potentially in the future. However, it is not just that the beliefs are true; these beliefs must be obtained in the "right way." When one obtains beliefs in the right way, epistemologists say that these beliefs are "justified" [1]. Moreover, "truth" and "justification" are independent conditions of beliefs [1]. However, one can have a true belief, which is justified, yet might be justified for the wrong reason and, therefore, does not constitute knowledge by epistemologists.[3] There are instances where something has "defeated" the individual's true and justified beliefs [1]. I find this last point particularly important in medical knowledge; physicians have had true beliefs that they had justified in the "right way," yet unknown defeaters have conspired not to make this knowledge. For example, in the account of peptic ulcer disease described in Chap. 5. The importance of this is that

[2] As I stated in Chap. 1, I am assuming for the purposes of this book that there is a physical universe that we perceive with our senses. I am not going to argue whether Descartes's "evil demon" exists or not. However, the idea of objective knowledge, that is, knowledge that is independent of the knower, is something that has received a great deal of attention many philosophers, including Hume, Kant, and Locke, among many others.

[3] This is known as the Gettier problem: Suppose there is a clock in the town square. Last night, at 11:58 pm, the clock broke, and the hands no longer moved past 11:58. If a person who has a noon appointment in an office in the town square walks by the clock at approximately 11:58 am in order to be on time for their appointment and sees that hands at 11:58, it is both true that it is 11:58 am, they would be justified in the belief that it is 11:58 am as the clock says because they expected to be at the square around that time, but the source of the justification, the clock, was not a reliable source because it was broken. Therefore, they truly did not have knowledge that the time was actually 11:58 am. The circumstances "defeated" their attempt to obtain knowledge.

if the same method of justification is used again, the belief may be false, even though it is believed to be true.

Although not intended to be a complete list, there are a few epistemological theories worth stating [1]:

Foundationalism: An asymmetric relationship between any two beliefs, such that A is based on B, B cannot be based on A. Basic beliefs must be "self-justified" from some nondoxastic sources, for example, sensory input (i.e., "seeing is believing"), and not purely reasoning about the beliefs.

Coherentism: Justification is a relation of mutual support among many beliefs rather than a series of asymmetrical beliefs. It is justified by being a member of a set of beliefs that fit together in the "right way." That is, the beliefs are like the beams in a frame of a building, in that they support each other. This will come up again later in the chapter.

Reliabilism: In this theory, one needs to consider the source of the belief. That is, is the process of obtaining the belief a reliable source or methods of acquiring a true belief? For this, we need to know the appropriate level of generality used to describe this process. A reliable cognitive process cannot yield a justification for the belief unless the believer is aware of the fact that the process is reliable (e.g., the Gettier problem as noted above). This is a specific issue in medical knowledge, both generally (i.e., about new diseases) and specifically (pertaining to individual patients).

Of importance is the concept that once knowledge is established, it can be passed on to others [1]. This is obvious as everyone receives the vast (nearly all?) of their knowledge via others—that's what our whole educational system is set up to do. Of course, the human brain has evolved to accept knowledge from others, as discussed in Chap. 3. The foundation here is trust in the source of the knowledge, as discussed in Chap. 4.

I would like to dispense with the bootstrapping problem. As previously noted in Chap. 4, bootstrapping is the issue of accepting information coming from a source based on the source providing such information. To judge the source reliability, we generally would like to have independent confirmation of its reliability. This is not an inconsequential issue in medicine, as much of the information a physician receives pertaining to a patient comes from tests—the processes of which physicians know very little. They trust that the methods used to determine the information are reliable. For example, government bureaus of weights and measures certify scales used to weigh objects. Other similar standards exist for other measurement instruments. (In fact, a whole field of metrology exists to study measurement.) However, how do we know these methods are reliable to test the instruments of measure? Surely, they have to have undergone some type of testing to determine if they are reliable to test the processes to determine the reliability of the index instruments of measurement. If we continue to ask for tests of reliability of the processes that are testing the reliability of the processes, we eventually come to our own senses, that is, our sight, hearing, touch, smell and taste. Our senses are our foundation of how we perceive the world. A few philosophers in the past have questioned whether our senses can be relied upon for knowledge, such as Descartes. In addition, although Melchoir [4], who was referred to in Chap. 4, gives a good defense of why, at least philosophically speaking, we are not bootstrapping when we use our senses, from a practical matter, it is all we have (and, for that matter, all other living creatures on this Earth have) of perceiving the world. We cannot exist otherwise. Although our senses sometimes deceive us, from a practical standpoint, as all knowledge comes from the senses in some form, I am going to assume that the information entering our minds from the senses is "reliable enough" to rationally analyze and make judgments. Corroboration with the observations of other individuals will lead to increased confidence in our sensory observations as a consequence of how our brains and minds evolved. It is not uncommon to hear the phrase "Do you see what I'm seeing?" as an example.

Similarly, much knowledge that we have has been told (or, more commonly now, written) to us by others. Although not all of this is true (as the example of peptic ulcer disease in Chap. 5 demonstrated), I am going to assume a certain amount of "baseline" truth upon which new knowledge is built. It would just be too impractical to go back in history and assess the voracity of all the information and knowledge that we now take for granted. Although I will acknowledge that much of the accepted "knowledge and facts" should be reanalyzed, it is beyond the scope of this book.

6.3 Medical Epistemology

Medical epistemology concerns itself with what clinicians, biomedical scientists and healthcare professionals know as individuals or as a professional group and how they come to know and use this knowledge [5]. In an editorial, ten Have and Gordijn [6] attributed the concerted study of the basis of scientific medical knowledge to the "philosopher and physician," Wladyslaw Bieganski (1857–1917). Interestingly, for Bieganski, as for myself, the purpose of scientific knowledge is not to understand the surrounding world (as it is for basic scientists) but to predict the future, with diagnosis being the foundation of therapy (i.e., another form of prediction).

Khushf has defined "epistemic practices" broadly as "activities associated with knowledge production and use" [5]. He then goes only to discuss four "frameworks" of epistemology in medicine. He ultimately rejects the first three, so, although this discussion is enlightening, I will not discuss these. Rather, his fourth framework, "epistemologies as compensations for heightened risks of error", appears most useful. In this framework, epistemology should be part of the epistemic practice that is oriented toward overcoming errors that emerge in antecedently given practices where knowledge is developed and used [5]. Such practices include (1) *descriptive epistemology*, which is empirical investigations into how people come to know things they know and how they use knowledge. (2) *Normative epistemology*, which is how people ought to arrive at the knowledge they accept and use. In addition, (3) *meta-epistemology* which are investigations into "higher-order" concepts that are used in descriptive and normative epistemologies, for example, the nature of knowledge and evidence, logics of justification, kinds of inference, etc.

Because medical epistemology is most usefully thought of as oriented toward providing a corrective mechanism for extant errors and problems that arise in existing practices of truth and justification in medical knowledge, there may not be one epistemology but several epistemologies [5]. It is interesting to me that this is analogous to the "pluralist" account of causation and causal attribution discussed in Chap. 5. In this sense, epistemologies are better understood as strategies for overcoming error, rather than as comprehensive accounts of how we attain justified true beliefs (as discussed in the section above). Khushf refers to Canguihem [7] that in the case of both medicine and epistemology, there is an ontic[4] priority of the "positive goods": health and knowledge. We become aware of both health and knowledge when we have a deficiency in either [5]. Hence, there is a need for epistemic corrective measures. This concept of using knowledge for good will show up later in a discussion of the importance of understanding and wisdom in the practical use of knowledge.

It has been my observation that medical knowledge is generated either "publically" through formal medical research, both observational and experimental, which then is published in some open forum and in the public domain, and "privately" through the focused practice, experience and reflection of the individual practitioner. de Cuzzani and Lie [8] discuss the importance of medical epistemology for clinical practice. For them, as for Bieganski, it is about justification of clinical interventions. They have noted that healthcare professionals may be prone to justify a clinical intervention based on premature acceptance of "knowledge." They identify a pattern, which I have certainly observed over the years, of initial enthusiasm for a new intervention, then this same intervention was later abandoned as useless (e.g., peptic ulcer disease). Others have documented this same phenomenon [9]. This, de Cuzzani and Lie [8] assert, demonstrates a lack of awareness of the limitations of knowledge, including the much-vaunted randomized clinical trial, as identified by Feinstein [10, 11]. With this as the background, I will address the public and private generation and acceptance of medical knowledge both descriptively and normatively.

6.4 Types of Medical Knowledge

First, we have to know what types of knowledge with which we are dealing. There are, of course, many ways to classify and categorize knowledge. This is no different in medical knowledge. The categories presented below are certainly not meant to be definitive or even representative. When one develops a classification system, however, it is usually for some purpose. To state clearly my purpose: It is simply the way

---

[4] "Ontic" is relating to entities and the facts about them.

that most physicians, healthcare professionals, and biomedical scientists think about how medical knowledge is organized. Therefore, this will be how I categorize this knowledge.

6.4.1 Basic Science

When those in the healthcare professions think of "basic science," they think of laboratories performing controlled experiments for no other purposes than to determine the functioning of biological systems. For example, Watson and Crick elucidated the structure of DNA. This is not to say that these scientists do not foresee the long-term practical usefulness of their work; only that for the present do they want to determine how the biological system works. These systems can be anything from the subatomic, for example, how electrons may be redistributed in a chemical reaction creating new molecules in medicinal chemistry, to the multicellular organism, for example, weight gain in mice with hormonal manipulations. In fact, much of the philosophy of science is dedicated to understanding this type of research. Nearly all of the examples of biomedical theories and the experiments associated with these theories in Schaffner's comprehensive book on theories, discovery and explanation are of this sort [12]. I do not mean this to be a criticism, because from "benchtop to bedside" is how many of our therapeutic breakthroughs occur, as the example on the acquired immunodeficiency syndrome (AIDS) below will attest. However, as the focus of this book is on persuasion in clinical medicine, I will not address issues of knowledge generation and acceptance in the basic sciences, although I suspect that the basic structure of such is not much different than clinical medicine.

6.4.2 Clinical Medicine

Clinical medicine is concerned with the health of the individual and the population. The practice of medicine, by an individual physician, is generally directed toward the care of an individual patient, very much like the clinical vignette in Chap. 1. Public health concerns itself with the health of populations, usually in conjunction with governmental agencies. As this book's focus is on the physician and the patient with how they accept medical knowledge, I will not address the public health aspects of medicine, although, clearly, public health officials must persuade members of the public about behaviors that would improve their overall health outlook, as was discussed in Chap. 4. What I will address will be limited to knowledge of diseases and their treatments.

It goes without saying that much of what the modern healthcare professional knows and applies in practice comes from textbooks, lectures, online sources, and other materials that simply state descriptions of disease, their diagnosis, and their treatments as established truths without the need for justifying these statements. In the physician's meta-cognitions of Fig. 1.1, the vast proportion of the physician's knowledge is of this sort. However, that knowledge, before being enshrined in the accepted biomedical cannon, was derived from observations of a biomedical nature, either serendipitously or through planned experimentation. This list following is a basic catalog of such knowledge as an introduction to the generation and acceptance of new knowledge.

Knowledge of Diseases

Illness has no doubt afflicted humans even as they evolved from earlier hominins. It is also most likely, although there is no record, that these afflictions were recognized and attempts made to ease the suffering of those afflicted. Anthropological investigations have suggested that human species, even before *Homo sapiens*, cared for one another. When particular individuals within a group have taken up the mantle as healers is also lost to time. It is only with the advent of the written record that we see medicine as a profession recorded. The earliest Egyptian papyruses date from 1900 BCE and were a clear treatise on diseases and their treatments, which was a domain reserved for educated physicians [13]. The basic medical paradigm is that of a patient afflicted with a disease and a physician treating a patient with a disease. Therefore, knowledge of diseases is the *sine qua non* of the physician. This then begs the question of "How are diseases identified?" In reality, this question has two parts. The first part is "What is a disease?" The second part is "Does this patient have a disease, and if so, which disease is it?"

The latter question is a question of diagnosis. This is the cognitive task of the physician to ascertain this diagnosis. This is the physician's cognition, as presented in Fig. 1.1. Although I will address the theoretical aspects of this process in this chapter, the actual process of diagnosis will be more fully addressed in Chap. 7.

The first question of "What is a disease?" is more complex than what it appears on its face. As has been my custom in this book, I will start with the *Merriam-Webster Dictionary* definition of "impaired normal functioning and that is typically manifested by distinguishing signs and symptoms" [14]. I would think that most people would not quibble too much with this definition; yet, it does fail in certain aspects. Because now we have to define "normal functioning" and "typically manifested by distinguishing signs and symptoms." And while these statements appear true, it does seem to downplay asymptomatic disease, and it also appears to give no room for mental illness. The World Health Organization (WHO) defined "health" as a state of "complete physical, mental and social well-being and not merely an absence of disease or infirmity" [15]. I would have to say, with this definition of health, I wonder if anyone is truly healthy by the WHO's standard of health. On the other hand, it does point to a more holistic definition of what the common Western, allopathic concept of disease suggests. Interestingly, the WHO does not seem to have a definitive definition of "disease," even though they produce the *International Classification of Disease*, now in the 10th edition (the ICD-10) [16]. In a very nuanced treatise, Scully [17] provides a very interesting account of "disease" in relation to cultural and historical attitudes, with some conditions going from being nondiseases to diseases, such as osteoporosis, while others have gone from being diseases to nondisease, such as homosexuality.[5] In other words, what is thought as a disease in a particular group of individuals is an agreed upon concept by members of that society and culture. This harkens back to what was discussed in Chap. 3 about social cohesion and cultural identity. Although clearly a fascinating subject, I will not further address it here. However, back to the point, what these definitions have in common is that there is some alteration in the individual's homeostatic state that leads to deteriorated function manifesting as the patient's symptoms and signs.

There are other definitions that appear to take the patient out of the disease definition. For example, Smart [18] asserts that diseases are causal processes best seen as simultaneously acting sequences of mutually manifesting dispositions (more on how he proposes that diseases are classified in the next section). Gagliardi [19] defines a disease in a physician-centric way: a disease is "an outcome of a diagnostic process performed by a physician using their knowledge and experience to assign the considered clinical case into a disease category."

Although all these definitions have some merit to them, I am going to use a working definition of a disease as an abnormal deviation of the homeostatically operational structure and function of a specific human body or mind, such that the individual will perceive adverse well-being or will have shortened survival, with or without intervention. In this definition, "abnormal deviation of the homeostatic operational structure and function" is the pathological process that leads to disease manifestations, either known or unknown. I have purposefully avoided the word "normal" because this implies more uniformity among humans than what actually exists. The term "body and mind" is to account for both physical and mental illness; "adverse well-being" is that the individual "feels ill" or is otherwise in distress; and "shortened survival" is that the individual may die sooner than that they would have if they did not have the disease with or without symptoms (note the counterfactual causation model here); and "with or without intervention" is to imply that some diseases are self-limiting, meaning that the individual will recover function without intervention, or that the individual may continue to deteriorate and die even with intervention. However, this definition is about categorizing a disease as a concept for physicians (and the lay public) in general. It is only a part of the disease process in an individual.

For an individual patient, the disease is both a subset of the category of disease described above *and* an overlap with other medical and nonmedical conditions or issues. When I say "subset" what I mean here is that the extent of the pathological

[5] Kenneth M. Boyd has also written a quite enlightening article on the difficulties of pinpointing with precision the terms "disease," "illness," "sickness," "health," "healing," and "wholeness" (Boyd KM. Disease, illness, sickness, health, healing and wholeness: Exploring some elusive concepts. J Med Ethics: Med Human 2000;26:9–17). He does quote Marshall Marinker proposal that (1) disease is a pathological process, most often physical…sometimes underdetermined…(with) an objectivity. (2) Illness is a feeling, an experience of unhealth, with is entirely personal, interior to the person of the patient. (3) Sickness is the external and public mode of health. This realm of disease and illness as a physical and social construct is important but a far too large and complex topic for this book.

abnormality will differ from patient to patient. The individual patient is an example, or a "token" to use Rizzi and Andur Pedersen terminology from the last chapter, of the disease. For example, if one takes the disease concept of "colon cancer," there is a range of pathological abnormalities within that disease category from carcinoma in situ to metastatic, stage IV cancer, with each stage having substantially different prognoses and treatment options. In addition, the disease will manifest differently in each patient. To continue with the colon cancer example, patients with colon cancer can present completely asymptomatically (e.g., cancer discovered by screening colonoscopy) or with the symptoms of pain, bleeding or obstruction. These are all different subsets of the disease category "colon cancer."

Additionally, patients will have associated conditions or issues. These can be physical conditions (such as other disease processes), mental/emotional processes (such as being able to understand their disease process), or social issues (such as family support or finances). These issues are not part of the disease category as defined above for the disease in general but may be crucial for the disease manifestation and medical decision-making for an individual physician confronted with an individual patient. Moreover, the disease, as a concept and physical phenomenon, the patient, and the patient's comorbidities all reside in an environment, which I use in the broadest sense of the term, encompassing the actual physical environment and social/cultural environment, which not only includes the patient but also the physician (Fig. 6.1). More on this in Chap. 7.

Biomedical scientists and clinical healthcare professionals, when assessing new information presented in the literature, are assessing information for the disease

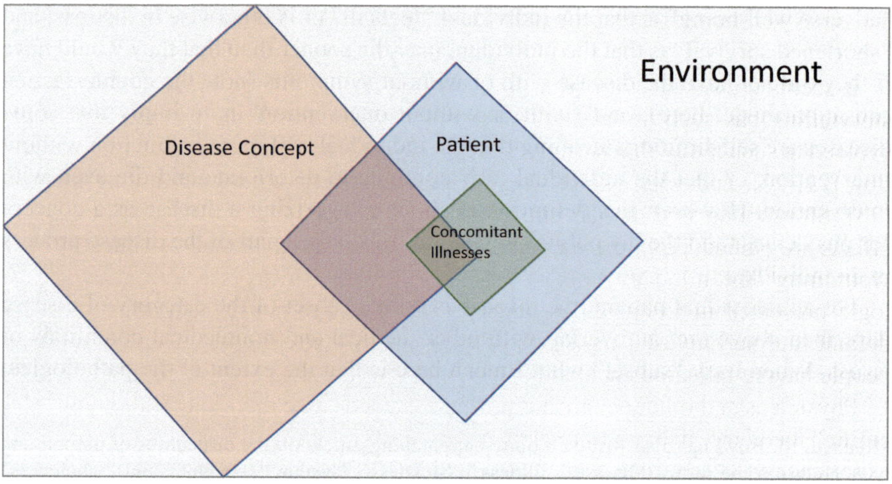

Fig. 6.1 The overlapping of the disease concept with the disease manifestation in an individual patient. The disease concept is the composite theory and accepted understanding of the disease in the general population. This will overlap to a greater or lesser extent in an individual patient, i.e., a patient may not manifest all of the items associated with the disease. In addition, a great portion of the patient will not be "involved" with the disease process. All of this is surrounded by the backdrop of the environment, social, medical, etc., that the patient is in

category, as a whole or in some subset. The application of this information will be addressed in Chap. 7. However, to understand how new knowledge is generated for disease categories, we must better understand how diseases are categorized and classified.

Classification of Disease

There are many ways that diseases are classified. Nosology is the branch of medical science dealing with disease classification. The ICD-10 mentioned above is an extensive nosology of known diseases (as determined by the WHO), for example. They can be classified by organ system (e.g., pulmonary or gastrointestinal); by pathological process (e.g., cancer or trauma); by symptoms (e.g., angina or dysuria); by disease vector (e.g., infectious or parasitic); by geographical location (e.g., tropical or wilderness); and by social or population effects (e.g., communicable or interpersonal). Of course, many diseases can be classified in multiple ways. The basic rationale for a nosology of disease is to provide a framework for medical research and practice [20]. Sometimes, this is not as helpful as we would hope [20], but that is not a subject for this book. Usually, the disease classification serves the need of the healthcare provider or researcher in their ability to predict patient outcomes.

Smart [18] argues that diseases should be "individuated" by their causes. I have dedicated Chap. 5 to understanding causation concepts, and it is in this setting of disease classification by cause that causal attribution becomes increasingly important. This can be considered the "ontological conception" of disease, such that distinguishing between the kinds of disease requires distinguishing between the kinds of "pathogen" within the patient as the identity of the disease is fixed entirely by the entity causing the disease [21]. This is in conjunction with the "monocausal model" which states that every disease has a necessary and circumstantially sufficient cause, and by this logic ensures (or nearly enough for practical purposes) that it will have a most one such cause [22]. Although, *prima facie*, this is naïve as it is well known that many diseases have more than one cause, what is meant is that *in toto* there is a single sequence of causal attribution for a given disease in a given patient. This is context, numerous causal conditions work jointly to create a sufficient causal sequence for the disease, which is a "multifactorial account."

Smart [18] then proposes a "Causal Classification of Disease," which, he emphasizes, is not an account of the causes disease but an account of how to individuate one disease from another. The main claim of this account is that diseases can be individuated by a "disjunction of conjunctions." That is, there is a conjunction of events (i.e., causal attribution) that leads to a disease; this conjunction of events is unique and different from other conjunctions of events for other diseases, i.e., there exists a disjunction between them, so that the diseases are unique and individuated. To this Smart adds the concept of "Dispositional Metaphysics of Disease," which states that from an ontological viewpoint, diseases are constituted by the simultaneous manifestation of reciprocal disposition partners. That is, the patient will have certain "predispositions" to allow for the "cause" of the disease to start the causal sequence leading to the disease within the patient. For Smart [18], therefore, the combination of the Causal Classification of Disease with the Disposition Metaphysics of Disease provides the "full-cause" of the disease and how to differentiate among diseases. I would say that this corresponds well to the disease-patient illustration of Fig. 6.1.

Although this framework was developed to account for diseases already known to medicine, as this chapter pertains to the generation and acceptance of new medical knowledge, the framework is applicable to the identification of "new" (or, perhaps more correctly, previously unidentified) diseases.

6.4.3 Identification of New Diseases

Humans, and probably all other living beings, exist in a constantly changing environment. This environment includes the physio-chemical milieu of the atmosphere, water and land (e.g., pollutants) or changes in other living organisms through evolution (e.g., microorganisms). As humans interact with these changes, the potential for a novel causal sequence leading to a new disease can occur. Recognition of this new disease and its causal attribution is creating new medical knowledge. New diseases are almost never recognized *en masse*, but rather, through reports of "unusual" case reports.

The Function of the Case Report in Medical Epistemology

Several medical journals publish case reports, and there are even a few now dedicated to publishing case reports.[6] These reports typically present unusual, rare or "never previously reported" cases [23]. These reports, when they truly present the "never before seen" case, can be seminal observations. Medical knowledge, ultimately, is derived from such observations [24]. Why are these, then, seminal observations? Medicine, like all sciences, is based on theories [12]. I will discuss Schaffner's account of biomedical theories later in this chapter. For now, however, observations of phenomena must "fit" into the explanatory framework of the theory. Kuhn [25] describes the "normal" aspects of scientific investigation as follows:

1. The class of facts that the paradigm (or theory) has shown to be particularly revealing of the nature of things.
2. The class of facts that can be compared directly with predictions from the paradigm.

[6] For example, the Journal of Surgical Case Reports, Journal of Medical Case Reports, ACS Case Reviews in Surgery, and BMJ Case Reports are just a few of the journals that publish case reports as their primary focus.

3. The class of investigations undertaken to resolve some of the paradigm's residual ambiguities and permit the solution of problems to which it had previously only drawn attention.

In this view, the theory predicts or explains particular observable phenomena. In Kuhn's parlance, this is "normal science." Tension occurs when there is an observed phenomenon that is not predicted or explained by the theory. This is what the case report does—it may be that the observation is unexplained by the extant medical theories and, therefore, may represent a new disease. The next section will present a brief history of one such new disease.

Acquired Immunodeficiency Syndrome/Human Immunodeficiency Virus

Acquired immunodeficiency syndrome (AIDS) and the subsequent discovery of human immunodeficiency virus (HIV) are good examples of the characterization of a new disease. The following account is based on the histories published by Gallo and Montagneir [26] and Greene [27]. Table 6.1 provides a timeline of the salient scientific biomedical events.[7]

The first case reports of young homosexual men with opportunistic lung infection caused by *Pneumocystis carinii* and rare skin malignancy, Kaposi's sarcoma, occurred in the summer of 1981. Both of these disease entities were exceptionally rare, and in the case of pneumocystis pneumonia, they were unheard of in immunocompetent individuals [28]. These cases did not fit the paradigm for these types of infections or malignancies. Because of this discordance with accepted theory at the time, this led to recognition that this may be a new disease process. As the cause was unknown, it was recognized by a syndrome with a constellation of findings, not only the previously mentioned opportunistic infections and rare malignancies but also "wasting" and the "young old" appearance. In 1982, it was bestowed the name AIDS by the United States Centers for Disease Control, based not on causation but on clinical presentation. This is a form of disease nosology that will be addressed below. Additionally, that year, the transmission was determined through epidemiological investigations, which were based on the probabilistic causal attribution model discussed in the last chapter. These included sexual intercourse and direct introduction into an individual's blood stream by either contaminated blood transfusions or contaminated needles. Much effort was spent to try to identify the causative agent leading to the pathogenesis of the disease. In 1984, the breakthrough of identifying a retrovirus in lymphoid tissue isolates of infected patients led to the determination that this was the infectious causative agent. Note how this fits quite well with Smart's Casual Classification of Disease (the viral introduction into the individual) and his Dispositional Metaphysics of Disease (the activities that predisposed these individuals to have the virus

[7] There were, of course, momentous social and political events around AIDS activities. These are beyond the scope of this book. However, Greene [27] does provide a nice account of these as well.

Table 6.1 The timeline of AIDS/HIV discoveries as an example of acceptance of new medical knowledge[a]

Year	Event	Medical knowledge concept
1981	First cases of a new immunodeficiency diseases associated with unusual opportunistic infections and malignancy (Kaposi's sarcoma)	Case reports identifying a disease syndrome not accounted for in existing medical theories
1982	Transmission by sexual contact and direct introduction in to blood stream documented	Beginning process of causal attribution at individual and population level
1982	Disease named "acquired immunodeficiency syndrome" by the United States Centers for Disease Control	Disease nosology in the absence of cause
1984	Retrovirus isolated from a "pre-AIDS" patient	Proposal of causative mechanism at cellular level
1984	This virus determined to be the viral "cause" of AIDS	Further evidence of causative mechanism
1985	Blood test for the "AIDS" virus approved by United States Food and Drug Administration	Causal attribution for predictability
1985	Genome of the "AIDS" virus reported	Further evidence of causal attribution
1986	The "AIDS" virus renamed from LAV and HTLV-III to the human immunodeficiency virus (HIV) by the International Committee of the Taxonomy of Viruses	Increasing precision of terms for use in research and clinical practice
1986	Three viral enzymes identified as essential in the replication of the virus	Causal attribution used to identify therapeutic targets
1987	AZT approved to target HIV reverse transcriptase as a therapeutic target	Therapy based on causal attribution
Years following and continuing	Continued identification of additional cellular receptors, patient-level risk and protective factors, and therapies and public health policies based on laboratory experiments, observational data and clinical trials	Continued inter-level and inter-field production of new medical knowledge as part of "normal" science

[a] Adapted from Greene [27]

introduced into their bloodstreams[8]) [18]. In 1985, a blood test for the virus was approved by the United States Food and Drug Administration. This allowed for improved diagnostic accuracy and, therefore, predictability. Additionally, that year, the RNA genome for the virus was sequenced. This allowed for the

[8] I want to be clear here that by this statement, I do not intend to infer any blame on these individuals for contracting AIDS. Of course, at the time, the disease was new and completely unknown. Therefore, their actions were not conscious activities knowingly infecting themselves or others. Of course, at the time, there was no blood test for the virus in the blood donated for transfusion; hence, those who became infected that way were also blameless. Subsequent public health efforts educating on safe sex practices and donor-specific blood speak to responsible behavior once these activities were identified as potentially transmitting disease.

possibility of finding therapeutic targets. In 1986, the virus, which until that time was referred to as the LAV or HTLV-III virus, was renamed by the International Committee of the Taxonomy of Viruses as the human immunodeficiency virus (HIV). This allowed for the development of a unified theory of the disease. Additionally, that year, three viral enzymes were identified as therapeutic targets due to their importance in viral replication. In 1987, AZT was approved as a treatment targeting the virus's reverse transcriptase enzyme. With this, the paradigm shift in theory was complete. Subsequent years had continued identification of additional T-cell surface receptors that were associated with viral access to the cell, patient factors that determine infection risk, and additional therapeutics, such as HAART therapy, which have turned AIDS from a universally fatal disease to a manageable chronic condition. In other words, this was now a theory in which Kuhn's "normal science" was functioning.

Although I have admittedly given a very abridged version of the history of AIDS as a manifestation of a new disease to now being incorporated into accepted biomedical theory, the illustrative point of how a new disease is recognized, then the causal sequence determined and attributed, with the main goals of predictability and identifying therapeutic targets is what is of importance.

6.4.4 Practical Clinical Knowledge

Natural History

The natural history of a disease is the course that the disease would have taken within the patient if no intervention occurred. Most of these descriptions come from older sources and have been enshrined in medical textbooks. It is presently unusual for a physician to observe the natural history of a disease if an effective therapeutic intervention is available. The only occasions where such an observation would occur is in those many diseases that are "self-limiting," meaning that the natural history is such that recovery is assured without intervention, for example, the common cold (although the alleviation of symptoms may be affected by treatment, the disease, itself, is not); if the disease is so far advanced that all forms of treatment are futile, for example, a patient with end-stage, metastatic cancer; or, last, if a patient refuses treatment. The only times where we see new medical knowledge generated in this realm is when a new disease is recognized, as in the cases of AIDS noted above.

Etiology

Etiology is the purported causative origin(s) or agent(s) of the disease. Identification of the etiology is considered of paramount importance as therapeutic interventions are generally directed toward eliminating the agent. For example, in the history of

AIDS, the etiological agent was determined to be HIV. However, there are numerous classes of etiological agents, from genetic alternations to environmental toxins. Many diseases have yet to have their etiologies be completely elucidated, such as Alzheimer's disease. Therefore, there is a great effort to determine the etiologies for many disease processes.

Pathogenesis

Pathogenesis is a description of how an etiological agent transforms the normal homeostatic mechanisms of the individual into the disease's pathological manifestations. The pathogenesis of AIDS includes the virus's abilities to enter a specific type of T-cell (CD4), which inactivates the cell's ability to provide the host a part of its immunological defense. This then leads to the ability of other opportunistic infections and malignancies to take root and lead to additional illness. The examples of cancer causation in the last chapter were truly elucidations of cancer pathogenesis. New knowledge is continually sought for this area of understanding disease.

Disease Incidence and Prevalence

Incidence is how often the disease occurs within a population, while prevalence is how many individuals within a population have the disease. Understanding incidence and prevalence are inherently probabilistic tasks of epidemiology. This is a stochastic form of knowledge, in that one is determining the frequency of the disease occurring in a given population over a given period of time (e.g., 5 per 100,000 individuals per year) or the frequency of an individual with the disease at a given time point (e.g., 500 per 100,000 individuals in 2020). This information is valuable for public health and health policy.

Risk Factors

A risk factor is a physiological, anatomical, genetic, mental, or behavioral predisposition to contracting a disease. This is what Smart [18] refers to as the dispositional metaphysics of disease. That is, using a counterfactual account, if the risk factor were not present, the individual would be less likely to contract the disease. As with incidence and prevalence, these are mostly probabilistic accounts, although there are examples of deterministic risk factors, for example Huntington's disease or a self-inflicted gunshot to the head. Much of what is published in the medical literature has to do with risk factors, with the goal of predictability and possible prevention by eliminating or mitigating the risk factor.

The Diagnostic Process

The diagnostic process, as exemplified in the clinical vignette from Chap. 1, as well as the blood test for HIV, pertains to increasing the probability that the disease bestowed upon the patient by the physician is correct. This process consists initially of the history and physical examination, then later with other "objective" testing.

Diagnosis through signs and symptoms is the initial step in the process. According to Giglari [19], there are two types of diagnostic processes: a pathophysiological diagnosis, also referred to as a causal diagnosis, and a nosological diagnosis. A nosological diagnosis is a diagnosis based on the identification of a clinical presentation without the need to explain the underlying etiology or pathology. On the other hand, pathophysiological diagnosis is based on understanding the causal sequence of the disease. We can see with the example of AIDS above that the diagnosis evolved from a nosological diagnosis (recognition of opportunistic infections/malignancies in immunocompromised patients of unknown cause) to a causal diagnosis (identification of HIV within the patient with blood tests). In both instances, medical knowledge is generated and then incorporated into the physician's cognition and metacognition (Fig. 1.1). More on how nosological diagnosis and pathophysiological diagnosis are applied in practice in Chap. 7.

After the history and physical examination, the physician orders tests. Although frequently in casual medical parlance, one will hear that the test "confirmed" a diagnosis, that is not often the case. Some tests absolutely can confirm a diagnosis, for example, a biopsy that on histology is a malignancy or the exploratory laparotomy that revealed the perforated ulcer. Nevertheless, it is more likely that the test increases or decreases the probability that the disease is present, usually consistent with Bayes's theorem. Diagnostic tests generally require a significant amount of research and, at least in the United States, require regulatory approval. This then becomes part of the physician's meta-cognition of evidence of theory (Fig. 1.1).

Therapeutic Intervention

After diagnosis, therapeutic intervention is another *sine qua non* of the clinical practice of medicine. Much medical research is dedicated to identifying therapeutic targets, and once these targets are identified, interventions can be developed to affect these targets. These targets can be anatomical, physiological, or molecular. Some interventions have been used for centuries, while newer interventions are continuously being tested.

Prevention of Disease

Disease prevention has been an undertaking of humans for some time [29]. The notion of prevention as a public health need was a consequence of the recognition of sanitation in mitigating the transmission of disease [30]. It is now an ingrained part of medical practice. It is a continuing area of medical research.

I do not intend to provide examples of all of these types of knowledge, only to inform the reader of the breadth of medical knowledge sought.

6.5 Medical Theories as a Starting Point for New Knowledge

Medicine, as a scientific discipline, contains a very large set of theories. Although the term "theory" can be vague (the *Merriam-Webster Dictionary* has six definitions [31]), what I think best encompasses what scientists think of when they think of theories is a coherent set of concepts that when taken together explain observed phenomena. Schaffner [12], whom I have quoted before, provides a very nice account of theories in biology and medicine. One of his important concepts is that the reason there are no "scientific laws" in biology, at least not in the deterministic sense as, say, classical physics, is because organisms and their environments are so complex that an identification and enumeration of all relevant factors in making such a law make it just too impractical a task. Moreover, there is even a debate on whether or not a theory can be considered "true" in a realism sense—that is, do theories actually correspond to something "real" in the universe, or are they just semantic constructs to help us explain observations or make predictions. Nevertheless, if all they are is the latter, this is still immensely helpful. In this sense, scientific "facts" are "socially constructed" by the interaction of the methods of observation and what is observed by the scientist. Therefore, there are some semantics involved in how words present phenomena and processes.

A brief word about the difference between theories and models. It appears at times that these two concepts are used interchangeably. However, I would like to make clear at least how I define and use them. A model is a mental representation of mechanisms of the occurrences of specific phenomena, while a theory is a bounded set of propositions, which may include models, to explain and predict the occurrences of these phenomena, including causal attribution.

Schaffner [12] further goes on to assert his idea of "generalized empiricism." There are several levels of control over the adequacy of scientific hypotheses and theories:

1. The scope of direct experimental or observational evidence.
2. The scope of indirect experimental or observation evidence.
3. The theoretical support (or, possibly, inter-theoretical discord).
4. Conformity to certain methodological desiderata such as simplicity and unity of science.

Theoretical terms do have meaning, but because they have meaning, that does not ensure their actual existence in the universe. They are, after all, the inventions from the imaginations of humans. This is an important point, in that, as will be discussed below and in the example of AIDS/HIV above, biomedical scientists at times have to create words and concepts to bridge the medical knowledge gap. These words and concepts will only have practical meaning if they provide a causal sequence that leads to improvement in predictability.

We must accept that all our observations of the phenomena in the universe are interpreted by us because of the theories that we already know and the models that we have created. That is, the facts never "speak for themselves," everything requires an interpretation. This is what Hanson [32] means when he says that all observations are "theory-laden," and there is no such thing as seeing with the "naked-eye" such that an individual can observe the world and report their observations completely objectively. To be able to report the observations requires a baseline understanding of the world. The world exists without independent meaning understandable to us. We provide meaning through our theories (scientific, social and cultural).

As Schaffner [12] further avers, it is not only the background theory but also various experimental (or observational) results and low-level generalizations that may not yet be systematized into any theory nor a part of any one specific theory that serve as parts of a premise set from which an inference into a new theory or hypothesis is made. That is, it will look something like:

Background theory

+

Experimental/observational results and/or low-level generalizations

≠

Not compatible

↓

New Hypothesis

The new hypothesis is generated through a cognitive process of abduction (discussed below) and creativity. This is illustrated by the example of AIDS presented above.

In the previous chapter, I presented Schaffner's observation of the "interlevel" and "interfield" construction of biomedical theories. In this, theories will frequently use concepts at different levels of physio-chemical or biological organization (atoms, molecules, organelles, cells, organs, organisms, population, etc.) and different fields (physics, chemistry, biology, ecology, etc.). Ultimately, these theories are only valuable if they help explain (or make understandable) observed phenomena and, more importantly, can predict the occurrence of future phenomena (or, at least, the phenomena we appear to observe). Usually, although not always, these theories are a combination of both mechanistic (deterministic) and probabilistic causation. Again, as illustrated in the AIDS example.

6.6 How Gaps in Medical Knowledge Are Identified

Admittedly, a "gap" in knowledge is somewhat an ambiguous term. Therefore, to be more specific, I am referring to a break of sorts between what is known and what is unknown. Alternatively, when a set a premises does not lead to the observed conclusion. What needs to be emphasized is that this gap may have not even been recognized as existing until a researcher "sees" it, perhaps in a moment of inspiration. Often, the researchers themselves cannot explain how the insight occurred. In the example of AIDS given above, the gap was the observation of otherwise healthy males falling ill with profound immunodeficiency and the cause of such immunodeficiency. This is just one example, as there are other gaps as well. The most common gap seen in the medical literature, in my opinion, is that between the outcomes of present treatment regimens and a better treatment regimen. This is an imagined gap, by which I mean that many believe already that the treatments we have are adequate. Someone has to believe that the method of treatment at present can be improved, and, hence, the gap.

In Chap. 2, I discussed abductive logic as espoused by Pierce. Simply speaking, a person recognizes that there are observations in existence (or an imagined existence in the future) that are in need of explanation. That person then infers a set of premises that would entail the existence of that observation. There has been a history of trying to understand the logic of scientific discovery, that is, how scientists generate new hypotheses to test. Schaffner gives a nice historical account, although the details of which are more than what is needed for this book. He finally quotes Hanson [33].

1. Some surprising, astonishing phenomena p_1, p_2, p_3, … are encountered
2. However, p_1, p_2, p_3, … would not be surprising were hypothesis of H's type to were to be true. They would follow as a matter of course from something like H and would be explained by it.
3. Therefore, there is good reason for elaborating a hypothesis of the type H; for proposing it as a possible hypothesis from whose assumption as true p_1, p_2, p_3, … might be explained.

As Schaffner notes, this appears identical to Pierce's abduction. However, the important point is the *recognition* of the gap *and* the creativity to *imagine* an explanation, which then becomes a hypothesis for testing, as was done with AIDS. In addition, unlike the basic physical sciences, but not unlike engineering, this gap can be simply a "better way of doing something." Here, the biomedical researcher must imagine a method, usually in the form of a treatment, which, when used, will lead to a causal sequence that will, most likely, result in an increased probability of a more favorable outcome for the patient. Once again, please note the epistemic counterfactual: since the imagined treatment is *not* used, our present (judged) poorer results are the consequence.

6.7 Hypothesis Development

All research is based on a hypothesis. That is, an idea that the researcher thinks is true *and* fills some gap in knowledge.[9] How a researcher (or group of researchers) comes up with this hypothesis is a matter of creativity, inspiration and intuition that probably the researcher themselves would not be able to explain. However, after the idea is generated, some form of abduction, as described above, must occur for the researcher to believe this new hypothesis is worth testing. That is, it must make some type of logical sense, whether from deduction, induction or informal logic.

Dragulinescu [34] calls this "inference to the best evidence." He starts by acknowledging that the predominate theory of scientific confirmation is the probabilistic theory, where the evidence raises the probability of the scientific conclusions being true, consistent with the theory of Bayes. However, there may be issues with probabilistic confirmation at times. For example, when the numerical data necessary for such Bayesian calculations are absent? (Quite frankly, as someone involved in medical research for over 40 years, I am not sure what these "numerical data" would be.) Going on, what if the sources of these data are not reliable [35]? In these types of settings, inference to the best evidence may be a viable alternative. Dragulinescu [34] emphasizes that inference to the best evidence and probabilistic theory are not competing but complementary. Moreover, inference to the best evidence should be consistent with probabilistic theory.

What inference to the best evidence entails is a method of confirming causal claims vis-à-vis medical evidence of the mechanism of causal attribution when scientists reason about choosing among potential hypotheses [34]. Psillos [36] provides the foundational concepts that we should choose the theory that best fits with the relevant background knowledge (consilience), explains more evidence or the total of it (completeness), does justice to the most important parts of the evidence (importance), makes use of fewer assumptions (parsimony), provides a unitary explanation for the diversity of evidence (unification) and articulates a mechanism when explaining (precision). This approach, although somewhat vague, seems consistent with what actual biomedical scientists do.

It is not enough to have imagined a potential hypothesis to account for a gap in medical knowledge; the research actually must create a coherent argument that this hypothesis is plausible and worth pursuing. This is what I have called the "Argument of the Hypothesis" [37]. This is generally the purpose of the "Introduction" section of the article or manuscript. (For those unfamiliar with the organization of a typical "original submission" medical research manuscript, there are usually four main sections: The "Introduction," which provides the background knowledge and theory of the knowledge gap to be addressed with the hypothesis that was tested; the "Methods

[9] This criterion of "filling some gap in knowledge" is not to exclude studies with the purpose of replicating prior studies. The scientific literature is replete with experiments and observations that have later been debunked by additional studies trying to replicate the first.

and Materials," which provides the actual methods that were used to produce the data which then become premises for the researchers argument in relation to the hypothesis; the "Results," which present the actual data; and the "Discussion" in which the researcher uses the data as premises in conjunction with existing knowledge and theory to refute or increase the probably truth of the hypothesis.) The research will gather extant knowledge (information and/or data), as well as the pertinent theory or theories, to construct an argument with its ultimate conclusion being the hypothesis to be tested.

6.7.1 An Example of an Argument of the Hypothesis

Because of the clinical vignette in Chap. 1 having to do with a patient with heartburn related to GERD, the randomized, controlled trial of medical versus surgical management of refractory heartburn seemed *apropos* as an example of an argument of the hypothesis. In the "Introduction" of their article, Spechler et al. [38] developed their argument. I will not quote the five-paragraph introduction word for word but paraphrase and order the salient premises of the argument:

Paragraph 1

1. The extent of GERD is a problem, both socially and financially.
2. Thirty percent of patients on proton pump inhibitors (PPIs) will have persistent heartburn symptoms.
3. Only 58% of patients on PPIs are completely satisfied with their treatment.

Paragraph 2

4. There are five possible mechanisms by which heartburn is refractory to PPIs:
   (a) The patient's abnormal acid reflux persisted despite PPI therapy.
   (b) The patient has reflux hypersensitivity such that even with normal acid exposure, "physiologic" reflux episodes (acidic and nonacidic) evoke heartburn.
   (c) The patient may have non-GERD esophageal disorders, e.g., achalasia.
   (d) The patient may have a nonesophageal disorder causing heartburn, e.g., cardiac disease.
   (e) The patient may have functional heartburn.[10]

Paragraph 3

5. For patients with persistent reflux-related symptoms (#4a and 4b, above), there is no proven medical therapy, with all available therapies based on expert opinion.

---

[10] Recall how these possibilities were carefully evaluated by our clinician in Chap. 1.

Paragraph 4

6. Antireflux surgery should improve symptoms of heartburn because it will eliminate both acid and nonacid reflux.
7. Antireflux surgery may not improve symptoms due to the following:
   (a) The cause of symptoms was not confirmed to be due to acid reflux.
   (b) Surgery was performed in patients with functional heartburn whose heartburn was not due to reflux.

Paragraph 5

8. Multichannel intraluminal impedance (MII)-pH monitoring may distinguish PPI-refractory patients from non-GERD patients.
9. MII-pH monitoring was not agreed upon by experts for patient selection for antireflux surgery.

Hypothesis (to quote word for word), "…if non-GERD and functional disorders were excluded by systematic work-up, then antireflux surgery would be superior to medical therapy for patients with PPI unresponsive heartburn that MII-pH monitoring identifies as being reflux-related."

Let us evaluate the illative core of this argument. I will place side by side a logical restatement of the premises with my interpretation of the premises paragraph by paragraph:

Premises	Interpretation
1. There exists a disease, D, such that D produces symptoms, S, and is a major health problem	D requires an effective treatment
2. Some patients with D treated with medication M will continue to suffer from S	M is not an effective treatment for all patients with D
3. Some patients with D treated with M with or without S will not be satisfied with treatment M	The conjunction of premise 2 and 3 demonstrated that M is not a universally satisfactory treatment of D (a treatment gap is identified
4. There exists a subset of patients with D, P_S, with persistent S on M. There are 5 causes of S in P_S, with 2 subsets of P_S, such that S is related to D, and 3 subsets such that S is related to not-D.	Causal attribution subset identified
5. For patients in P_S, there are no alternative medical treatments for M	Identification of a subset treatment gap
6. There exists a treatment A that negates D	Potential alternative treatment to M based on causal attribution derived therapeutic target
7. There exists a subset of P_S treated with A with persistent S, such that A would negate S, P_{SA}, if P_{SA} can be identified	A is not a universally satisfactory treatment for all P_S. Additional subset treatment gap identified, with implicit treatment population target identified
8. There exists a test, T, which may identify P_{SA}	Predictive method potentially identified

Premises	Interpretation
9. T not definitively proved to be predictive of P_{SA}	Diagnostic gap identified which is needed for predictive purposes. This now identifies a medical knowledge gap for a very specific problem
Conclusion from background premises: For P_S a treatment gap exists For the subset of patients, P_{SA}, a treatment gap exists For the subset of patients, P_{SA}, a diagnostic gap exists	The main conclusions of the illative core identifying treatment and diagnostic gaps in a group of patients, requiring closure.
Hypothesis from abduction: For T-identified P_{SA}, such that S in P_{SA} patients treated with A, $P_{SA}(S\|A)$ is less than S in P_{SA} patients treated with M, $P_{SA}(S\|M)$, or, more formally, $P_{SA}(S\|A) < P_{SA}(M\|A)$	Treatment based on predictability of T to identified the groups of patients most likely to have improved S with A

Therefore, in this argument, the authors identified a treatment gap in the population of patients with heartburn, which is a substantial health care issue. The standard medical therapy fails a substantial portion of patients (they give prevalence of 30% with persistent symptoms and 42% dissatisfied, to support this claim). They identify that there are 5 causal subgroups for these patients in the treatment gap, with only two related to a specific disease that is the therapeutic target of the medication. (Left unsaid, the 3 other subsets of patients have also identified one or more treatment gap(s), but those patients are not the subjects of this study.) Surgical treatment based on the causal attribution of patients in these two subgroups has been identified, yet this surgical treatment is not universally successful in relieving symptoms. This failure could be because the surgical treatment is applied to patients outside this subset and therefore would be predictably ineffective. This is another treatment gap specifically for this subset of patients. To better apply the surgical treatment, identification of the subset of patients in whom the treatment would address the cause of the symptoms would reduce the failure rate. This is a diagnostic gap, with the aim of improving predictability. There is a test which does just that, but not all agree as to its predictive value for this purpose because of lack of evidence. This identified a gap in medical knowledge for now a very specific problem. Therefore, proving that surgical treatment is superior to medical treatment in this narrow subset of patients would provide such evidence.

My assertion is that all medical research articles that purport to create new knowledge will (or should) have such an argument for their hypothesis. That is, the researcher needs to justify why we should believe why a medical knowledge gap exists and why the hypothesis is plausible.

6.8 Argument of the Experimental Protocol

Once the hypothesis is asserted, the researcher must now devise a study to produce data (that is, additional premises) that have some relation to the hypothesis to either refute the hypothesis or increase the confidence that the hypothesis is true. This is what I have called the "Argument of the Experimental Protocol" [37]. I use the term "experimental" in the broad sense of either gathering information through observations or creating new information through conscious manipulation of relevant factors in the subjects in question, that is, experiments. To better understand how this is constructed, we must first understand the armamentarium of study design types, the data that they create and how the data are analyzed.

6.8.1 Types of Studies

There are many types of study design methods from which new medical knowledge is generated. The following will be a brief overview of the types and the information that is produced. These study designs are generally divided into "observational" and "interventional" designs [39]. Again, for the purposes of the argument of the experimental protocol, I view all of these types as "experimental."

Observational

Observational studies entail a researcher "observing" phenomena while not actively trying to control the environment in which the phenomena occur. That is, they are not experimenting. The data they gather about the phenomena has already occurred, or will occur as part of the natural history, and they try to associate other occurrences of different phenomena to determine possible causal attribution. By their very nature, these studies are stochastic and probabilistic. However, how they are designed bears great weight on the voracity of their conclusions. A list and description of these types of study designs follows (Tables 6.2 and 6.3) [39]:

Ecological Study Design

This type of study compares clusters of people, usually grouped based on geographical location or temporal associations, then assigns one exposure level (a potential causal agent) for each distinct group and can provide a rough estimation of disease prevalence.

Proportional Mortality Ratio Design

This type of study utilizes the distinctly-defined, well-recorded outcome of death and subsequent records that are maintained regarding the decedent to be able to identify potential relationships between exposures, for example, geographical location, occupation, or age and cause of death.

Table 6.2 Observational study design: strengths and weaknesses[a]

Study design	Strengths	Weaknesses
Ecological	Easy to assign exposure levels	Inaccuracy of data Inability to control for confounders
Proportional mortality ratio	Death outcome well captured	Utilizes deaths only Inaccuracy of data (death certificates) Inability to control for confounders
Case-crossover cohort	Reduces some types of biases Good for acute health outcomes with a defined exposure Cases act as their own controls	Selection of comparison time point difficult Prone to recall bias No demonstrated temporality
Cross-sectional cohort	Individualized data Ability to control for multiple confounders Can assess multiple outcomes	No temporality Not good for rare diseases Poor for diseases of short duration
Case-control	Individualized data Ability to control for multiple confounders Good for rare diseases Can assess multiple exposures	Cannot calculate prevalence Can only assess one outcome Poor selection of controls can introduce bias No demonstrated temporality
Retrospective and prospective cohort	Temporality demonstrated Individualized data Ability to control for multiple confounders Can assess multiple exposures Can assess multiple outcomes	Not good for rare diseases

[a] Adapted from Thiese M. Observational and interventional study design types; an overview. Biochem Medica 2014;24:199–210

Table 6.3 Standards for study design and reporting[a]

Guideline name
Consolidated Standards of Reporting Trials (CONSORT)
Strengthening the Reporting of Observational Studies in Epidemiology (STROBE)
Standards for Reporting Studies of Diagnostic Accuracy (STAD)
Quality Assessment of Diagnostic Accuracy Studies (QUADAS)
Preferred Reporting Items for Systematic Reviews and Meta-Analyses (PRISMA)
Consolidated Criteria for Reporting Qualitative Research (COREQ)
Statistical Analysis and Methods in the Published Literature (SAMPL)
Consensus-Based Clinical Case Reporting Guideline Development (CARE)
Standards for Quality Improvement Reporting Excellence (SQUIRE)
Consolidated Health Economic Evaluation Reporting Standards (CHEERS)
Enhancing Transparency in Reporting the Synthesis of Qualitative Research (ENTREQ)

[a] Adapted from Thiese M. Observational and interventional study design types; an overview. Biochem Medica 2014;24:199–210

Case-Crossover Study Design

This type of study uses the individual to act as their own control for comparison issues. Cases are assessed for their exposure status immediately prior to the time they become a case and then compared to their exposure at a point where they did not become a case.

Cross-Sectional (Prevalence) Study Design

This type of study assesses a population by a study sample at a single point in time to measure the prevalence of the outcome in question.

Case–Control Study Design

This type of study design compares groups with and without the exposure for the outcome in question while matching for as many confounding variables as possible.

Cohorts

This type of study design includes subjects based on exposure status and assesses the outcome of interest [39]. There are a variety of these types of studies, and the above study designs can also be considered cohort studies. The different types of cohort studies include the following:

Retrospective. In retrospective studies, the cohort has already experienced the exposure and may or may not have experienced the outcome of interest. This type of study is based on a review of existing records. It is subject to several types of bias, mostly based on how precisely the exposure, the level of exposure and the outcome were recorded.

Prospective. In prospective studies, the cohort with the exposure of interest is identified, and then this cohort is followed into the future for the occurrence of the outcome of interest. This has the advantage of being able to precisely record both the exposure and the outcome, thereby reducing the potential errors that retrospective studies may suffer.

Single cohort. These may be either retrospective or prospective studies of a single group of subjects. Although this can provide information on the occurrence of the outcome of interests, there is no comparator group. These are sometimes referred to as "case series."

Cohort comparisons. As with the single cohort, these can be either retrospective or prospective studies. However, more than one cohort is studied for comparative purposes, i.e., two or more. The advantage of these types of studies is that some information is provided comparing two or more exposure levels.

Observational studies, for the most part, are stochastic studies using probabilistic causal attribution, although not exclusively. The most concerning issue with observational studies is the validity of the study [40]. Grimes and Schulz [40] identify two types of validity: internal and external. Issues in internal validity include biases such as selection bias, information bias, and confounding, which are present to some degree in all observational studies. Attempts to mitigate these biases are usually made with choice of statistical methods, more on this below. External validity has to do with the ability to generalize from the study to actual patients in clinical practice. This will be further addressed in Chap. 7.

Interventional

Interventional studies are experiments. The group of patients with a particular disease is subjected to an intervention, and the effects of that intervention on the disease process are measured as the outcome. By their very nature, these studies are prospective, with the population of interest (individuals with the disease) chosen, the exposure (intervention) controlled, and the outcome of interest carefully recorded.

Pre-Post Study Design

This type of study measures the occurrence of an outcome before and again after a particular intervention [39].

Nonrandomized Trial Study Design

This type of study compares a group where the intervention was performed with a group where the intervention was not performed [39]. Importantly, in this type of design, the individuals in the group chose whether to have the intervention; that is, whether they received the intervention was not randomly allocated.

Randomized, Controlled Trial Study Design

In this type of study design, a "homogenous" group of individuals is randomly divided into groups with an independent randomization process assigning which individuals will receive the intervention which will not. The purpose is to ensure as much as possible that the potential confounding factors are evenly distributed between the groups so that any difference between them is due to the intervention [39].

Cross-Over Randomized, Controlled Trial Study Design

This type of study design is the same as the randomized, controlled trial design, except at some time point, the individuals who did not receive the are allowed to "crossover" and receive the treatment. In this way, they act as their own control group and to act as a control of sort with the individuals initially receiving treatment because any difference between the groups will disappear if the difference was in fact due to treatment. In some types of interventions, the group that initially received the treatment will have to treatment stopped if they showed an improvement in their disease. If they returned to their baseline status, then the change is additional evidence that the treatment was the cause of their improvement.

Laboratory Study Designs

These types of studies would be considered "classic" experiments. They include a wide range of materials and methods, such as molecular biology, tissue culture, animal experimentation, and even human experimentation under very strict conditions. Recently, these types of experiments have used advanced computer simulations, such as decision analyses and artificial intelligence. There is now the concept of "translational" research, with the specific purpose of using the conclusions of these types of studies to generate human-based studies. Much of the philosophy of science and biology is in understanding these types of experiments and the theories underlying them. I chose not to address these types of studies, as most of the practical medical literature published and used clinicians are of the observation and interventional types.

6.9 Types of Data

To be specific, what I mean when I refer to "data" is the information generated by the observational, interventional and experimental methods. This information is generally quantitative in some manner, although there is a whole methodology of "qualitative" research that attempts to analyze the nonquantitative responses of their human subjects. This is a quite active and fruitful methodology that does eventually quantitize their data. I will not address it further here.

Frequency (Categorical). Frequency data are an enumeration of the number of phenomena occurring by the total number of episodes that the phenomena could have potentially occurred for a particular period of time. This is also referred to as "categorical" data because the data are from specific categories of subjects. These phenomena are usually, but not exclusively, categorial events or objects. The general formula is the number of events/total number of subjects at risk. For example, if one observes 8 surgical site infections in 64 patients after a particular operation, the frequency is 8/64 = 0.125. When this is multiplied by 100, we then obtain a percentage of 12.5%, which is often how frequently data are reported in medical research articles.

Of course, when a researcher observes that "12.5% of patients developed a surgical site after an appendectomy," this is an absolute correct account of that particular group of patients at that particular time and location. However, a historical account of one particular group of patients at a particular time and location is not the aim of the research. The researchers want to use that frequency as an estimate of the probability of future similar patients suffering a surgical site infection.

There are many issues with this which I will address, but for now, I want to address the issue of frequencies used as point estimates of probability. Probability is based on the following foundation: The event in question is inherently stochastic, or, at least, not all the causal sequence is known to make it deterministic; and probability of the event occurring is an intrinsic property of the event, that is, its probability (or chance) of occurrence is an inseparable feature of the event. For example, a "fair" coin, when flipped without skill,[11] has a 50% chance (0.5 probability) of landing heads. This 50–50 chance is an intrinsic property of the coin, unless the coin is manipulated in some way. Let us assume a world where coins do not have the inherent property of a 50–50 chance of turning up heads. For example, some coins could be 60–40, others 90–10, etc. However, if we find ourselves with a coin and we do not know what its inherent probability of landing heads *a priori* is, how can we determine this? This is done by flipping the coin a certain number of times and counting the number of times it comes- up head, that is, the frequency of heads in a particular sample of flips. If this is done over many flips over a long period of time, this is called the "long-run frequency," and this frequency is a point estimate of the actual intrinsic probability property of the phenomenon.

Hacking [41] quotes the von Mises definition as follows:

The frequency or probability for any kind of event E from the collective group K (containing k number of individual events/items/observations, etc.) is considered the proportion of times in which events of this kind occurs in the first n members of K (where $n < k$). Call this $P_n(E)$. If $P_n(E)$ approaches a limit as n becomes large *without bound* (emphasis mine, that is, as n approaches k), it represents the limit by P(E). This is the probability property of the collective K. Presumably, it is a property of some part of the world that it would generate a collective with certain P(E) for some E. Hacking [41] emphasizes that P(E) is von Mises's explication of frequency in the long run.

There are points worth emphasizing. When speaking of collectives, n is a sample of the entire population K. We frequently do not know how well n represents K. It is K that has the property of P(E), and each member, k, presumably will either be or not be the event. However, this is not known *a priori*; therefore, we assign the event a P(E) chance of occurring. However, because P(E) is unknown, and the frequency

[11] What I mean here is that the person flipping the coin has not determined a way to flip the coin just to reliably land heads. Although I would imagine this to be a very difficult skill to acquire, it is not impossible to believe that it could be.

of the event in the sample is a point estimate of the probability. For example, I performed a computer simulation of randomly generating the numbers 0 and 1, with each a 0.5 frequency of occurring, that is, "a flip of a fair coin." Figure 6.2 shows the results of the simulation of the first 100 flips. We see that there is variation in the point estimates of P(E) = 0.5 which does approach, but only infrequently actually give 0.5. When the simulation was taken to 1000 flips, 0's occurred in 51.3% of the flips (i.e., a frequency of 0.513). To continue, when taken to 10,000 flips, 0's still predominated at 50.65%. That is, after 10,000 flips, there were 130 more 0's than 1's, even though the *a priori* probability would have predicted no difference. If I performed the simulation again, most likely I would get slightly different results. Therefore, it is unlikely that in any actual series of observations, a sample would approach the "without bound" criteria of von Mizes. However, this is the best that any researcher can do and is a natural bound of medical knowledge.

Continuous Data. Continuous data, as the name suggests, are data on a continuum. Such data include measures such as weight, height, hemoglobin level, etc. This type of data can be envisioned as a "number line," with the "space" in between the number having meaning. For example, the space between 1 and 2, it also contains the numbers 1.4 and 1.5. Between these, there are the numbers 1.45 and 1.46, and between these, 1.452 and 1.453, *ad infinitum*. However, when collecting continuous data, each datum is discrete. Moreover, this datum is a property of the phenomenon being observed. However, how much this value represents an intrinsic property is quite different than frequency as a point estimate of probabilities. Let us take the example of weight. Everything on Earth that has mass has a weight. Therefore, weight is an intrinsic property of everything with mass on Earth. However, if an object has a weight of 5 kilograms, 5 kg is a property of that individual object, but is it an intrinsic property of all such objects? If we take humans as an example, there is certainly no one weight that is an "intrinsic property" of humans. However, when one weighs a certain number of humans, these values

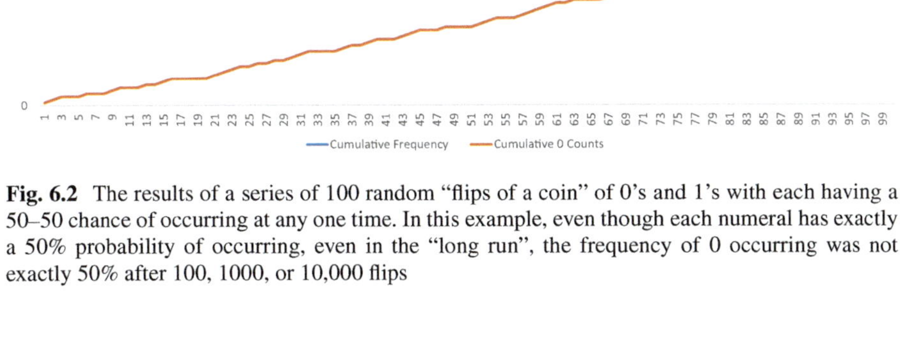

Fig. 6.2 The results of a series of 100 random "flips of a coin" of 0's and 1's with each having a 50–50 chance of occurring at any one time. In this example, even though each numeral has exactly a 50% probability of occurring, even in the "long run", the frequency of 0 occurring was not exactly 50% after 100, 1000, or 10,000 flips

provide some level of information about the average (or mean) weight of that group of humans. This information can then be applied to an individual or to a population. There are various ways that these data can be analyzed.

Ordinal. Ordinal data are numerical hierarchical categories but without meaning in between the categories. For example, cancers are commonly staged from 0 to 4, and each successive stage is defined by worsening disease. That is, stage 1 is more advanced than stage 0, and stage 2 is more advanced than stage 1. However, there is no such stage as stage 1.5, as the patient is either stage 1 or stage 2. As with continuous data, the ordinal rank tells us a great deal about the subject within that rank, but there is no intrinsic ordinal rank value that defines a population. Information that we obtain for a population is the distribution of the ranks for that population. There are various ways that these data can be analyzed.

Relationships/Correlations. Relationship data correlate the numeric values of one set of phenomena with the numeric values of another phenomena. In this manner, we can see how the values of one phenomenon change with the values of another phenomenon. This relationship can be either deterministic or probabilistic. These relationships can be determined at any level of biological organization. They can also be analyzed by various statistical methods.

6.9.1 Choice of Outcome to Be Measured

Of course, the purpose of the study is to generate data. However, this requires the researcher to identify what type of data can be used as premises in their eventual "Argument of the Hypothesis's Judgment" (described below). The outcome measured needs to be relevant to the hypothesis in some manner (recall the relevance criteria of Johnson for informal logic discussed in Chap. 2). How this relevance is determined is a matter of judgment of the researcher given the existence of the background information available and overarching biomedical theory, as asserted by Schaffner [12]. This choice is vitally important, as the acceptance of these data as premises in any subsequent argument by the researcher's audience will determine the persuasiveness of their argument.

In the study on medical versus surgical treatment of refractory heartburn mentioned above [38], these investigators have chosen several outcome endpoints, which is not unusual in medical studies. However, their main outcome measure was "treatment success", for which they had a very specific definition of "an improvement (decrease) in the GERD-HRQL[12] score by 50% from baseline to 12 months." Since the hypothesis was specific about the superiority of surgical to medical

[12] The GERD-HRQL is a patient-centered quality of life instrument that measures the severity of the typical symptoms of GERD. The best possible score is 0, and the worst possible score is 50. If a patient's score at baseline was 24 and at 12 months it was 12, then this would be a reduction of 50%.

treatment for refractory heartburn, a specific measure of heartburn severity is clearly relevant to the hypothesis.

6.9.2 Samples and Sample Representativeness

Ultimately, any medical research article is a type of logical induction (see Chap. 2) in that the researchers are inferring attributes to a general population (i.e., all individuals with a specific characteristic, in the case above, all patients with PPI refractory GERD) from examples of specific individuals (i.e., the sample of patients with refractory GERD who agreed to participate and completed the study). Using the notations of von Mises, K would be the collective of all patients with PPI refractory GERD. An important concept, however, is that in medical research, there is a presumption that K will include *all future patients with PPI-refractory GERD.* The importance of the limitations of this concept will be further discussed in Chap. 7, but for now, the assumption is that attributes found in population K will remain static, now and into the future. In this example, n is not von Mises's "first n members" but a sample of n members from K. This leaves the question of how well does n actually represent K?

Ideally, the standard is to obtain a "random" sample from the population. This implies that "all members of the population" have an equal chance to be chosen. Even with this, if there is a population, K, with k members, if one member is chosen at random, then the chance of the next member being chosen is 1 in k – 1, which is better than the first chosen member, which was 1 in k, and so on. That is, as a member is chosen, the remaining members' chances of being chosen are better than the preceding members, going against the concept of having "equal chances" [41]. The theoretical solution for this is to "replace" each selected member with a new member of the population. However, if the entire population is already eligible for selection, it is unclear from where these new members will materialize, other than the member just chosen is put back into the pool of K. Therefore, from a practical standpoint, this is simply an issue that we will have to live with and, moreover, it is probably relatively inconsequential.

A bigger and more relevant issue is whether the sample n of k which was chosen is representative of K? Again, if we take our example study [38], the sample came from Veterans Affairs patients referred to Veterans Affairs gastroenterologists with GERD. These patients then underwent screening and had to meet specific selection criteria, not the least of which all patients had to be approved for surgery by a surgeon performing the operation. Although these "inclusion criteria" provided a relatively homogenous group of patients who were subsequently randomized to the tested treatments to evenly distribute any confounding variables, how representative this group is of the entire population is a relevant question for the generalizability of the data, or "external validity" to use the term of Grimes and Schulz [40]. This becomes quite important when applying the results of this study to an individual patient who may or may not have met the inclusion criteria. More on this in Chap. 7.

6.10 Statistical Analysis

As previously mentioned, although there are biomedical studies that are deterministic in nature, the majority will present probabilistic data in the form of frequencies, continuous or ordinal data, or relationships and correlations. It goes without saying that statistics is a large and well-developed field of study, and at present, there are several computer programs that perform all the complex calculations necessary. My purpose here is not to go into all that technical detail, but to describe how statistical analysis is used in medical research pertaining to increasing the confidence that the data generated by the study is true, or, at least, true enough, to be used as premises in the argument of the hypothesis's judgment.

Without becoming too technical, any biomedical study is generating data from a sample of individuals from the entire population of interest. If the study included all of the populations of interest, there was no need for statistical analysis because we would know exactly the data we would wish from the population. However, this is usually impractical, hence the need to study samples of the population. As we have seen in Fig. 6.2 of a long-run frequency, where the sample is chosen and how large the sample is can give varying results. This implies that there is no guarantee that the sample chosen for study is reflective of the entire population, although the larger the sample, the more likely our point estimates will be close to the actual population. Statistical analysis tries to quantify this imprecision.

In most biomedical research, there are two broad types of imprecisions. There is the imprecision of how the sample reflects the population. There are statistical techniques to estimate this, such as the "95% confidence interval," "standard deviation," "standard error of the mean," etc. The second type, one more crucial for research, is comparisons of two or more samples. For example, in the study of Spechler [38], two treatment strategies were compared to determine which one would have the highest frequency of a "successful" outcome. (Recall the arguments constructed for inguinal hernia repair from Chap. 2). This frequency difference is then used as a point estimate of the efficacy of one treatment over the other. Much foundational statistical theory and practice has gone into how best this difference should be determined to be true or not [42]. Although this topic is far too great for my purposes here, the basic issue is that the researcher wants to avoid two main types of errors: accepting that a true difference exists when there is not a difference (referred to as a type I or alpha error) and rejecting that a true difference exists when one does exist (referred to as a type II or beta error). It is important that of the menu of statistical tests available, the one which is appropriate for the data (and there are numerous criteria for this) be chosen. The results of this statistical analysis further solidify the confidence in the data to be used in the argument.

6.11 The Argument of the Experimental Protocol

Once the researcher proposes a hypothesis, they must create a study design that will generate data relevant to their hypothesis. If the hypothesis predicts a very specific outcome, then that outcome needs to be sought by the methods of observation or experimentation. Some outcomes, especially in clinical medical research, are more general. In these settings, more than one outcome may be sought to provide a preponderance of evidence for the hypothesis. (Recall the description of conductive informal logic in Chap. 2). For example, if the hypothesis is that treatment *x* is better than treatment *y* for disease *A*, the researcher may choose several endpoints to prove this, such as longevity of the patients, their quality of life, the cost-effectiveness of the treatment, ease of administration, and so forth.

In a medical research article, this comes under the section usually entitled "Methods and Materials" or just "Methods." This section will describe the subjects of the study, what exposures these subjects had, what endpoints was collected and how, and how this data was analyzed. This section has to be constructed in a way that the data can be reliably used in the premises of the argument of the hypothesis's judgment. Let us continue to use the article by Spechler [38] as an example, section by section and paragraph by paragraph, but again, not word for word.

Section 1. Trial Oversight

1. Statement of ethical compliance.

Section 2. Trial Design

- Pre-randomization trial procedure.

2. Source of patients to be entered into the trial identified and inclusion criteria presented.
3. Identification of eligible patients by initial screening.
   Additional survey forms were completed.
   Physiological testing was performed, including MII-pH, among others.
   Patients not meeting the inclusion criteria were excluded.
4. Additional inclusion criteria of surgeon approval were described.
   Protocol revision was performed intratrial due to slow accrual.

Section 3. Randomization

5. Randomization procedure described.

Section 4. Medical Treatment Group

6. Investigators and patients blinded to active medical treatment vs placebo.
   Medications and dosages explained.
   Definition of treatment failure given.

Section 5. Surgical Treatment Group

7. Surgical treatment explained.

Definition of treatment failure given.

Section 6. Follow-Up

8. The time period of data collection is described.

The GERD-HRQL questionnaire was administered every 3 months as the main outcome measure.

Section 7. Statistical Analysis

9. Statistical analysis described.

Primary endpoint: Treatment success defined at >50% improvement of GERD-HRQL at 12 months.

Secondary endpoints: frequency of non-GERD disorders and frequency of anxiety and depression.

Statistical tests used.

Let us evaluate the illative core of this argument. I will place side by side a logical restatement of the premises with my interpretation of the premises paragraph by paragraph:

Premise	Interpretation
Section 1. Trial Oversight 1. Statement of ethical compliance	This is not part of the how the data is generated, just an assurance that patients are treated in an ethical manner
Section 2. Pre-randomization Trial Procedure 2. There exists a group of patients, P, with symptoms, S, that may participate in the trial if they meet certain inclusion criteria 3. Potentially eligible patients of P were identified Additional survey forms completed Physiological testing done Ineligible patients of P removed 4. Additional inclusion criteria described Therefore, this leaves an eligible group of P_S patients treatable by A, $P_{SA\text{-}E}$ Protocol revisions explained	Identification of source of subjects for the trial, such that these subjects have characteristics relevant to the hypothesis of the study Note that the eligible group of patients, $P_{SA\text{-}E}$, is a subset of all P_{SA} patients, but may not necessarily be a representative sample of P_{SA}
Section 3. Randomization 5. Randomization procedure described	The type of study, randomized controlled trial documented. Type of randomization to evenly distribute confounding factors and treatments described.

Premise	Interpretation
Section 4. Medical Treatment Group 6. There exist within eligible $P_{SA\text{-}E}$, a subset receiving active medical treatment, M, and another subset receiving placebo treatment, N, such that neither the patients or investigators knew which treatment P's were receiving Medications and dosages explained Definition of treatment failure explained	To determine if M was responsible for the outcome, a comparison group received an inactive agent, N. Because no one knew what P was receiving, knowledge bias was eliminated as cause of outcome. Description of M as evidence that subsequent outcome data relevant to hypothesis Definition of outcome as evidence that subsequent outcome data relevant to the hypothesis
Section 5. Surgical Treatment Group 7. The exist within $P_{SA\text{-}E}$ a subset receiving surgical treatment A Definition of treatment failure given	Description of A as evidence that subsequent outcome data relevant to hypothesis Definition of outcome as evidence that subsequent outcome data relevant to the hypothesis
Section 6. Follow-up 8. Time period of data collection described	Description of follow-up and data collection as evidence that subsequent outcome data relevant to hypothesis
Section 7. Statistical Analysis 9. Primary endpoint described Secondary endpoints described Statistical tests used	Description of data analysis as evidence that the data are relevant to the hypothesis and differences seen are not due to chance or bias

This study is a randomized controlled trial of a very specific group of patients. Three interventions will be compared: "active" medical treatment, "placebo" medical treatment and surgical medical treatment. The patient eligibility criteria tried to ensure that no known disease-related confounding factors were present in the group. However, this may then affect the representativeness of this sample. Descriptions of medical and surgical therapies were presented to persuade readers that relevant accepted treatments within the existing theory of GERD were used; that is, the treatments themselves are not confounding factors. The method that the data were collected, using a validated symptom severity questionnaire at 3-month intervals to a final outcome at 12 months, was presented to persuade the readers that the most relevant outcome to the hypothesis was obtained. Last, the statistical tests used were presented such that any difference in this interventional comparison was not due to chance or bias; therefore, these data can be used as truthful premises for the next argument.

6.12 Argument of the Hypothesis's Judgment

The final part of a medical research article I have named the argument of the hypothesis's judgment. Each study was performed to determine the possible truth of the hypothesis. The experimental or observational protocols were developed and executed to generate data relevant to the hypothesis. Efforts were made to make the data as reliable and relevant as possible, that is, to reduce bias and confounding. All this was done so that the data can be used to judge the hypothesis. In a medical research article, this is generally done in the "Discussion" section.

To once again use the Spechler [38] article as an example, I will go through the Discussion section paragraph by paragraph.

Paragraph 1

1. A minority of PPI-refractory patients were found to have GERD.
2. In that group, antireflux surgery in the form of a laparoscopic Nissen fundoplication was superior to active medical therapy and medical placebo.

Paragraph 2

3. Discussion as to why some patients with PPI refractory GERD improved with education and a standardized PPI regimen.

Paragraph 3

4. Discussion of the proper evaluation of patients with PPI-refractory GERD, including MII-pH monitoring.

Paragraph 4

5. Discussion of the potentially surprising success of laparoscopic Nissen fundoplication with patients with esophageal hypersensitivity.

Paragraph 5

6. Discussion as to why the researchers did not test for a particular gene mutation associated with PPI metabolism.

Paragraph 6

7. Discussion as to limitations of the study—specific patient population of Veterans Affairs patients, no "sham" surgery performed.

Paragraph 7

8. Limitation and explanation resulting from need to adjust protocol intra-trial.

Paragraph 8

- Conclusions

9. Systematic evaluation revealed that heartburn was both truly PPI refractory and reflux-related in a minority of patients.
10. In that group, laparoscopic Nissen fundoplication was superior to medical therapy.
11. Systematic evaluation can identify patients with PPI-refractory heartburn who would benefit from laparoscopic Nissen fundoplication.

Let us evaluate the illative core of this argument. I will place side by side a logical restatement of the premises with my interpretation the premises paragraph by paragraph:

Premise	Interpretation
1. Minority of P with S had D In this subset $P_{SA}(S\|A) < P_{SA}(M\|A)$	With the primary endpoint of $P_{SA}(S\|A) < P_{SA}(M\|A)$, the confidence that the hypothesis is true increases. Closure of previously identified treatment gap.
2. Some P with S and M, P_S were not truly this subset as M negated S when administered properly	A secondary endpoint of identifying causal attribution of a subset of patients which was not initially the outcome of interest. Closure of previous unidentified treatment gap.
3. Importance of T in identifying D in P	A secondary endpoint of the importance of proper patient diagnostic evaluation. Closure of previously identified diagnostic gap.
4. Importance of an in subset P with cause 4b	A subset of the primary endpoint. Closure of a treatment gap.
5. There is a subset of P_S that may be part of an untested subset	This may be a potential bias and a possible future study. Potential knowledge gap identified
6. The study P_S subset may not represent the population of P_S	Identification of potential bias and applicability to larger population.
7. Study plan and execution altered	Potential decrease in the reliability of the truth of the premises
8. Conclusions The frequency P_S related to D < the frequency of P_S related to not-D $P_{SA}(S\|A) < P_{SA}(M\|A)$ T increases predictability of $P_{SA}(S\|A)$	The judgment of the hypothesis is that there is increased confidence of it to be true.

My purpose here is not to assess the quality of this particular study but rather to use it as an example of how biomedical articles are organizationally presented from a logical viewpoint. Although there is still controversy over how theories are constructed and accepted as true [12], for the more limited area of a single hypothesis, what is considered is how well the data "support" the hypothesis [41]. This concept of "how well the data support the hypothesis" is quite vague, although Hacking and Schaffner apply a Bayesian approach to this. This has quite a bit to do with the underlying belief network that the reader may already have. In fact, I aver that scientists, physicians and other health care professionals have something similar to the social umwelt with respect to accepting the conclusions of studies generating new information, based on their training and social/professional interactions with other professionals in their own field, which I refer to as the professional umwelt. One approach is that of Levi [43], which he calls "direct inference": at any time *t*, an investigator *X*, who has a cognitive state characterized by a body of knowledge, a confirmational commitment and a credal state. *X*'s credal state is the system of *personal* (emphasis mine) or credal probability judgments at time *t*. *X*'s confirmational commitment at *t* is the criterion endorsed at *t* for evaluating revisions of *X*'s credal state due to changes in a body of knowledge. *X* should revise their credal state with changes in knowledge. This approach has appeal, at least to me, because it acknowledges how personal beliefs can affect a healthcare professional's scientific judgments. This has certainly been my personal observation in 40 years of being involved in medical research.

A schematic diagram, therefore, of the general structure of a medical research article will look something like Fig. 6.3. The first, the hypothesis's development, the

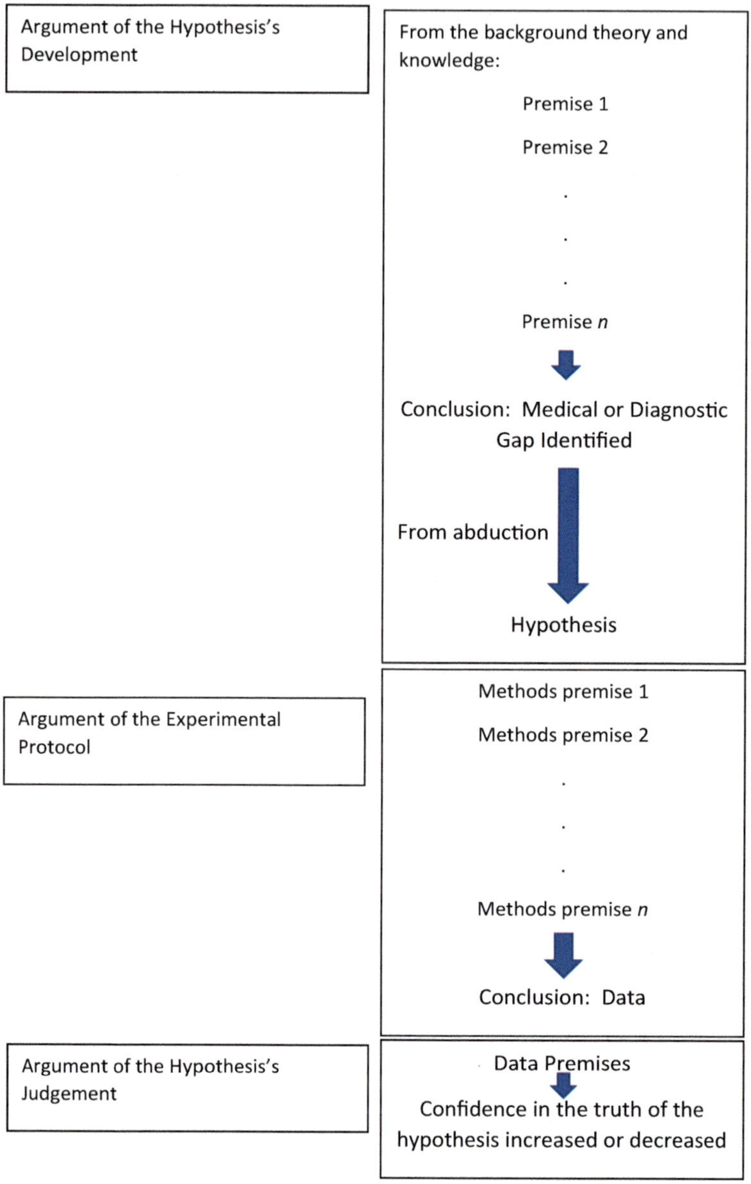

Fig. 6.3 Schematic of the illative core of the general structure of the arguments in a medical research article

background knowledge premises are used to come to conclusions related to medical knowledge gaps, whether of biomedical fact, treatments or diagnostics. The second, the experimental protocol, uses the methods and materials to generate data, which has some logical relation, in a physical or theoretical sense, to the hypothesis. Last, the hypothesis's judgment is use of the data generated as premises to increase or decrease confidence of the researcher (and later journal referees and, if published, readers of the article—a form of manifest rationality).

6.13 Data Interpretation in the Context of the Strength of Evidence

Presently in medicine, there is a whole field dedicated to "evidence-based medicine." This field attempts to integrate the evaluation and application of the "best evidence" available for a clinical question [44]. It is centered around assessing the "strength (or quality) of evidence." In fact, a hierarchy of data quality was devised (Fig. 6.4) to supposedly help practitioners, both clinical and scientific, easily identify the "best evidence." Ironically, the currently accepted hierarchy of evidence was determined by expert opinion and not by the performance of the actual evidence. What I mean by this is that the criteria to determine what is thc based evidence was produced using the weakest methodological criteria. To my knowledge, there is no study that proves when this hierarchy has been applied to a group of patients, that these patients actually had better outcomes. This hierarchy is also not universally accepted, and some have suggested revisions [45]. The "quality of evidence" hierarchy has more to do with quality of evidence in the context of theoretically reducing bias and confounding, rather than predictability for an individual patient. That is, it strives to ensure as best as possible that statements about exposure effects reflect the magnitude of the exposure effects and not some other potential factors. There have been a number of proposed study design grading criteria that help researchers, editors, peer-reviewers, and readers assess the quality of the study presented (Table 6.3). However, it is still an open question whether the best evidence for an individual patient corresponds to the best quality evidence in the hierarchy (Fig. 6.4).

Nevertheless, bias is an important issue in whether the data generated can truly be used as premises in the hypothesis's judgment. Issues in bias and confounding can greatly affect the premises of a medical research argument [40]. The data from the study are used as premises in the argument such that the researchers are trying

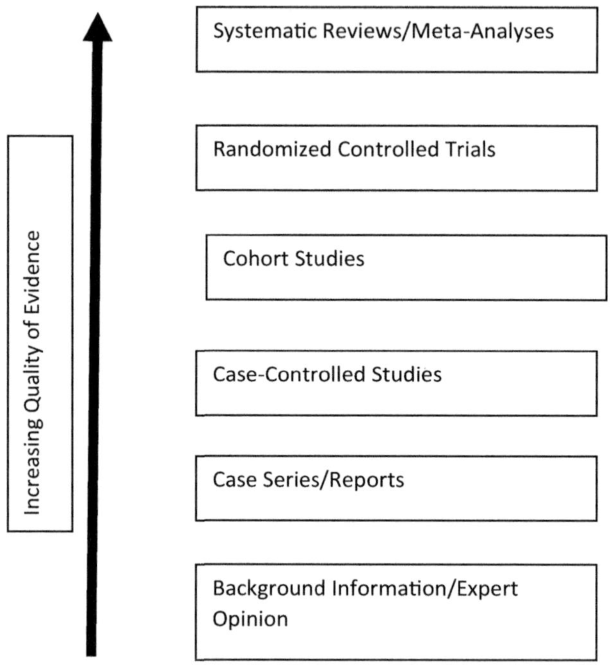

Fig. 6.4 The presently accepted hierarchy of evidence. However, other variations exist

to persuade their audience of the truth of their conclusions. If the data-premises are in error because of bias, then the soundness of the conclusion is questionable. Selection bias is an absence of comparability between the groups being studied. An obvious example is when comparing the effects of daily exercise to no exercise in older patients, having a group that is preponderantly young would bias the results. In the article analyzed above by Spechler [38], the researchers made great efforts to create homogenous groups as much as possible except for the treatment exposure. Information bias has to do with incorrectly determining the exposure, outcome or both. For example, if the outcome of interest was myocardial infarction occurrence, but the investigators also included exertion chest pain into that outcome, this will lead to an inaccurate accounting of the number of myocardial infarctions. Last, confounding occurs when factors, knowingly or unknowingly, result in a mixing or blurring of effects. The researcher attempts to relate an exposure to an outcome but actually measures the effects of a third factor, the confounding variable [40], as the above example of having a preponderance of young individuals in a comparison of exercise in older patients illustrates. I would point out that these "confounding variables" are what the practicing clinician has to contend with and may actually be important in decision-making. Again, more on this is Chap. 7.

One of the rationales of randomized, controlled trials is to eliminate bias by distributing potential confounding factors, known and unknown, among the groups being compared so that the magnitude of the treatment effect observed is the actual magnitude of the treatment effect. Therefore, it follows that data from randomized, controlled trials should show different treatment effects compared to observational studies. However, in a summary of the results of methodological studies, Angelmeyer et al. [46] showed that the results of randomized, controlled trials and observational studies did not have significant effect estimate differences between them. They concluded that factors other than study design *per se* need to be considered when exploring reasons for lack of agreement between these types of studies. In other works, randomized, controlled trials are not necessarily better evidence than observational studies. This mostly has to do with what purpose the evidence is intended to be used.

The last issue I want to address in this section is what I like to refer to as the "sports score" approach to clinical trial results. In any sporting event, one side wins at the end of the game whether they won by the slimmest or greatest of margins. In other words, the magnitude of the win is irrelevant to the win being recognized. In randomized, controlled trials, the size of the treatment affect is frequently treated in the same manner. For example, if there is a randomized, controlled trial comparing two treatment options, X and Y, for a specific condition, and the results of the trial are that treatment X produces outcome O at time t at a frequency F, while treatment Y produces outcome O at time t at a frequency of F-0.01, and the results reach statistical significance by the appropriate statistical test, then it would be judged that X is superior to Y. However, the margin is quite narrow, implying that almost as many patients had outcome O. Therefore, this implies that there were a number of patients who achieved O while being treated with Y. This then begs the question of if these patients were treated with X, rather than Y, would they have achieved O at F? Moreover, even though there is a statistically significant difference, is it a "clinically important" difference? Are there other issues, such as patient choice/autonomy, quality of life, and financial considerations, that need to be addressed when devising a treatment plan in which treatment Y is more desirable than treatment X? These are questions that require more interpretation than simply acquiescing to the "final score."

6.14 How Medical Research Is Peer-Reviewed

After the researcher completes their study and writes the manuscript, they usually submit it for publication.[13] The researcher will choose a journal in which they would like to have their study published. There are a number of factors that go into the researcher's choice, such as whether the focus of the journal is consistent with the topic of the study, how prestigious the journal is, its target audience, its circulation,

[13] Often, the researcher will submit an abstract to a meeting so that they can present their study at a meeting. This will generally be reviewed by the program committee of the organization sponsoring the meeting. These abstracts either be accepted or rejected by the program committee without the research receiving commentary by the committee. In this way, submission to journal with formal peer-review is different.

etc. Once the researcher submits the manuscript, the editor(s) will make a determination on whether the topic fits in with their journal. If it does, then the editor will send it for peer review. Although this can lead to acceptance or rejection of the manuscript without comment, more typical is that the researcher will receive a list of criticisms or suggesting for improving the manuscript from the reviewers. The researcher then has to respond to these criticisms before the paper will be considered for publication.

This process is, in essence, the dialectic of manifest rationality, as described by Johnson [47] in Chap. 2. Typically, at least one, but usually two or three, sometimes more, peer reviewers chosen by the journal editor will review the manuscript. Some journals allow for the researcher submitting the work to suggest reviewers or request that other reviewers not be used. The reviewers will read the manuscript, and, if there is interest in the manuscript, will provide a series of criticisms of the argument posed in the manuscript usually in the form of questions to the researcher. The reviewers are anonymous, although some reviewers will reveal themselves. The researcher is then allowed to answer the criticisms either by revising the manuscript to satisfy the reviewers' criticisms or by directly challenging the reviewers' criticisms in a response to the editor. If these criticisms are answered to the satisfaction of the reviewers and editors, the paper is generally accepted for publication. Figure 6.5 demonstrates a flow diagram of how medical knowledge is created, how it is subjected to manifest rationality, and how it is disseminated and accepted or rejected by other professional and lay people.

These exchanges are almost always a private matter among the researcher, reviewers and journal editor. However, with the consent of all parties, the editor of the journal *Surgery* published the reviewers' criticisms with the responses of the researchers, who were myself, and my coauthor, Adham Saad, of our paper "Toward a Unified Theory of Occurrence and Recurrence of Hiatal Hernia" [48–50]. Although a reiteration of the entire text of the criticisms and responses is much too long for the space in this book, as the researcher who submitted the work and answered the criticisms, this is a good example of the dialectic that goes on in medical journal peer-review to reach a type of manifest rationality as proposed by Johnson [47].

This type of dialectic to improve the argument and increase the confidence of the conclusions of a medical research article is dependent on an honest exchange with integrity by both the reviewers and the researcher. Unfortunately, this may not always be the case. Mahoney [51] identified possible prejudices in the peer-review review process. This may be one of the reasons that some journals allow researchers to request that some individuals not review their work. Sadly, despite science purported "objectivity," rivalries exist, which may affect the peer-review process. This, in my opinion, reflects humans' natural tendency to approve of propositions that the already hold and disapprove of the ones that they do not, as discussed extensively in Chaps. 3 and 4. This, I believe, also reflects the particular social umwelt that biomedical scientists and healthcare professionals have. Moreover, the cautionary tale for the reader is that peer review is not an omniscient process and that the reader should apply their own judgment of the illative core of a medical research article.

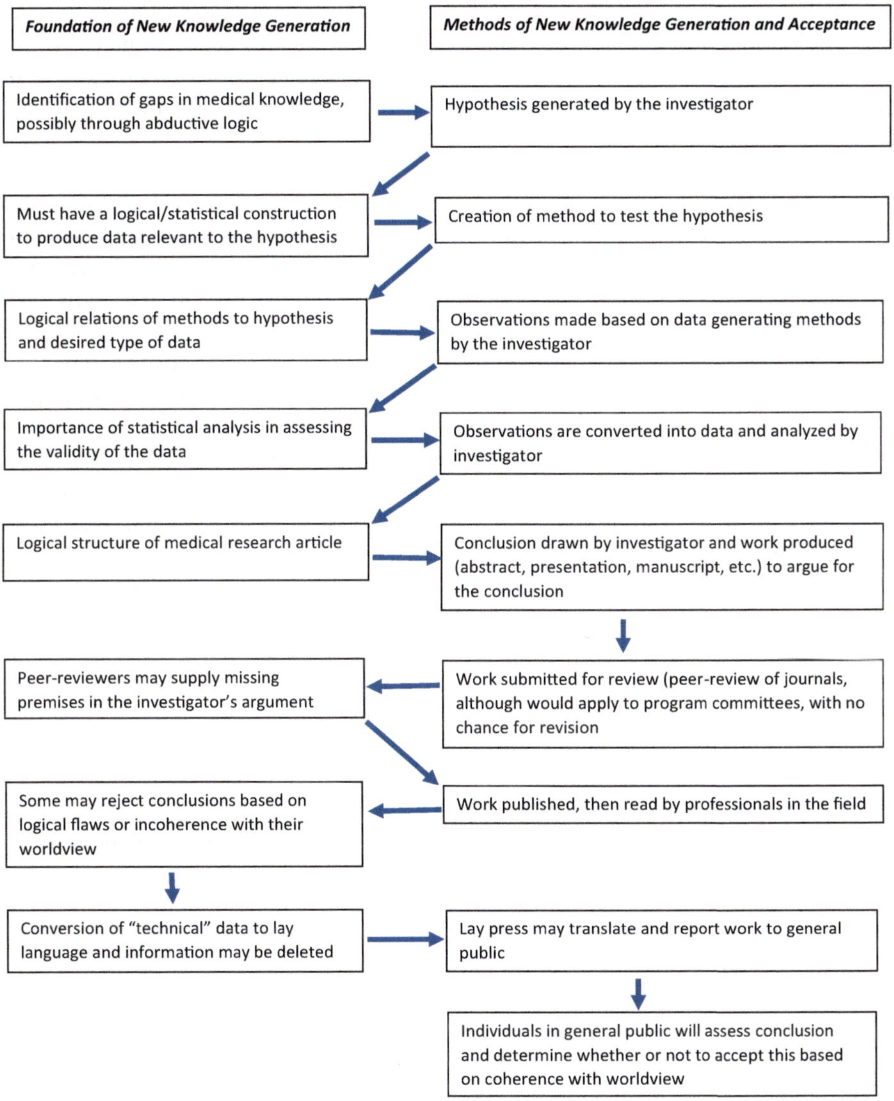

Fig. 6.5 Flow diagram of how medical knowledge is created and accepted

6.15 Knowledge Derived from the Practice of Medicine

I have spent much of this chapter discussing how medical knowledge is generated and argued as a scientific biomedical process. This is how physicians, biomedical scientists and healthcare professionals increase the corpus of their knowledge, which they then apply. When specifically addressing the delivery of care by a physician to a single patient, this fits into the model of the physician's cognition and metacognition, as presented in Fig. 1.1. However, when discussing rationality and logic in Chap. 2, I acknowledged that a portion of physician decision-making is due to intuition, particularly in experienced physicians. This draws from a reservoir of experience and deliberation. At this point, I would like to address the physician's personal medical knowledge.

Knowledge as derived in the typical biomedical publication or presentation is directed at generalized knowledge pertaining to a category of individuals or a category of disease processes. In practice, many patients will not fit into these categories. Their presentations may include factors that are not "studiable" in the sense of medical science. However, they are a source of knowledge to the individual practitioner.

Knowledge that the clinician acquires in the course of their practice is somewhat maligned as "anecdotal" or "unscientific." Maltrend [52], on the other hand, argues that clinical knowledge, including the complexities of human interactions, is simply not available for inquiry by means of biomedical scientific approaches. Therefore, there is a gap between medical research and clinical practice [52]. If what I have described in the preceding discussion of how medical knowledge is created, its objective is to make generalized propositions with as few confounding factors as possible. However, in my clinical practice, as I am sure in every other physician's clinical practice, the confounding variables, especially the patient's attitudes, are an inescapable part of practice. This is also the part of clinical practice that appears not to be well studied scientifically.

This type of knowledge gained through experience and focus reflection is what Maltrend [52] refers to as "tacit knowing." That is, the physician may be accumulating knowledge without consciously realizing that is what is happening. This comes in the form of subtle patient clues such as a wayward look or a change in the tone of voice, "data" that the entirety of human evolution has formed our brain and mind to understand (Chap. 3); yet, it is impossible, or nearly so, to scientifically quantify. Matrend [52] emphasizes that within medical culture (i.e., scientific biomedical professional umwelt), knowledge can be empirically verified by scientific and biomedical methods. The human interactions and interpretations that constitute a considerable element of clinical practice cannot be investigated from this epistemic position.

Clinical problems presented by patients may not be "compatible" with "textbook" knowledge of medicine [52]. Excluded from the realm of inquiry are issues involving human interaction, mind or experiences; the "art of medicine," including elements of clinical interaction and judgment, are outside of scientific medicine. The diagnostic process is complex and includes interpretations related to pattern recognition, moral judgments and intuition [53]. When medical knowledge generated from groups is applied to individuals, careful negotiations with the specific patient and situation are essential for adequate understanding and management [54]. Human knowing is characterized by the fact that we know more than we can tell, but people are not able to articulate how they come to their decisions and actions because their knowledge is tacit [55]. This ability to know without being able to articulate is what intuition is. Perhaps it is this way because there is no corresponding language that can be used to articulate the insight. Johanneson [56] proposes that the practice of rule-following requires situational understanding and judgment power, which constitutes concepts and can be incompletely articulated by verbal means. I believe that this personal knowledge is a consequence of physicians reflecting on their patient care experiences and the nuances of the individual patient. Schon [57] refers to this as "reflection-in-action"—practitioners can reflect on their intuitive knowing in the midst of action. The practitioner's repertoire of examples, images, understandings and actions, rarely made explicit in action, comprises a capacity for dealing with unique cases. This is very compatible with Abernathy and Hamm's [58] description of intuition, as described in Chap. 2.

With knowledge acquisition and practical experience, expertise develops. Dreyfus and Dreyfus [59] propose that "expert competence" is characterized by context dependency, producing knowledge from the interaction of the expert's repertoire of cognitive patterns and environmental cues. These "artistic" patterns of behavior are difficult to explicate, let alone teach.

Kvale [60] discusses "communicative validity" and "pragmatic validity" for validity discourses of clinical epistemology. That is, knowledge must be validated through use (i.e., the pragmatic) and through the ability to communicate (i.e., the communicative). "Reliability" is accounted for by communication of programs that describe action and cognitive patterns that have effectively accomplished their intended ends.

6.15.1 Understanding and Wisdom

In the preceding sections, what has been discussed is the creation and acceptance of new medical knowledge in both descriptive and normative terms. I have been treating this knowledge as axiomatic propositions, that is, bits (or, bytes, for the more computer oriented) of information from which we form beliefs, as opposed to Johnson-Laird's mental models as previously discussed. I have quoted epistemologists that the goal is to obtain "justified true beliefs." However, this is an incomplete assessment. Zagzebski in her book *Virtues of the Mind* [61] sought to link the attainment of knowledge to moral virtues. There are intellectual virtues, such open-mindedness, and intellectual vices, such as closed-mindedness. For her, simply seeking knowledge is not by itself a virtue. There are two concepts that again have deep common usage, although quite ill-defined: understanding and wisdom. However, both are essential to the practicing physician, as well as other healthcare professionals. Simply having accumulated a vast store of "bits of knowledge" does not mean that one understands this knowledge.

Considering knowledge as purely bits of "justified true beliefs" does not take into account these belief relations to other beliefs. As Kvanvig puts it, the focus on a single belief of a single person at a single time with the object of a discrete proposition cannot be separated from other beliefs [62]. That is, one's beliefs are not in isolation. They mutually support the individual's entire belief structure and how the individual manipulates these beliefs into new beliefs and actions. To me, this appears to be a form of epistemic coherentism mentioned in the section on the tenants of epistemology. This brings us to the concept of *understanding*. Zagzebski [61] quotes Julius Moravcsik: "Understanding is more than just the reproduction of facts, it is possessing the right concepts, and the intuitive insights of the connection that makes the parts of the proof to be the proper parts of a sequence." To make an analogy, bits of knowledge are like the gears, springs and belts, but understanding is the ability to see their relations in a working machine. Zagzebski [61] sums this up as "one understands a proposition as part of and because of one's understanding of a system or network of truths, that is, as a pattern of a whole chunk of reality." I cannot think of a better way to sum up how healthcare professionals understand their patients, nor how biomedical scientists understand theories and models, for example, the understanding of AIDS and HIV as recounted above.

Subsumed in understanding is *wisdom*. Again, a concept that is both familiar and vague. Like understanding, Zagzebski [61] asserts that "wisdom is an epistemic value qualitatively different from the piling up of beliefs that have the property of justification, warrant or certainty…Wisdom is a matter of grasping the whole of reality." She further goes on to say, "Wisdom takes a different form in each individual case and resists analysis that does not make essential reference to the standpoint of the individual." In other words, how, when and why an individual accumulates wisdom is difficult to elucidate and probably impossible to replicate. One can accumulate knowledge (or rather bits of information), but that does not amount to wisdom. She emphasizes the aphorism of the difficulties attaining wisdom: (The sum of) Human knowledge has increased (over time), but (the sum of human) wisdom has not [61]. She further points out two essential features of wisdom: it is a result of experience, and it cannot be taught. Hence, as was pointed out in Chap. 2, it is the experienced physician who can access their intuition *because* that physician has understanding and wisdom.

Wisdom is the use of knowledge and understanding in the service of doing what is good. Wisdom, unlike knowledge, cannot be misused because it unifies knowledge, desires and values in a way to produce beneficial thought and action [61]. Moreover, the judgment to use knowledge selectively because there are nuanced differences from situation to situation so that good is maximized, rather than applying knowledge uniformly, in the way that Evidence-Based Medicine advocates, is wisdom. I would assert that the underlying foundation of Evidence-Based Medicine rests on rejecting wisdom in the service of uniformity (or, in the parlance of "quality improvement," reduction in the variation of care[14]) because their understanding of the "evidence" is based on the disease concept (as illustrated in Fig. 6.1) and not necessarily on the whole of the specific disease, in a particular patient, with possibly an assortment of comorbidities, in the overall environment that the patient *and*

[14] I want to point out that I am not rejecting quality improvement efforts in medical care, nor that variation in care may be detrimental. My contention is that an *unwise* application of protocols or algorithms will lead to a certain number of misapplications of these protocols and algorithms.

physician find themselves. This wise application of personal knowledge will be discussed further in Chap. 7.

It is also apparent to me that when the researcher comes to a hypothesis, the logical process of abduction used is a mixture of wisdom, understanding and creativity. Having such a spark of inspiration requires an underlying deep understanding of the relevant whole, the wisdom to "see" the missing section(s) of the whole, and the creativity to imagine the bridge across this gap. Quite frankly, this is a poorly understood and not often explored part of the research process.

6.16 Acceptance of Medical Knowledge as a Form of Persuasion

Ultimately, once the proposed new knowledge is publicly presented, either through presentation at a medical conference or through publication, the desire of the researcher is that the audience (or, as I have previously identified, the "listener" of the argument) will be persuaded that the new knowledge proposition will be accepted. I submit that this form of persuasion is no different from any other form of persuasion (see Fig. 4.2).

6.16.1 In Relation to Healthcare Professionals

For the publicly presented medical research article to be persuasive, the listener must determine that the illative core is sound *and* that there are no negating counterfactuals in their corpus of medical knowledge and theory. If the article is at odds with their corpus, then they must decide whether their corpus needs revision, either through an intuitive Bayesian model or through Levi's direct inference route [43]. It is unlikely that any clinical professionals actually consciously think in Bayesian terms and what threshold Bayesian probabilities these are quantitatively. In fact, this is the great difficulty in Bayesian accounts of accepting a hypothesis or theory (see Hacking [41]) or the Bayesian persuasion models discussed in Chap. 4. I assert that under most conditions for the average healthcare professional, such revisions are done intuitively. Realistically, there may be other determinates on whether the professional will be persuaded by the article, perhaps because of their own self-interest, but this is a topic that I do not wish to address in this book.

What I provided above is a description of how new medical knowledge is accepted as true by a healthcare professional, but I have not provided a normative account of whether this knowledge *should* be accepted.

What are the criteria for new knowledge to be accepted? Going back to the illative core of the three arguments of the medical research article, the first would have to do with the background knowledge and theory that led to the identification of the medical knowledge gap. This knowledge has to be true. However, all theories are potentially provisional, so it is up to the listener as to whether or not to accept the background knowledge as providing true premises for the subsequent conclusion. Most of this background knowledge is built upon other medical research, which is usually referenced in medical research articles. If these references are from reliable sources, then the premises could be considered at least potentially true by the listener. As noted in Chap. 4, there is also a matter of trust in the sources of these references. Therefore, the normative criteria here are trustworthy references of the medical knowledge used as premises in an illative core that is logically sound, either deductively, inductive, or informally leading to a conclusion that identifies the medical gap.

The conclusion identifying the medical gap is not the hypothesis. The leap from the gap to the hypothesis requires abductive creativity. Although the creative aspects of conceiving of a hypothesis are probably not subject to logical analysis, after the hypothesis is proposed, it certainly should make logical sense that if true, it would close the medical gap. In this sense, a counterfactual test would be to consider that the hypothesis was true, and therefore, in its absence, the medical gap will still persist, which seems to be a reasonable position to accept that, at least, the hypothesis deserves to be tested.

The second argument is that of the experimental protocol. This requires determining what type of data is needed to test the hypothesis. In some studies, this is relatively easy, for example, in the Spechler [38] article analyzed, proving the hypothesis is simply determining whether there was better treatment success with surgical therapy in that very selected group of patients or not. Sometimes, this is not such a straightforward process. Next, after determining what type of data is needed, the sources from which the appropriate data can be obtained need to be identified. For the vast majority of medical research, this source is patients, either directly (i.e., direct experimentation on patients, as in the Spechler article [38]) or indirectly (i.e., from their medical records). In basic medical science research, these sources can be animals, cell cultures, molecules, etc. After the source is determined, what is done to generate the data needs to reliably result in the data desired. Again, for example, Spechlar and his co-researchers wished to create data on the treatment success of laparoscopic Nissen fundoplication; therefore, the protocol must include patients who underwent laparoscopic Nissen fundoplication. What variables are chosen to be included in the study matters a great deal, especially in understanding the difference between explanatory and predictive modeling [63]. Management of confounding variables is of great importance. This can be consciously addressed in prospective studies; however, in retrospective studies, addressing confounding variables needs to be a part of the data analysis. The methods that address these confounding variables need to be appropriate.[15] Last, the data need to be statistically analyzed to determine if what is observed is due to chance

[15] Although too big of a topic for this chapter, there are many statistical methods to address these confounders, such as case–control study design, multivariate analysis, propensity analysis, and machine learning methods, such as artificial neural networks.

or if the point estimates generated are a reliable estimate of the intrinsic probability of the population in question. Much of the peer-review process, in my experience, deals with these issues.

Last, once the data are generated, how does it relate to the hypothesis? This is what I have termed the argument of the hypothesis's judgment. In a hypothetico-deductive model [12], the hypothesis can be falsified but never confirmed. As Schaffner [12] points out, this is considered an outmoded approach. Nevertheless, if the data do not "support" the hypothesis, using Hacking's terminology [41], the hypothesis can be proven to be false. More often, the data support, at some level, the hypothesis. To what extent, is a matter of Bayesian or direct inference positions of the listener.

To correlate this with physician's meta-cognition (Fig. 1.1) framework in Chap. 1, this fits into the physician's meta-cognition of evidential theory. That is, the physician has to accept, through whatever process they have, that the new knowledge generated if true enough to use in their metacognitions and cognitions. The normative account I have given above, admittingly, still requires a great deal of personal judgment by the listener (Fig. 6.5).

6.16.2 Patients and the Lay Public

How the nonhealthcare professional general public accepts new medical knowledge is similar to healthcare professionals (Fig. 6.5) but with the use of different criteria. In Chap. 4, I discussed how individuals are persuaded with respect to healthcare information. However, suffice to say, individuals do receive healthcare information and have to interpret this information.

How the message is delivered and by whom influences to what extent health knowledge is accepted by individuals. When the new knowledge is delivered by a healthcare professional, particularly the patient's personal physician or another healthcare professional personally known to the patient, there is a better chance that the information will be accepted. This may be simply a matter of trust in the messenger. In general, when healthcare professionals provide new knowledge to patients, it is filtered and reformatted in a way as to be as understandable as possible to the patient. As with other forms of persuasion, trust in the source of the information is an important factor in the acceptance of the new information. Nevertheless, all the issues previously discussed in Chap. 4 with respect to their social umwelt and cultural identity still apply.

Healthcare professionals are not the only means by which the general public hears of new medical knowledge. Journalists and the news media also report new medical knowledge (Fig. 6.5). This information is clearly filtered so that perhaps the main point of the new knowledge is presented, usually with a patient with the issue in question as an example. Even more so than with information coming from healthcare professionals, trust in the source of the information can be even more problematic.

Last, for some, there is a suspicion of the medical-industrial establishment. Although it is not within the scope of this book to discuss the causes of this suspicion, it suffices to say that events perpetuated by many in the past (and perhaps even now) gave many individuals and groups cause to be suspicious. This is part of the greater trust requirement of accepting new knowledge.

6.17 Summary and Conclusions

In summary, epistemology is the philosophical study of how knowledge is acquired and used. Medical epistemology is the subset of this field related to knowledge in scientific and clinical medicine. Epistemologists have focused on the normative criteria for accepting "justified true beliefs." These beliefs are required to be true and their acquisition justified. The criteria by which some beliefs are justified and others are not, even though they may be all true, are far from agreed upon. In medicine, knowledge is acquired through education (i.e., knowledge that has been agreed upon by prior trusted sources, usually in textbooks or lectures), through research (i.e., the creation of new knowledge based on preexisting theoretical structure and the identification of gaps in medical knowledge), and experience (i.e., through the individual practice of medicine).

Knowledge through education requires the learner to trust what the educator has written or said. This type of knowledge is generally presented as an accepted fact (quite frankly, whether it is justified or not). Given where we are in the history of medical knowledge, this knowledge is the foundation for the acquisition of all subsequent knowledge. It is unhelpful, in my opinion, to be such a skeptic as to reject this knowledge on the grounds of bootstrapping, as it has served humanity fairly well, although not infallibly so.

New knowledge is generated first by the researcher when the researcher identifies a gap in medical knowledge. They must then produce an argument where this gap is, at least, a plausible conclusion of the premises. Using the logical technique of abduction (in my opinion, a mixture of wisdom, understanding, and creativity), the researcher develops a hypothesis. I have demonstrated, on a logical basis, using an example of a medical article in a prestigious journal, how this process of developing the hypothesis is done by researchers, as well as creation of the methods of the study to produce relevant data to compare to the hypothesis, and the logical structure of judging whether the hypothesis should be rejected or if the confidence in it should increase, both from a descriptive and normative viewpoint.

Knowledge generated through clinical practice by individual healthcare professionals tends to be underappreciated by biomedical scientists, medical academicians and philosophers. It is my contentions that this is a vital store of practical knowledge. Moreover, it is through this practical knowledge that incorporation of new knowledge is operational. The value of knowledge as a part of a greater cognitive state of understanding and wisdom with increasing experience is important and underappreciated.

Once we understand medical knowledge in the context of making it operational for practical ends, we are better equipped to understand how and why this knowledge can and should be applied to clinical practice.

References

1. Truncellito DA. Epistemology. Internet Encyclopedia of Philosophy. https://iep.utm.edu. Last accessed 25 Aug 2022.
2. Steup M, Neta R. Epistemology. In: Zalta EN, editor. The Stanford encyclopedia of philosophy. Stanford: Stanford University; 2020. https://plato.stanford.edu/archives/fall2020/entries/epistemology. Last accessed 25 Aug 2022.
3. Ryle G. The concept of the mind. Chicago: University of Chicago Press; 2002. (Originally published 1949)
4. Melchoir G. The persuasiveness puzzle about bootstrapping. Ratio. 2020;33:27–36.
5. Khushf G. A framework for understanding medical epistemologies. J Med Philos. 2013;38:461–8.
6. ten Have H, Gordijn B. Medical epistemology. Med Health Care Philos. 2017;20:451–2.
7. Canguihem G. The normal and the pathological. New York: Zone Books; 1991.
8. de Cuzzani P, Lie RK. The importance of epistemology for clinical practice. Theor Med. 1991;12:87–90.
9. Prasad V, Vandross A, Toomey C, et al. A decade of reversal: an analysis of 146 contradicted medical practices. Mayo Clin Proc. 2013;88:790–8.
10. Feinstein AR. The scientific tribulations of randomized clinical trials. Clin Res. 1978;26:241–4.
11. Feinstein AR. Clinical biostatistics XLVII: scientific standards vs statistical association and biological logic in the analysis of causation. Clin Pharmacol Ther. 1979;25:481–92.
12. Schaffner KF. Discovery and explanation in biology and medicine. Chicago: University of Chicago Press; 1993.
13. Clendening L. Source book of medical history. New York: Dover Publications; 1960.
14. Disease. The Merriam-Webster Dictionary. https://merriam-webster.com. Last accessed 4 Sept 2022.
15. Constitution of the World Heal Organization. https://who.int. Last accessed 12 Sept 2022.
16. Mellor D, Merali S. What exactly is a disease? https://theconversation.com. Last accessed 4 Sept 2022.
17. Scully JL. What is a disease? EMBO Rep. 2004;5:650–3.
18. Smart B. On the classification of diseases. Theor Med Bioeth. 2014;35:251–69.
19. Gagliardi F. Nosological diagnosis, theories of categorization, and argumentations by analogy. J Med Philos. 2022;47:311–30.
20. Saracci R. Nosology expansion: not always for health's sake. Eur J Epidemol. 2019;34:621–3.
21. Whitbeck C. Causation in medicine: the disease entity model. Philos Sci. 1977;44:619–37.
22. Broadbent A. Causation and models of disease in epidemiology. Stud Hist Philos Biol Biomed Sci. 2005;40:302–11.
23. Velanovich V. The function of the case report in medical epistemology. Theor Surg. 1992;7:91–4.
24. Bench RJ. Health sciences, natural science, and clinical knowledge. J Med Philos. 1989;14:147–64.
25. Kuhn TS. Logic of discovery or psychology of research? In: Lakatos I, Mugrave A, editors. Criticism and the growth of knowledge. Cambridge: Cambridge University Press; 1970.
26. Gallo RC, Montagnier L. The discovery of HIV as the cause of AIDS. N Engl J Med. 2003;349:2283–5.
27. Greene WC. A history of AIDS: looking back to see ahead. Eur J Immunol. 2007;37:S94–102.

28. Centers for Disease Control (CDC). Kaposi's sarcoma and pneumocytitis pneumonia among homosexual men—New York City and California. MMWR Morb Mortal Wkly Rep. 1981;30:305–8.
29. Becker DM. History of preventive medicine. In: Becker DM, Gardner LB, editors. Prevention in clinical practice. Boston: Springer; 1988.
30. Terris M. Evolution of public health and preventive medicine in the United States. Am J Public Health. 1975;65:161–9.
31. Theory. The Merriam-Webster Dictionary. https://merriam-webster.com. Last accessed 5 Sept 2022.
32. Hanson NR. Observation and explanation: a guide to the philosophy of science. New York: Harper and Row; 1971.
33. Hanson NR. Is there a logic of scientific discovery? In: Feigel H, Maxwell G, editors. Current issues in the philosophy of science. New York: Holt, Rinehart and Winston; 1961.
34. Dragulinescu S. Inference to the best explanation and mechanisms in medicine. Theor Med Bioeth. 2016;37:211–32.
35. Feduzi A. On Keynes's conception of the weight of evidence. J Econ Behav Org. 2010;76:338–1.
36. Psillos S. Simply the best: a case for abduction. In: Kakas AC, Sadri F, editors. Computational logic: from logic programming into the future. Dordrecht: Springer; 2002.
37. Velanovich V. The logic of the medical research article. Theor Med. 1993;14:257–63.
38. Spechler SJ, Hunter JG, Jones KM, et al. Randomized trial of medical versus surgical treatment for refractory heartburn. N Engl J Med. 2019;381:1513–23.
39. Thiese M. Observational and interventional study design types; an overview. Biochem Med. 2014;24:199–210.
40. Grimes DA, Schulz KF. Bias and causal associations in observational research. Lancet. 2002;359:248–52.
41. Hacking I. Logic of statistical inference. Cambridge: Cambridge University Press; 1965.
42. Stigler SM. Statistics on the table: the history of statistical concepts and methods. Cambridge, MA: Harvard University Press; 1999.
43. Levi I. Direct inference. J Philos. 1977;74:5–29.
44. Guyatt G, Rennie D, Meade MO, et al., editors. User's guide to the medical literature: a manual for evidence-based clinical practice. 3rd ed. New York: McGraw-Hill; 2015.
45. Murad MH, Asi N, Alsawas M, Alahdab F. New evidence pyramid. Evid Based Med. 2016;21:125–7.
46. Angelmeyer A, Horvath HT, Bero L. Healthcare outcomes with observational study designs compared to randomized trials. Cochrance Database Syst Rev. 2014;(4):MR000034.
47. Johnson RH. Manifest rationality: a pragmatic theory of argument. New York: Routledge; 2012.
48. Velanovich V, Saad AR. Toward a unified theory of the occurrence and recurrence of hiatal hernia. Surgery. 2020;168:1170–3.
49. Sarr MG, Behrns KE, Harken AH, Wexner SD. Editors' introduction to: toward a unified theory of occurrence and recurrence of hiatal hernia. Surgery. 2020;168:1169.
50. Authors response to peer reviews of: toward a unified theory of occurrence and recurrence of hiatal hernia. Surgery. 2020;168:1174–7.
51. Mahoney MJ. Publication prejudices: an experimental study of confirmatory bias in the peer review system. Cogn Ther Res. 1977;1:161–75.
52. Malternd K. The legitimacy of clinical knowledge: toward a medical epistemology embracing the art of medicine. Theor Med. 1995;16:183–98.
53. McGuire CH. Medical problem solving: a critique of the literature. J Med Educ. 1985;60:587–95.
54. McWhinney IR. An acquaintance with particulars…. Fam Med. 1989;21:296–8.
55. Polyani M. The tacit dimension. Gloucester, MA: Peter Smith; 1983.

56. Johannessen KS. Rule following intransitive understanding and tacit knowledge. An understanding of the Wittgensteinian concept of practice as regards tacit knowing. In: Hoibraaten H, editor. Essays in pragmatic philosophy. Oslo: Norwegian University Press; 1990.
57. Schon DA. The reflective practitioner. How professionals think in action. London: Avebury; 1991.
58. Abernathy CM, Hamm RM. Surgical intuition: what it is and how to get it. Philadelphia: Hanley & Belfus, Inc.; 1995.
59. Dreyfus HL, Dreyfus SE. Putting computers in their place. Soc Res. 1986;53:57–76.
60. Kvale S. To validate is to question. In: Kvale S, editor. Issues of validity in qualitative research. Lund: Studentitteratur; 1989.
61. Zagzebski LT. Virtues of the mind: an inquiry into the nature of virtue and the ethical foundations of knowledge. Cambridge: Cambridge University Press; 1996.
62. Kvanvig J. The intellectual virtues and the life of the mind. Lanham, MD: Rowman and Littlefield; 1992.
63. Sainani KL. Explanatory versus predictive modeling. PM&R. 2014;6:841–4.

Chapter 7
Adoption into Clinical Medicine and Application of Medical Knowledge to Patient Care

7.1 Introduction

The prior chapter dealt with the production and acceptance of medical knowledge. For medical practice, however, knowledge is the penultimate goal. The ultimate goal is to provide *useful* knowledge that can be incorporated into patient care decisions. In this way, medicine is a practical pursuit. It is similar to other practical professions. For example, engineers use their knowledge of physics to create machines and other structures to fill a variety of needs; lawyers use their knowledge of law and legal theory to achieve the best legal outcomes for their clients; architects use their knowledge of physics and materials to create buildings; similarly, physicians use their knowledge of biology to address health issues in humans. Whether one wishes to call this an "applied science" or a "craft," I am not going to debate. Nevertheless, it is the physician's task to apply their knowledge to improve the health of their patients. This chapter addresses the application of biomedical knowledge to patient care.

The application of knowledge to practical problems, of course, is not limited to medicine. This is a pursuit of nearly all the professions and trades. Unlike the "pure" sciences or the academic humanities, which pursue knowledge for its own sake, the practitioners of these practical vocations seek useful knowledge that can be applied to the concrete problems that humans face. These concrete problems in medicine are the health of the patient, in general, and cure of disease, in particular. To provide a basis for this chapter, let us review the salient aspects of the physician's cognition and metacognition (Fig. 1.1) from Chap. 1.

Please recall the clinical vignette from Chap. 1—that of a patient with heartburn. The physician's cognition is their focus on the patient's complaints, plus eliciting any other pertinent information that the physician requires to narrow their differential diagnosis. As the physician hears and thinks about what the patient is telling them about their symptoms (i.e., the physician's cognition), the physician is

V. Velanovich, *Medical Persuasion*, https://doi.org/10.1007/978-3-031-30371-5_7

beginning the process of sorting the possible diagnoses based on which of these diagnoses best matches the patient's symptom complex (Fig. 1.1). The physician makes the assumption that the patient's symptoms are a patient-perceived manifestation of some disease state. This is the physician's theoretical framework of their metacognition (Fig. 1.1). In this process, the physician is using their knowledge of disease, which was acquired through their education and training, additional instruction through reading or conferences, and their experiences as a practicing physician. I will refer to this as "accepted medical knowledge," which is the bulk of the corpus of knowledge of a practicing physician. However, the physician will not accept all information presented to them as reliable (or, at least, not reliable enough) to be used in clinical applications, that is, the evidence for the underlying theory of the physician's metacognition (Fig. 1.1). Physicians, as discussed in Chap. 6, will have a variety of criteria, at various levels of rigor, to accept this new knowledge, which are the techniques of evidential foundational appraisal (Fig. 1.1); that is, how the evidence the physician may use was generated and, therefore, how reliable it is. Nevertheless, most knowledge that physicians come from what they perceive to be trusted sources.

The main theme of this chapter is the rational basis for how that physician chooses among the possible diagnoses for a particular patient and how they come to treatment decisions. My contention is that the physician will create a logical argument, perhaps unconsciously, to themselves, unless they are forced to defend their diagnostic and therapeutic decisions to others. As discussed in Chap. 2, I defined rationality as a "human mental framework that leads to the adoption of processes that result in well-founded beliefs and practices." I certainly think that most physicians meet this definition of rationality and that most are rational agents. Additionally, in Chap. 2, after reviewing the types of logical systems, I determined that the informal logical system best describes how physicians come to conclusions in everyday practice and, for the most part, how patients accept these conclusions. However, I did not attempt to determine a set of normative rules because it is unlikely that these rules would be followed as prescribed. Rather, as I have throughout this book, I will try to take a practical approach, coupled with ideas and theories of other writers on this subject.

7.2 Proposed Methods of Reasoning by Healthcare Professionals

How physicians and other healthcare professionals reason about patients' problems has been the source of much thought. What I will provide here are several theories about this reasoning to which may be pertinent to how physicians incorporate medical knowledge into their decision-making and how physicians come to a diagnosis and treatment recommendations. These will be presented in the most relevant sections below.

7.3 How a Physician Determines Which Diagnostic Tests or Treatments Should Be Incorporated into Medical Practice

7.3.1 Conceptualization of Disease

Although I have acknowledged that the physician's task also includes prevention, the physician's traditional and still ongoing role is in addressing illness in a given patient. Specifically, the physician is tasked with diagnosing the patient's disease and recommending the most appropriate treatment. For this, they must have a concept of disease in general and of a specific disease that afflicts a particular patient. I have discussed biomedical theories in Chap. 6, and medicine certainly has an overarching theory of disease, which I defined in Chap. 6 as "an abnormal deviation of the homeostatically operational structure and function of a specific human body or mind, such that the individual will perceive adverse well-being or will have shortened survival, with or without intervention." Within this overarching theory, each disease as known to Western medical science has its own theory, as the examples of AIDS/HIV from Chap. 6 or peptic ulcer disease in Chap. 5 illustrate. However, we must acknowledge the limitations of the universality of biological theories pertaining to medicine. That is, biomedical theories tend to be bounded by disease type and/or pathophysiology. This may not account fully for the patient's perception of their illness from a personal, cultural or social level and may affect the physician's ability to persuade the patient. Nevertheless, there are two notions at work here. One is the conceptualization of the disease in the physician's mind that they can manipulate while thinking. The other is the actual physical pathophysiology occurring in the patient. The physician must approximate their mental abstraction as close to the physical manifestation as possible to be able to effectively reason about what, on a practical level, should be done for the patient to achieve their healthcare goals.

7.3.2 Initial Foundation of a Physician's Medical Knowledge

As previously mentioned in Chap. 6, most of a physician's knowledge of medicine comes from formal education in medical school, textbooks, conferences, and the like. It is very likely that the physician accepted this information *prima facie*. The volume of information that a medical student must learn in a relatively short period of time is tremendous. This information is presented through lectures, laboratory demonstrations, textbooks, and the like as accepted knowledge by the medical community. Of course, what is accepted as uncontested medical knowledge now may prove to be false later, as the example of acid and peptic ulcer disease in Chap. 5 illustrates. However, the student is in no position to mount such a challenge. Therefore, it is rational for the student to accept some information or knowledge on authority because no one can learn everything from primary sources [1]. The student merely accepts their teachers and textbooks as trusted, perhaps authoritative, sources of knowledge. This is true for the student-teacher relationship as well as the doctor–patient relationship.

Evidence and Evidence-Based Medicine

The current mantra of evidence-based medicine has been defined as the "conscientious" and "judicious" use of the "best evidence" in making medical decisions [2]. However, "conscientious" and "judicious" represent terms of virtue derived from virtue ethics and virtue epistemology [3]. The implication is that even though evidence-based medicine strives to be as "data-driven" as possible in the assessment of the "best" evidence, there is an invariable component of judgment involved. Below, I will discuss this judgment as *phronesis* or practical wisdom. Nevertheless, it does appear that the proponents of evidence-based medicine desire to abandon the traditional clinical approach to practice, which couples knowledge of pathobiology (pathophysiology) and scientific mechanisms with individual experience and personal intuition with approaches based on research studies and available "scientific" evidence [3]. This acceptable scientific evidence is based on population-level studies, especially randomized, controlled trials [4], eventually producing the evidence hierarchy [5], which was introduced in Chap. 6.

It is important to understand that evidence represents a way to justify or validate propositions or premises in an argument that will be used to support a conclusion. Evidence does have a scientific context but also a human context possessing a social and personal dimension [6]. As was made clear in Chap. 3 about the evolution of the human mind, it truly cannot be otherwise. Evidence can only be interpreted in the context of the individual's social/cultural or professional umwelt. Mike [6] further asserts that evidence needs to be used in the best possible way acknowledging uncertainty. This, I aver, requires a certain wisdom and humility in the individual using the evidence to construct, because of the uncertainty, an informal, but inductive, argument. Therefore, evidence has a scientific factual facet and a more personal, contextual facet. These factual and personal facets affect the two categories of medical evidence—one for specific medical evidence from the patient and one for general evidence that reflects upon the physician's past experience, views and values [7]. It will affect how physicians use the evidence and how patients receive the evidence.

Evidence from Observational or Randomized Controlled Studies

As discussed in Chap. 6, observational studies are certainly one of the most common, if not the most common, medical research studies published. In these types of studies, data from one or more patient cohorts are generated for the purpose of determining disease causation, risk factors, diagnostic accuracy, or treatment outcomes, among other purposes. These generally produce data based on frequencies, means or medians, or correlations and regressions. These data are usually analyzed, most often statistically, to assess how well they support the hypothesis. There are several considerations that a physician needs to assess to determine if the evidence should be incorporated into their corpus of medical knowledge and used in any clinical decision-making.

The first consideration is that inferences from observational, as well as randomized trials, are based on "bounded" populations from which the sample size was obtained. Specifically, what I mean by a bounded population includes such factors as the geographical area that the sample size comes from, racial/sex distribution, and restrictions due to inclusion and exclusion criteria. As our clinical vignette from Chap. 1 was for a patient with GERD, let us look at an example of observational studies related to the use of Nissen fundoplication for the surgical treatment of GERD. The study published by Peters et al. [8] of Nissen fundoplication analyzes a sample of patients from their practice in that particular location. This then bounds the sample to a specific group of individuals at a specific time period. Therefore, the physician must decide how "generalizable" these data are. What I mean here is: Are the patients in this study similar enough to humans in general that the data can be extrapolated to all humans? If not, then to which subset of humans? If just to a subset of humans, does that subset include the patients in a particular physician's practice. This becomes an induction problem. For example, in the study by Peters et al. [8] pertaining to Nissen fundoplication, the study population probably reasonably reflects patients with GERD referred to a university practice. Similar considerations are also relevant for randomized, controlled trials. For example, in the study presented by Spechler et al. [9] in the last chapter, the sample was chosen from a pool of patients referred to gastroenterology clinics within the United States Veterans Affairs medical facilities. How well these samples reflected all patients within the Veterans Affairs medical system and how well the population of the Veterans Affairs system represents the general population is a judgment that has to be made by physicians trying to determine the generalizability of these conclusions. In other words, this becomes an issue of categorization.

One of the themes of this chapter is that precise categorization of a patient is the *sine qua non* task of the physician. There are several factors that will make up the characteristics of a category of patients. It is vital to determine which of these characteristics are essential for placing any one patient into that category. In addition to the characteristics mentioned above, other characteristics, such as additional comorbidities, medication allergies or adverse reactions, patient preferences and values, and, unfortunately in some jurisdictions, insurance coverage can affect whether a particular patient or group of patients is in the same category of patients as in the study.

Next, as mentioned in the last chapter, are there problems associated with bias and confounding in the study? There are several issues here due to accurate and relevant measurements, comorbidities, and types of treatments. Of particular importance in procedural studies is the level of skill required to perform the procedure. For example, a study advocating a particularly difficult procedure would be completely unapplicable to a physician not trained in that procedure. Therefore, this would affect whether the physician incorporates this knowledge as relevant to their practice. The issues surrounding operations or procedures will be discussed later in the chapter.

A physician trying to determine whether a diagnostic test or treatment should be incorporated into practice based on observational studies will need to address several issues. The first issue has to be due to the validity of the conclusions of the study. This was discussed in Chap. 6. Next, is the preponderance of evidence. For a physician to incorporate new techniques, whether diagnostic or therapeutic, usually requires more evidence than a single study. Most practical physicians would like to see several studies from other investigators before incorporation. Logically, these can be considered conjunctions of premises that support the conclusion. Using the example of the Nissen fundoplication, this operation has been in practice since the mid-1950s, is described in all general surgical and gastrointestinal surgical textbooks, and has been taught to generations of general and gastrointestinal surgeons. A literature search in PubMed[1] using the phrase "Nissen fundoplication" returned 7608 articles. There is much evidence (with some, admittedly, having different interpretations) for this treatment. Other evidence may also include approval from state/national regulatory agencies. That is, if the treatment is not approved for use in a given patient population or for a particular purpose (sometimes this is referred to as an "off-label" use), the physician may not incorporate it into their practice because the lack of regulatory approval will lower the confidence in the treatment by the physician.

However, this is certainly not a uniform consideration by all physicians or other healthcare professionals. Individuals naturally vary in their enthusiasm to adopt innovations and will have different criteria and motivations to do so (more on "non-patient" motivations of physicians below). There is the "Rogers's bell curve" of the diffusion of innovations where approximately 2.5% of professionals who are the "innovators" of new medical practices, the 13.5% who are the "early adopters," the 34% who adopt as the "early majority," the 34% who adopt as the "late majority," and finally, the 16% who are the "laggards" [10]. There may be a number of reasons why this distribution is like this, including physician awareness of the innovation, the physician not being persuaded that the evidence warrants adoption, general lack of physician education leading to a misunderstanding of the innovation, possible unforeseen consequences when the innovation is applied generally, not wishing to use "experimental" treatments, or other practical matters. The point is that physicians and other individuals will vary in their adoption of new innovations, and, in my opinion, this is related to their social/cultural/professional umwelt rather than strict normative criteria.

Even a well-executed controlled trial can lead to unforeseen consequences when the conclusions are applied to the general population. An example of such was the drug class of COX-2 inhibitors. A randomized trial of celecoxib (Celebrex[R]) versus

[1] There is a very good account of the rise of the political dominance of allopathic medicine in Paul Starr's The Social Transformation of American Medicine: The Rise of a Sovereign Profession and the Making of a Vast Industry.

nonsteroidal anti-inflammatory drugs was published in 2000, showing fewer episodes of gastrointestinal toxicity with equivalent pain relief [11]. This was followed quickly with aggressive marketing by the pharmaceutical company, with subsequent widespread use of the drug. Within a short time, reports of the increased occurrences of cardiovascular complications with not only this drug but also others in the same class (e.g., Bextra^R and Vioxx^R) led to the withdrawal of Bextra^R from the market [12] and restrictions of the others by regulatory agencies [13]. This is an example showing that the original samples that formed the basis of these studies may not have reflected the general population. This is also a problem of inductive argumentation. That is, a set of particular observations were made that were extrapolated in a general conclusion, which, in this case, was materially false, even though the logical construction and the premises of the study were true.

One of the practical matters is the question that a physician may have of "Can I institute the diagnostic test or treatment in my practice?" The corollary question is "Is my practice or institution capable of performing this test or treatment?" There are a variety of reasons why a particular practice or institution cannot incorporate a diagnostic or therapeutic innovation into their armamentarium. Such limitations include financial limitations, lack of expertise, lack of demand, lack of interest, etc. My purpose here is not enumerate all the potential reasons, but simply to state that even if a physician feels that the evidence points toward incorporation, it may simply not be possible to do so. In fact, these considerations become part of the reasoning process pertaining to the adoption of a new technology. I will discuss more below on other "nonpatient" considerations that physicians will use in an argument like this.

The above considerations pertaining to how well a particular treatment works are examples of the difference between "efficacy" and "effectiveness." *Efficacy* pertains to whether an intervention produces a difference under "ideal" circumstances; efficacy trials (otherwise also known as "explanatory trials") are the means to determine this. *Effectiveness* measures the "degree of beneficial effect" under "real world" clinical settings. Effectiveness trials (pragmatic trials) are the means to determine this [14]. These authors say, in addition, that to be clinically "meaningful," the results must be relevant to specific patient populations in specific settings [14], that is, a specific diagnostic category of patients. Moreover, can an individual physician use the results in their reasoning about their patients? This is a practical matter. In Chap. 6, we previously discussed the "internal" and "external" validity of a study. To reiterate, external validity is a study's generalizability or applicability [14]. For the physician, is the knowledge asserted by a study general knowledge that can be applied to humans as a whole or some defined subset of humans? Factors that determine this include, some of which were previously mentioned, patient characteristics, the condition under investigation, drug regimens, costs, compliance, comorbidities, and concomitant treatments [14]. To this, I would add procedurally related factors such as type of procedure, who is doing the procedure and patient-to-patient and surgeon-to-surgeon variability of the procedure. Trials may not always take these factors into consideration. The trade-off when investigators try to increase generalizability is that internal validity may suffer [14]. Many trials are keen on determining the magnitude of the treatment effect of the intervention. That is, they are interested in testing the intervention. These investigators do everything possible to reduce confounding and bias. This does not necessarily determine how patients respond to the treatment. The former is efficacy, and the latter is effectiveness. This is a nuanced but important difference. Therefore, the hypothesis of the study is vital—is the aim to determine the precise treatment effect in a group of patients, or is the aim to determine the treatment outcome in day-to-day clinical practice. One is not necessarily better than the other, only that the information is not exactly interchangeable. The discerning physician just needs to understand what the conclusion is so that they can use it as a premise in a future argument correctly.

Systematic Reviews/Meta-analyses

At the top of the "evidence pyramid" (Fig. 6.4) are systematic reviews and meta-analyses. The reason that these are considered the "best evidence" in the framework of evidence-based medicine is that they supposedly provide an analysis of "best" data on a particular topic. A systematic review, as opposed to traditional literature reviews, "aims to comprehensively identify all relevant studies on a specific topic and to select appropriate studies based on explicit criteria. ...the methodological quality of the studies included is assessed by on the basis of explicit criteria..." [15]. All this is supposed to lead to a review that "is transparent, verifiable, and reproducible, and, as a result, the likelihood of bias is considerably smaller" [15]. There are very specific guidelines pertaining to how a systematic review should be performed, for example, the "Preferred Reporting Items for Systematic Reviews and Meta-Analyses (PRISMA)" (Table 6.3). The goal of these guidelines is to obtain the "best" information in the most transparent way. Then, criteria are set as to which of these studies is included in the systematic review. The ultimate purpose is to improve the quality of the evidence by including only "high-quality studies" and eliminating the judgment of the author(s) as to what is the most important or impactful evidence for the sake of "reducing bias." The value is that systematic reviews probably do provide the *best* evidence of efficacy, but they do so at the expense of the most *appropriate* evidence of effectiveness. In addition, a few of the pitfalls of systematic reviews, as with meta-analyses below, is that there is a publication bias for "positive" studies, i.e., those showing a treatment effect, negative studies are frequently never published, and it is common not to be able to identify or obtain the data for unpublished studies.

A meta-analysis is a statistical method that is used to combine the data of individual studies "to arrive at a more accurate estimate of (exposure) effects" [15]. As meta-analyses are frequently performed for treatments, the effects in question are generally differences between treatment and placebo or between two or more treatments. The theoretical statistical foundation of meta-analysis is worth discussing. It is essential to use statistics to determine a characteristic value of any population or to compare populations. Briefly, there exists a theoretical imaginary population of studies comparing treatment A, T_A, to treatment B, T_B, and these studies each have a true difference between the treatment outcomes, O, such that $T_A - T_B = O$. For example, if there was a treatment A for a particular disease that had an absolute true outcome of 80% survival, while treatment B had an absolute true survival of 30%, O would be 50%. This value of 50% is the true difference, and each trial within the imaginary population will be a point estimate of this true difference. Each actual study comparing T_A to T_B is a randomly chosen member of the theoretical imaginary population, and all of the actual studies are a random sample of the entire theoretical imaginary population. Please note the distinction: The actual population of studies done *is not* the population from which the sample is drawn; *it is* the sample of an imaginary population that would exist if we indeed had access to all of those imaginary studies freely (according to the principles of sampling as discussed in the prior chapter). Therefore, if there were *n* studies, the members of the sample of treatment differences would be $O_1, O_2, \ldots, O_n$. It is assumed that this sample of O's will follow a Gaussian distribution (normal bell-shaped curve) and that the mean of O's will be the point estimate of the true treatment difference O.

A very important assumption is that the population of studies of T_A compared to T_B are methodologically the same (or, at least, close enough the same as not to make a material difference). This is an essential feature in which theory differs from practice.[2] From a practical standpoint, it is rare for studies, especially randomized, controlled trials that take significant time and resources, to be replicated exactly, as discussed in Chap. 6. There are several reasons for this: There is a research and publication bias for "new" results or information. Replicating a study simply does provide "novel" results. There is also a publication bias against "negative" result trials. Therefore, frequently, studies that did not show a statistically significant difference between treatments will not be published or event submitted for publication.[3] Therefore, we can see possibility that the studies actually completed and published may not, in fact, be representative of the theoretical, imaginary true population of such studies. Hence, determining how much difference is tolerable is a matter of judgment by the individuals performing the meta-analysis. This can be addressed by these individuals with tests of heterogeneity, but once again, it is left to the investigators performing the meta-analysis as to how much heterogeneity is too much.

There are two consequences to this. First, the meta-analysis point estimate may not truly reflect the true treatment difference. In fact, we truly have no way of determining how close the point estimate is to the actual difference. Second, because of techniques to reduce heterogeneity, applicability to any one patient or physician practice is limited. That is, with attempts to increase homogeneity and "large numbers," there is a loss of granularity. In other words, we have once again the issue of improving the point estimate of efficacy as the expense of

[2] I have two aphorisms that are consistent with this point. One is "The longer I go on in this business, the less confident I am in predicting what's going to happen." The other is "Just when you think you know it all, something happens to prove that you don't."

[3] I am quoting Toulmin directly here. Perhaps a more inclusive moniker would be a "religious advisor."

understanding the effectiveness of the treatment. This then becomes a problem of with the category of the patient match the category for which the treatment is effective.

Loss of granularity is a broad, but sometimes poorly recognized, problem in population-based studies. A significant amount of patient detail is either not recorded or ignored. This is exactly the opposite of what the clinician does. The clinician attempts to accumulate as much relevant detail as possible about an individual patient, knowing that any of these data points may eventually be a key premise in any clinical argument about a patient's care. However, such granularity in a study may be difficult to gather and even more difficult to quantify for statistical analysis purposes.[4] The only types of publications where such granularity and detail is the *sine qua non* of the study are case reports. Therefore, although a meta-analysis may provide the best-possible point estimate of the true treatment effect, it does not provide the wisdom of how to apply the point estimate to an individual patient.

Systematic Reviews vs. Narrative Reviews

I explained above what a systematic review is; however, I did not give an account of what a "traditional" narrative review is. In common practice until the advent of the systematic review, a narrative review is the review article in a journal or even book chapter summarizing and synthesizing the extant information on a specific subject. These reviews are generally performed by either experts in the field or those with intense interest in the subject. Usually, the authors are already quite knowledgeable about the literature and are intimately familiar with the field's challenges and knowledge gaps. They do not approach the task with the primary purpose of "reducing bias" but, rather, to increase understanding—one can rightly say, to provide a modicum of wisdom. They may not have a "systematic" method of choosing articles for review, but rather, they value studies for the importance of their conclusions in understanding the field. They interpret the content of the article in relation to what is known and what needs to be known. In other words, the process is that of practical (and professional) wisdom of understanding effectiveness, perhaps at the expense of efficacy (although I am not convinced that this latter assertion is true).

Are all narrative reviews also the epitome of wisdom? Of course not. These authors are potentially subject to the same foibles as the rest of humanity, such as being overly critical of those who have a differing opinion and too confident in their own. The physician reading such articles should be on the alert for such problems. Nevertheless, to lambast narrative reviews as hopelessly bias and, therefore, to be dismissed, is, in my opinion, unjustified.

---

[4] The reader will recall that this is the very same Charles S. Peirce who proposed the logic of abduction.

Evidence-Based Medicine and the Duhem-Quine Problem

Evidence-based medicine, in its quest for the "best" evidence, is open to shortcomings in understanding. Specifically, in comparing the tenets of evidence-based medicine to the tenets of medical understanding more broadly, evidence-based medicine creates a problem of underdetermination of theory by evidence as expounded by the Duhem-Quine thesis/problem [16], which was previously discussed this problem in Chap. 6. As a reminder, the Duhem-Quine thesis/problem is that it is impossible to test a scientific hypothesis in isolation because an empirical test of the hypothesis requires one or more background assumptions, for example, background theories and prior observations; thus, the test of the hypothesis is also a test of the test. What "underdetermines" means in this sense is that the data presented as evidence are not enough to determine the conclusion. A simplistic, but good, example of this is the aphorism: "Correlation does not prove causation." Simply because two phenomena are frequency, or even exclusively, found together does not prove that one caused the other, as the example of day always following night in Chap. 5. There are two types of underdetermination, holist and contrastive [17]. Holist underdetermination arises when our inability to test hypotheses in isolation leaves us underdetermined in our response to some disconfirming evidence. This is because a hypothesis has empirical implications or consequences only when conjoined with other hypotheses and/or background beliefs. Contrastive underdetermination is that for any corpus of evidence confirming a theory, there might well be other theories that are also confirmed by that very same body of evidence [17]. Therefore, when evidence-based medicine claims that particular methods of obtaining evidence are the "best" methods, it frequently fails to acknowledge all of the background theory, much of which was not obtained by "best-evidence" means. For example, the evidence-based dogma of hierarchies of evidence privileges clinical research over basic science, exacerbating the problem of underdetermination [16]. That is, probabilistic population-based comparisons over mechanistic explanations or causally attributive sequences. Evidence-based medicine is contained within a "black box" of causal attribution, and is accepted as best evidence based solely on its statistical significance. Moreover, I would add that evidence-based hierarchies actually prioritize certain types of clinical research, namely, randomized, controlled trials and meta-analyses, such that only the results of these types of studies are worthy of belief. Because of creating homogenous groups of patients for bias and confounding reduction purposes, it reduces the number of patients for which the data are applicable. It also "confounds" decisions for the clinician by reducing potentially relevant granular data. Therefore, evidence-based medicine is unable to meaningfully test core medical beliefs that form the basis of our understanding of disease and therapeutics [16]. This is because such causal attribution through mechanism, although very appealing to both healthcare professionals and the lay public, is not even in the evidence hierarchy explicitly, although it may be present implicitly as "expert opinion"—at the lowest level of evidence. I agree with Chin-Yee [16] that evidence-based medicine prevents the development of a theoretical framework required for understanding mechanisms of disease and new therapies.

Evidence-Based Medicine and Tacit Knowledge/Clinical Epidemiology

In the prior section, I discussed the problem of underdetermination of the "evidence" in evidence-based medicine. In this section, I will discuss how it also fails to account for "tacit knowledge", which was previously discussed in Chap. 6. Evidence-based medicine does not account for tacit knowing as developed by Polanyi [18]; rather, it wants to eliminate tacit knowing from clinical medicine [19]. This is because there is a dichotomy between clinical and statistical intuition in clinical reasoning [19]. This has led to clinicians finding that evidence-based medicine has not improved but has hindered clinical judgment [20–22]. In my opinion, the foundational issue is that evidence-based medicine uses population-based comparative studies as "best evidence" that are done using homogenous groups to eliminate confounding, but it is exactly those confounding factors that the clinician must use in their clinical reasoning. In addition, because of an emphasis on confounding reduction through study design and statistical methodology, the "explanatory power" of the study is almost irrelevant.

Tacit knowledge cannot be ignored because clinicians use "tacit knowing" in clinical practice [23]. This is compatible with intuition, as discussed in Chap. 2, and the techniques for evidential appraisal, as shown in Fig. 1.1. For Polanyi [18], tacit knowing is equivalent to "practical intuition" (I am not sure there is any other kind of intuition but practical. But that opinion is irrelevant for my purpose here). In Chap. 2, I discussed the account of Abernathy and Hamm [24] of the intuition of the experienced physicians. This account dovetails almost seamlessly with Polanyi, in that physicians not only have a great deal of medical knowledge but also have a wealth of experience (and, hence, not only data but also personally tested evidence appraisal methods) with how actual human patients interact with them. Specifically, physicians, especially those who are experienced, perceive nonverbal information from the patient, often unconsciously produced by the patient and received by the physician, in making their assessment as how ill a patient may actually be. Moreover, tacit knowing and evidence-based medicine are diametrically opposed in their epistemological foundations [19]. This is exactly the type of "soft data" that evidence-based medicine discounts with the scientific slur of "anecdotal evidence." Evidence-based medicine dismisses individual knowledge without transforming it into another theory [19]. In other words, it is as if these data do not exist, let alone deserve epistemological status.

"Clinical epidemiology," on the other hand, is the application of statistics to clinical reasoning without sacrificing the fluidity of the clinical context [19]. One sees this in observational studies or case series which generally have more clinically relevant detail in their analyses, by my observations, and, therefore, more helpful granularity. Although I have emphasized experienced physician intuition and practical wisdom, it also must be acknowledged that this does not consistently produce the "right answer" to clinical problems. As observed by Elstein [25], "Expert clinical judgment is not as expert as we thought it was." Sadly, even the best of clinicians make errors. These errors require some type of explanation. I wonder how much these errors are due to lack of physician knowledge, errors in reasoning, or not thorough enough thinking due to time pressures of their clinical practice (which will be discussed below). An increased reliance on randomized, controlled trials will not improve this situation, as, according to Braude [19], such a reliance is not entirely warranted epistemologically.

There is a danger of overreliance on statistical methodologies that paint illusions of precision. The great statistician Ronald Fisher was skeptical that we could reach absolute certainty about facts based purely on statistical analysis [19]. There is an issue with the insistence on statistical certainty at the expense of clinical reasoning. Every physician knows that knowledge obtained in the clinic is always contingent and embodied [19]. That is, a physician during the iterative process of coming to a conclusion about a diagnosis is open to revising the level of confidence they have in the evidence based on continually accumulating additional evidence (perhaps through tacit Bayesian qualitative calculations). This is an important point in that much of clinical decision-making is time-dependent and is a judgment made with a quantum of uncertainty. Even proponents of evidence-based medicine [26] acknowledge that without clinical expertise, clinical practice risks becoming tyrannized by external evidence. For Feinstein [27], clinical epidemiology, as opposed to evidence-based medicine, is characterized by its use of epidemiological and statistical analytical methods to enhance clinical reasoning. Feinstein [27] believes that evidence-based medicine ignores the subtlety of the clinical context. In my opinion, it appears that evidence-based medicine actually takes the patient out of the decision-making argument because the patient does not represent the "best evidence."

What should we make of clinical experience? It is very common to hear physicians, especially seasoned physicians, say "In my experience..." with the implication that they have a great deal of credence in this evidence. According to Feinstein in his classic work, *Clinical Judgment* [28], clinical experience is the accumulation of clinical wisdom or knowledge through the experience gathered over time of treating individual patients. Moreover, "clinical judgment" is not the knowledge of causes, mechanisms or names for diseases but a knowledge of patients [28]. I would also add, for physicians, and especially for surgeons, knowledge of oneself. What I mean by this is that knowing one's capabilities and capacities is no small part of practical wisdom and clinical judgment.

The type of logic employed in structuring an argument leading to a diagnosis has been assessed differently by different authors. For example, Feinstein [28] assessed that deductive logic is employed to establish a diagnosis, an etiology, or a pathogenesis of a patient's disease. I am not completely convinced that deductive logic is the correct form to describe this process, but I will acknowledge that others assert it is as well. It is not just arriving at a diagnosis, I would also add the "degree" of disease, or, even within a particular patient, severity and "clinical or personal" impact of the disease, that is, how the disease impacts the patient personally, is a matter of diagnostic interest to the physician. In another series of works, Feinstein [29–31] further asserts the physician's "sensory organs give a clinician the power to make many observations of which no inanimate instrument is capable ..." This has implications for artificial intelligence in medicine because artificial intelligence relies on data input, in the form of numbers, words or pixels, not direct observation in a social context, more on this in Chap. 9. Statistical techniques are mere adjuncts to the huge range of data that the good clinician should use in forming clinical judgments. Nevertheless, there has not been adequate attention given by serious investigators to clinical judgment [32].

Feinstein [28] thought that clinical judgment required logical discipline; he also asserted that "intuition" based on "hunches" or "nebulously defined" clinical experience also lacked logical discipline. Others have thought the same, which will be addressed below. Nevertheless, he acknowledged intuition in medicine but implored it to be more explicit: "without intuition, imagination or esthetics, the 'scientist' is a dullard. Without rationality, discipline or logic, the 'artist' is a dawdler" [28]. That is, having an intuitive spark of inspiration is one thing, but it must be supported by valid argumentation. By itself, intuition is insufficient as explicit knowledge, yet it is an inherent part of the process of linking tacit knowing with explicit knowledge [19]. Intuition is an inescapable practical cognitive element of clinical reasoning by many physicians that incorporates tacit elements of clinical knowledge in a rational manner, albeit one that resists explicit formulation [19]. More on this below.

7.3.3 *Phronesis* and Medical Practice

The concept of *phronesis* comes, like many things in Western philosophy, from Aristotle. He defined *phronesis* as practical wisdom that guides the achievement of the good human flourishing using the "right" means [33, 34]. One can assert, particularly given the World Health Organization's definition of health quoted in the prior chapter, that a concept of *phronesis* in medical practice is needed. Medical decisions and recommendations in routine clinical practice can follow accepted protocols and guidelines. That is, the "easy" decisions that make up the bulk of clinical practice, which physicians practice almost habitually. However, in more complex cases, these deliberations require more than just the "best evidence," institutional protocols, or professional society guidelines. Because of these complexities and nuances, some authors have advocated "alternative ways" of coming to the "best" rather than the "right" decision, where "best" equates to good and "right" equates to correct in the sense of true or approved [35] (please note that this usage of the word "best" is different that the way it is used in evidence-based medicine. It is more akin to its usage in "virtue theory" [33]). In this sense, the "right" recommendation would be the evidence-based recommendation. However, in this context, *phronesis* involves the ability to know and deliberate about the goals that are worth pursuing and the "right means" most likely to accomplish those goals [36]. Medical decisions require clinical knowledge, understanding of patients' social circumstances, patients' or caregivers' values and beliefs, and the available resources [37]. Kaljian [37] developed a five-stage theory related to goals, concrete circumstances, virtues, deliberation and motivation to act. It is reasonable to expect, although this is done mostly out of professional habit than overt thought, for physicians to behave in this manner because of the need to make practical decisions about their patients.

These practical decisions are the stuff of the physician's work. In their daily activities, physicians are not typically in search for the truth but are trying to choose among alternative actions [38]. Practitioners learn their craft as a set of more or less general principles implemented and augmented by certain "tricks of the trade," self-discovered or copied and adopted from respected teachers [38]. However, as these practitioners become experienced, they internalize these principles so that their application and their modification through experience become largely subconscious. A skilled practitioner will rely heavily on the subconscious choices and will strenuously resist any attempt to focus consciousness upon them because it would lead to a loss of efficiency [38]. This is another description of the physician's tacit knowledge and intuition in the framework of practical wisdom or *phronesis*.

Physician's Need to Evaluate Evidence and Act Despite Uncertainty

Physicians have a deep and perhaps unrealized connection to the fundamental means by which to gain certainty, that is, reasoning [39]. For Montgomery [39], medical errors are due to poor reasoning. Examples of poor reasoning by some authors include "nonanalytic" decision-making processes such as intuition, emotional intelligence [40], and the "dual process theory of cognition" [41]. I am not necessarily convinced that all medical errors are due to "poor reasoning." I have previously discussed in Chap. 2 that one can have a completely sound argument with a valid conclusion based on the available premises thought to be true but may be materially false either because the heretofore presumed true premises were actually false (or, at least, not true enough) or crucial premises were not included in the argument because they were simply unknown at the time. We have also discussed in Chap. 3 how the human mind evolved to actually effectively use emotion in decision-making. As mentioned in the section pertaining to intuition in Chap. 2, physicians may "feel uneasy" because they sense that "something is not right" with their patient, which is simply a form of self-emotional intelligence. However, to be clear, being attuned to the emotions of oneself or others is not the end of the rational process; it merely points to maybe where to start. The physicians still must sort through and evaluate evidence to increase certainty but must act in the face of uncertainty. Kassirer [42] noted that physicians tend to overvalue diagnostic certainty prior to coming to a decision, leading to over-testing and sometimes under-action. For clinicians, according to Montgomery [39], accumulating relevant facts is insufficient to make medical decisions, and other factors come into play. To this, I would add that there are "external" factors with which all health care professionals must contend, such as time constraints, competing pressures with other patients, need for income generation, administrative issues, etc. These practical external pressures, quite frankly, are mostly ignored by theoretical accounts of medical decision-making, but I will discuss them below.

Physicians, and probably most people, understand evidence can only be evaluated in the context of other background information and frameworks. For example, it is not enough that a randomized, controlled trial produces a "score" (as discussed in Chap. 6) of one treatment over another and pronounces a "winner," these data need to fit into a larger theoretical framework of disease, such as causal sequence or mechanism, and the patient's social/cultural context. Such dovetailing to other forms of evidence not only increases the weight of the evidence but also increases understanding by the physician and the patient.

This social context applies not only to the patient in terms of their social/cultural umwelt but also to the physician in terms of their professional umwelt. Montgomery [39] makes a distinction between the predominantly allopathic medicine as practiced in Western societies and other empiric approaches to medical care. He makes the salient observation that the allopathic approach became dominant over other approaches, such as homeopathic medicine, due to wins in the political arena.[5] One theoretical distinction is how human variability is viewed. Allopathic medicine views variability among humans as variability of a specific human archetypal form, while homeopathy, as an example of an alternative theory, views each human as ontologically distinct, with just a diversity of these distinct types. That is, each human is their own archetype [39]. Because of this theoretical difference, allopathic physicians seek "economical" explanations for variety, such as seeking a "general principle" to explain variety. One of these general principles is the reference to "dichotomizing" forces and entities to achieve a great economization of underlying mechanisms and principles [39]. However, human health is more complicated, which makes comprehensive theories impossible to universally apply.

One such theory is the statistical principle of the "central limit theorem." The central limit theorem states that the distribution of a mean of sample values is approximately normal, regardless of the distribution of the values used to calculate the mean, and grows closer to normal as the sample size increases [43]. Let us take the example of a randomized, controlled trial that might establish the "mean effect" for a treatment for a particular disease, but Montgomery asserts that this is not the "real effect" of the treatment [39]. He goes on to say that these data are based on the statistical central limit theorem, which has an ontological status of its own—namely, that the mean becomes "the measure of any individual subject" [39]. That is, what we think of as "normal" is what falls within the 95% confidence interval. More to the point, if, say, the odds ratio for cure of a disease based on a randomized, controlled trial is 1.5, this is sometimes interpreted that *each individual patient* has a 50% greater chance of improvement with the treatment than without. However, this is clearly not the case; even though the process might, in fact, be stochastic in nature, we cannot make the *a priori* assumption that each individual patient has that chance, only, on average, that the entire population of such patients will have that chance in aggregate. Therefore, it is crucial for clinicians to recognize when the mean does not provide sufficient information for their own or the patient's decision-making [39]. This is an assertion with which I agree.

---

[5] There are many aphorisms in medicine for this concept: "Common diseases are common." "When you hear hoofbeats look for horses, not zebras." "It is more common to have an atypical presentation of a common disease rather than a typical presentation of an uncommon disease.", etc.

7.4 How a Physician Determines Which Diagnostic Tests or Treatments Would Be Appropriate for an Individual Patient

7.4.1 Medical Diagnostic Reasoning

Diagnosis serves not only as a basis for treatment decisions but also to explain a patient's symptoms and signs. This explanation requires a causal mechanism in which the "cause" of the disease produces the symptoms. This mechanistic understanding comes not from the diagnosis itself but from the "theoretical framework" in which the physician operates [44] (note that this is a similar idea to the physician's meta-cognition of Fig. 1.1). There is a bidirectional relation between patient data (signs, symptoms, test results, etc.) and diagnosis: The diagnosis is inferred from the patient data, and the patient data are explained by the diagnosis [44]. Diagnoses are explanatory because they pick out the actual cause of the patient data in each individual case [45]. Blaxter [46] states that diagnosis is an ambiguous term that can refer to either a category or process. Several categories and processes of diagnosis and diagnostic nosology are discussed in Chap. 6.

The concept of diagnosis is a type of *covering law explanation* that appeals to laws or regularities, which presuppose "repeatable types" [44]. However, being a "repeatable type" (as the discussion of Hume and Mill in Chap. 5 illustrated) is not enough. For a repeatable type to be explanatory, the "causal model" of explanation requires that one should provide some information about its cause [47–51]. As discussed in Chap. 5, I have emphasized that the attributed causal sequence to be useful must provide an acceptable level of confidence in prediction. Even though Hempel [52] describes "causal regularities" as "laws of succession," in biomedical theories, these are truly not "laws," but probabilistic causal mechanisms that serve as explanations. Nevertheless, according to Maung [44], "covering law" treats symptoms as repeatable types. Maung [44] views the explanation of an individual case as a "token" of a homogenous type. That is, the patient is in a category of patients with that disease and other distinguishing factors. What is crucially important about individual cases in medicine is what is distinctive about them as particulars [53]. This may not always work in that the likeliest cause of a clinical presentation in the relevant reference class may not be the actual cause of the clinical presentation in an individual case [44]. Between the statements of Gorovitz and MacIntyre [53] and Maung [44], I would say that there could be a myriad of confounding factors which would cast doubt on whether a particular case in a such a "homogenous type." This is because "disease" is a concept meant to provide both meaning and explanation to patient's symptoms and the observed pathology/pathophysiology.

A complete description that achieves absolute concordance between the reference class and the correct diagnosis may not be possible [54, 55]. In fact, physicians must judge which aspects of an individual patient they must ignore to achieve some practical categorization. Each step in the diagnostic process is a matter of successive categorization, which is based on probability calculations, perhaps subconsciously, by the physician, with some tests, such as a biopsy, being nearly 100% certain but most not so (see discussion below). Ultimately, the key function of a diagnosis is to determine the correct treatment for the patient [44]. That is, matching the category the patient is in with the category of appropriate treatments.

Mechanistic explanations, which are considered more intellectually satisfactory by physicians (no doubt, as a remnant of their education, and, perhaps, because it is a type of story), require items to deliver an acceptable causal sequence. Mechanistic explanations should include (1) component parts and (2) their activities organized in such a way that they produce the phenomenon, which is a useful way to think in medicine [56–58]. Mechanisms can provide grounds for prediction about what would happen to a phenomenon of interest given a specific intervention [59]. That is, the importance of causality in predictability. The diagnostic process aims for the degree of identification to achieve the best outcome for the patient [60]. That is, it is a practical matter such that decisions must be made. For those decisions not routine or obvious, practical wisdom was also involved. Mechanisms linking a given diagnosis and patient data may cross a number of overlapping models [44], which are the interlevel and interfield models of biomedical theories that were previously discussed. A theoretical understanding of how cause and effect are linked can consist of knowledge about mechanism malfunction and knowledge about pathological mechanisms or both [58]. This provides the underlying framework for a physician to interpret how probabilistic study results are applicable to their patient.

7.4.2 How Physicians Learn About Disease Presentation

As previously mentioned, physicians (and, for that matter, anyone else) do not primarily learn information and knowledge from assessing original sources. They are usually presented with well-accepted biomedical theories and facts through their education from textbooks, lectures and other educational materials. This provides the overarching framework within which the physician understands all other information presented to them (see the discussion of underdetermination above). New knowledge is then presented to the physician via journal articles, conferences, webinars, etc., and the physician then judges the voracity of these new arguments and whether to adjust their corpus of knowledge (as discussed in Chap. 6). However, for now, let us provide an example of a textbook description of a common disease, GERD, which was our clinical vignette from Chap. 1.

An Example of Textbook Description of a Disease Presentation

This is an example of the presentation of the symptoms of GERD from a standard medical textbook, *Maingot's Abdominal Operations*, 13th ed. [61]:

> Symptoms of gastroesophageal reflux can be categorized as "typical" or "atypical". Typical symptoms include heartburn, regurgitation, water brash, and, when advanced, dysphagia. While considered a typical symptom, dysphagia warrants investigation for potential complications, including an underlying motility disorder, stricture, ring, or malignancy. Atypical symptoms, on the other hand, include cough, globus sensation, hoarseness, throat clearing, asthma, aspiration pneumonia, pulmonary fibrosis and atypical chest pain.

What we see with this description is a qualitative enumeration of the symptoms of GERD. What this description attempts to do is provide the physician with a list of not only what they may hear when a patient recounts their symptoms but also what additional information to elicit from the patient to better complete the "history of present illness" (Fig. 1.1). From this, the physician starts their diagnostic task.

7.4.3 Diagnosis as a Matter of Semiotics of Signs and Symptoms

Nessa [62] proposes understanding the patient's signs and symptoms through the concept of semiotics. Semiotics is the theory of signs and their meaning. A sign stands for something. That is, it is a name we use when referring to something in the world. Wc communicate through signs and interpret the world through the meaning of signs. The subject matter of semiotics is messages and their relation to interpretation, meaning and reference. The "meaning" of a message is given by what the receiver understands by the message. The "reference" of a message concerns the relation between the message and the objects of the world to which the message refers [62]. Nessa [62] refers to the works of Ferdinand de Saussure, the linguist, in whose theory a linguistic sign (e.g., a word) consists of the "signifier" (i.e., the actual word) and the concept that it corresponds to, the "signified" (i.e., the actual phenomenon in the world). For example, in the clinical vignette, the patient and physician use the word "heartburn" to signify the entire process that leads to the patient perceiving that particular symptom. To expand on this, medical symptoms and diagnoses are conceptualizations of ideas and, therefore, are linguistical signs [62]. Nessa [62] then goes on to summarize the theory of Charles S. Peirce[6] in this regard. In Peirce's theory, a "sign" is something that stands for somebody about something in some respect or capacity. It addresses somebody, that is, creates in that person's mind an equivalent sign, or perhaps, a more developed sign. The sign that it creates in the mind is the "interpretant" of the first sign. This sign stands for some actual phenomenon. Therefore, in this theory, there are three elements: the primary sign (the actual word or symbol), the interpretant (the secondary sign created in the mind of the receiver when the primary sign is address toward them), and the actual phenomenon in the world. In this sense, diagnoses are not primarily facts belonging to the "real world" but interpretations and ways of structuring reality, hypotheses

[6] The search was performed on September 27, 2022.

and conjectures. When a patient tells a physician what their symptoms (the actual phenomenon as perceived by the patient) are, the words (the primary sign) they use will be interpreted by the physician (interpretant or secondary sign) to understand what the patient is experiencing and then use this in their assessment. The concordance of the primary sign and interpretant is vital to proceed down the correct diagnostic path.

7.4.4 The Patient's Presentation as a Story or Script

In seeing how a typical description of a patient's presenting symptoms and understanding this as signs in the semiotic sense, what we see is the patient's presentation as a "story" or as a "script." These stories have a qualitative rather than a quantitative feature. It, of course, is not surprising that the patient's symptoms would be fashioned into a story. As discussed in Chap. 3 on the evolution of the human mind, humans have an affinity for stories—it is a human universal. Moreover, it is one of the primary, if not *the* primary, ways that humans communicate with one another.

This History of Present Illness as Clinical Story-Telling

Bowen [63], from a more pedagogical viewpoint, put forth suggested strategies to teach diagnostic clinical reasoning by teaching faculty to clinical trainees. My interest in this work is not in the educational aspect, although there is much to be lauded on this account, but for her description of clinical reasoning. She avers that clinicians "transform" the patient's presentation in a "story" that is a "meaningful" clinical problem [63]. Please note that understanding the world and events around us in story form is a human universal, most likely a direct consequence of human evolution, as described in Chap. 3 and above. In these clinical stories, there is actually very little quantitative analysis, such as Bayesian calculations. From the story formed, the clinician creates a mental abstraction of the patient's information to use to discriminate among the potential diseases afflicting the patient [63]. The first step in diagnostic reasoning is "data acquisition" based on the physician's knowledge, experience and other "contextual factors" [64]. Although not said specifically, what appears to have been meant by "knowledge, experience and other contextual factors" is in the same vein as what I have referred to as the "physician's theoretical framework meta-cognition" in Fig. 1.1. Therefore, "knowledge, experience and other contextual factors" is the overarching theoretical framework, and with this, the process proceeds in a nonlinear, iterative way as follows: patient's story bidirectionally moves to data acquisition to accurate patient "problem representation" to hypothesis generation to search for and selection of illness scripts to diagnosis, with the search for and selection of illness scripts also contributing to additional data acquisition needs [63]. Another way to interpret "knowledge, experience and other contextual factors" is that this also encompasses aspects of wisdom and understanding of the seasoned clinician. "Data acquisition" includes the patient's history, physical examination, and any objective tests. I interpret "hypothesis generation" as creating a differential diagnosis. The "problem representation" is the physician's mental abstraction that is rarely articulated but transforms patient-specific details into abstract terms [65–67], perhaps for easier mental manipulation. These mental abstractions help with the retrieval of information from the working memory of the physician [68], again as a consequence of human brain/mind evolution. Within these mental abstracts, clinicians use "semantic qualifiers", which are paired, opposing descriptors (e.g., high-low, normal-abnormal, etc.) which are paired, opposing descriptors that can be used to compare and contrast diagnostic considerations. One can see how this corresponds to the "dichotomized" thought process as stated by Montgomery [39] above, or to Johnson-Laird's description of rationality by mental models discussed in Chap. 3. Unfortunately, although intellectually easy, such dichotomization leads to a reduction in granularity, which may affect reasoning.

Expert clinicians store and recall knowledge as narrative descriptions of diseases, conditions or syndromes—that is, "illness scripts"—that are connected to problem representations as mental abstracts [65, 69–71]. These representations trigger clinical memory to apply to the patient's particular presentation [63]. This is where the number of categories that the physician can recall works in the diagnostic process. Illness scripts have a predictable structure, almost as a story arc: the disposing conditions, the pathophysiological insult and the clinical consequences [63]. This mental abstraction of "illness scripts" is very similar to the structure of "surgical scripts" as described by Abernathy and Hamm with respect to surgical intuition [24]. Note also the implicit importance of mechanism (the pathophysiological insult), causal attribution (the pathophysiological insult and clinical consequences) and predictability (the clinical consequences) in how physicians understand how the disease process in a particular patient's presentation, which I assert is how most physicians think about clinical medicine. It is also somewhat contradictory to the evidence-based medicine ethos of applying the "best evidence" based on meta-analyses of clinical trials. This process, however, probably does use an unconscious qualitative Bayesian calculation as evidence accumulates revising prior probabilities.

Experience leads to a store of patient cases that the physician can use to recognize nuance and subtlety [63]. This is the basis of Abernathy and Hamm's [24] view of intuition and that of Feinstein's [28], although the latter is somewhat more circumspect about intuition. Additional data gathering is purposeful. It is a search for the defining and discriminating features of each illness script under consideration [63]. This is much different than a series of quantitative Bayesian adjustments of prior probabilities based on each accumulated quantum of evidence. Both analytic and nonanalytic reasoning strategies are effective and can be used simultaneously in an interactive fashion [72]. The nonanalytic fashion is that of pattern recognition (i.e., the illness or surgical scripts), developed through clinical experience, while deliberative analytic reasoning is saved for complex, unusual or rare diseases for which the physician may have little experience [72].

The history, including the history of present illness, past medical, surgical, social and family history, as well as allergies/adverse medical reactions, the review of symptoms, and, finally, the physical examination starts the process for the physician of creating a differential diagnosis, that is, a list of possible diseases that the patient may have. Or, rather, explain their symptoms. These are the first premises the physician uses when starting their reasoning pertaining to this particular patient. This is a process of narrowing the possible categories in which the patient's presentation can be conceptualized by the physician, that is, abstracted in a manner for further rational manipulation. Alternatively, to use the terms of semiotics described above, the patient's primary signs are interpreted by the physician as secondary signs from which they reason. The next step for most, but not necessarily all, cases is that the physician will order additional "objective" testing to further narrow these categories. More precisely, increasing the likelihood that the patient's presentation can be explained by certain categories and decreasing the likelihood that it is explained by others. All this will eventually achieve the goal of having enough confidence that the patient presentation fits in a disease category that matches well enough to an effective treatment.

7.4.5 *Information Through Objective Testing*

Objective testing is used to increase the confidence that a particular patient has a particular disease. That is, they add additional premises to the argument, or another way of understanding it is that they increase the weight of evidence. What is meant by "objective testing" is that the information is not obtained through communications between the patient and physician, nor through a physical examination by the physician (although some would say that a physical examination is objective, but I am not going weigh in on this assertion one way or the other). These tests are processed in a way that is repeatable, and the results are permanently incorporated into the patient's medical record. These include blood and other bloodily fluid tests (usually providing some type of quantitative data), imaging[7] (such as radiographs, ultrasounds, computed-tomographic scan, etc.), physiological tests (see footnote 7) (such as electrocardiographs, manometry, etc.), enhanced visualization technologies (see footnote 7) (such as endoscopies, ophthalmoscopy, nonwhite light wavelengths, etc.) and tissue samples (see footnote 7) (histological examinations, electron microscopy, genetic analysis, etc.). This is not meant to be a comprehensive list but merely to document a sample of what is available as objective tests.

To understand how these objective tests are then incorporated into the physician's diagnostic reasoning, an understanding of the precision of the tests in

[7] This makes one recall the famous Yogi Berra saying, "In theory, there should be no difference between theory and practice; but in practice, there is."

providing reliable (or, at least, reliable enough) information to use as premises in a diagnostic argument will provide a basis.

Sensitivity, Specificity, Positive Predictive Value, Negative Predictive Value, Accuracy

The way that diagnostic tests are determined to be of value is through determining their rates of true positives, true negatives, false positives and false negatives. A true-positive (TP) is defined as the test showing that a disease is present and the disease is present in an individual; a true-negative (TN) is defined as the test showing that the disease is absent and the disease is absent in an individual; a false-positive (FP) is defined as the test showing that the disease is present, but the disease is absent in an individual; and a false-negative (TN) is defined as the test showing that the disease is absent, but the disease is present in an individual. It is assumed that there is some "gold standard" that confirms the presence or absence of the disease (this can be problematic, but I will not address this issue). With this, the *sensitivity* of the test is defined as TP/(TP + FN); that is, the frequency with which the test is positive for the disease when the disease is actually present. The *specificity* of the test is defined as TN/(TN + FP); that is, the frequency with which the test is negative for the disease when the disease is actually absent. The *positive predictive value* of the test is defined at TP/(TP + FP); that is, the frequency at which the test is correctly positive. The *negative predictive value* is defined as TN/(TN + FN), that is, the frequency with which the test is correctly negative [73]. The *accuracy* of a test is defined as (TP + TN)/(TP + TN + FP + FN); that is, the frequency of correct test results in the entire number of tests administered.

Therefore, to be clear, these measures of test performance from the standpoint of test administration. They *do not* reflect the frequency of the patient having or not having the disease based on the test. This is a common error in clinical interpretation. An even more common error is to accept the results of the test in a dichotomized fashion; that is, if the test is negative, the patient does not have the disease, and if the test is positive, the patient does. This is a diagnostic fallacy and can lead clinicians to dismiss possible diagnoses and accept others in error. From the standpoint of creating an argument toward a conclusion, which is the diagnosis, what can occur is that physicians will use premises that are false (or, at least, not true enough) in their arguments, leading to a conclusion that is logically valid but materially false.

Bayesian Probabilities

One of the essential features in correctly interpreting a test is assessing the underlying prevalence of the disease.[8] This is where understanding the Bayes theorem is essential [74]. The foundational concept of the Bayes theorem with respect to

[8] I personally have been involved in two randomized, controlled trials that produced negative results and were never submitted for publication or presentation.

diagnostic testing is that the chance of an individual patient having the disease with a positive or negative test is related to their probability of having the disease prior to testing. This is, in fact, what the physician truly wants to know: What is the chance that this particular patient has the disease in question, given that they have either a positive or negative test. The relevant formulas are as follows:

For the chance of having the disease, given that the test is positive:

$$P[D+|T+] = (P[T+|D+] \times P[D+]) / \{(P[T+|D+] \times P[D+]) + (P[T+|D-] \times P[D-])\}$$

where P[D+|T+] is the probability of having the disease (D+) given that the patient has a positive test (T+); P[T+|D+] is the probability that the test is positive given that the patient has the disease (i.e., the sensitivity); P[D+] is the probability of the patient having the disease prior to any testing (i.e., the *a priori* probability); P[T+|D−] is the probability of a positive test given that the patient does not have the disease (i.e., 1 – the specificity); and P[D−] is the probability of not having the disease prior to testing.

For the chance of having the disease, given that the test is negative:

$$P[D+|T-] = (P[T-|D+] \times P[D+]) / \{(P[T-|D+] \times P[D+]) + (P[T-|D-] \times P[D-])\}$$

where P[D+|T−] is the probability of having the disease given that the patient has a negative test (T−); P[T−|D+] is the probability of a negative test given that the patient has the disease (i.e., 1 − the sensitivity); P[D+] is the probability of having the disease prior to any testing; P[T−|D−] is the probability of a negative test, given that the patient does not have the disease (i.e., the specificity); and P[D−] is the probability of not having the disease prior to any testing.

Let us compare two hypothetical examples, with a test having what would be considered very good sensitivity and specificity of 0.9, i.e., 90%, with the only difference being the *a priori* probability of having the disease.

Example #1: Let P[D+] = 0.1; P[D−] = 0.9; sensitivity = 0.9; specificity = 0.9; P[T+|D+] = 0.9; P[T+|D−] = 0.1; P[T−|D+] = 0.1; P[T−|D−] = 0.9, then P[D+|T+] = 0.5 and P[D+|T−] = 0.012. That is, if given the chance that the patient has the disease is only 10%, then if that patient has a positive test, then their chance of actually having the disease is only 50%. More likely than the background prevalence, but still only a coin flip. On the other hand, their chance of having the disease if the patient tested negative was only 1.2%. That is, far less likely than the background prevalence.

Example #2: Let P[D+] = 0.9; P[D−] = 0.1, with everything else being the same, then P[D+|T+] = 0.988 and P[D+|T−] = 0.5. That is, given the chance that the patient has the disease is 90%, then if the patient has a positive test, their chance of having the disease is 98.8%, while if the test is negative, they still have a 50% chance of having the disease.

Therefore, even though the sensitivity and specificity are the same, the underlying probability of the disease being present (i.e., the prevalence) makes a substantial difference in the level of confidence of the test. In example #1, although the chance of the patient having the disease increases with a positive test from 10% to 50%, if a physician would treat this patient, they have a 50–50 chance of treating someone who does not have the disease. If the treatment has any substantial adverse events, this is not insignificant. That is, there is a potential for the physician to cause harm, rather than help, the patient. On the other hand, with a negative test, the physician can be very confident that the patient does not have the disease. Alternatively, in example #2, the situation is the opposite.

What this means, is that to increase the confidence that a positive test actually means that the patient has the disease (in the parlance of doctors, increasing the "yield" of patients with the disease), the physician should apply the test to those patients for whom it is already more likely to be present. Practically speaking, this is done through the history and physical examination. Conversely, to increase the confidence that the patient does not have the disease when the test is negative, it should be applied to patients who already have a low probability of the disease. However, this latter situation is generally not what either the physician or patient wants because the goal is to get to a diagnosis that will be associated with an effective therapy.

Objective Test Development

Diagnostic test development is a complete subject by itself, and it is not my intention to go into this in great detail [75]. However, the basic tenets are worth reviewing because these tests are used as premises in how a physician reasons about a patient's diagnosis. The process is complex and includes issues related to the burden of proof in establishing the scientific validity of and clinical usefulness of a new test; regulatory hurdles; issues surrounding costs, insurance coverage, and ensuring appropriate compensation for the work that goes into the development and delivery of a new test; preference among physicians for traditional diagnostic methods that are often less formal and require a higher degree of expert analysis and interpretation; among other concerns [75]. None of which I will discuss here.

Example: The Development of the 24-h pH Monitoring for Pathologic Esophageal Acid Reflux

In keeping with the clinical vignette of Chap. 1, one of the main diagnostic tests to "prove" that a patient has pathological esophageal acid reflux is 24-h pH monitoring.[9] The device was developed and tested by Johnson and DeMeester [76]. I do not

[9] Some would argue that imaging, physiological tests, enhanced visualization technologies and some tissue sample examinations are not truly objective because they require the interpretation of a physician, e.g., a radiologist, endoscopist, or pathologist. As true as this is, and I will not argue the point, these are still considered objective tests by most healthcare professionals.

intend to go into great detail in describing its development, but simply to give the salient features.

The idea of measuring the pH (i.e., a measure of acid concentration) of intraesophageal fluid is based on the premise that gastric acid is the primary physiological cause of esophageal acid reflux producing the symptom of heartburn. This connection between esophageal acid exposure and its effects on the esophagus began with Tileston first observing "peptic ulcer of the esophagus" in 1906, and then Winkelstein first correlated the symptoms of heartburn with acid regurgitation and reflux esophagitis [77]. This was the beginning of developing a new disease model, as illustrated in the AIDS/HIV example of Chap. 6 or the *H. pylori*-peptic ulcer disease model of Chap. 5. Approaches to relieving acid reflux, including medical and surgical therapies, followed [78] based on reducing the exposure of the esophageal mucosa to acid, but these approaches were not always successful. Johnson and DeMeester recognized the gap in medical knowledge of not being able to accurately determine if acid reflux was the cause of the patient's symptoms. Hence, through abduction, determined the need to develop an instrument to do just that.

The device that was developed consisted of an antimony pH electrode, a silver-silver chloride cutaneous reference electrode and a portable solid-state memory unit. The monocrystalline antimony pH electrode had a diameter of 2.1 mm and a response time of 90% within 30 s, which was at the end of a long probe. After calibration in buffer solution at pH values of 1 and 7, the electrode was introduced through the nose, and its tip was placed 5 cm above the distal margin of the lower esophageal sphincter previously located by manometry. The reference electrode was placed on the chest, and the digital memory box was worn on the waistbelt. The patients were instructed to spend 12 h ambulant and 12 h recumbent. They were encouraged to maintain their normal activities and eat normal meals with the exception of acidic foods and beverages. GERD medications were discontinued 1 week prior to the test. The pH monitorings were analyzed by a computer program. pH cutoff limits of 2, 3, 4, and 5 were set for the variables of number of reflex episodes, mean number of reflux episodes per hour, number episodes longer than 5 min, length of the longest episode, mean length of reflux episodes, percentage of time spent with a pH below the chosen cutoff limit, frequency duration index = mean number of reflux episodes per hour × mean cumulative duration of reflux episodes per hour. In the ambulatory setting, 30 patients with GERD were compared to 30 volunteers with no symptoms of GERD. Sensitivities and specificities were determined for each cutoff value as well as the 95% confidence interval for the normal controls. It was determined that a pH cutoff of 4 was most discriminatory [79]. Further studies showed that a percent time of pH <4 of >4% and a composite "DeMeester score" of >14.7 were indicative of pathologic acid reflux [76].

Subsequent studies and practice have repeatedly shown the value of pH monitoring in determining the presence of pathologic acid reflux and identifying patients who would benefit from treatment. It is now considered an essential part of the evaluation of patients with symptoms of GERD [61]. In other words, when pH monitoring demonstrates pathological reflux, the physician can be quite confident that pathological reflux is occurring. Because of such innovations as the symptom index or symptom associated probability, the physician can also be confident that the patient-perceived symptoms of heartburn actually correspond to episodes of acid in contact with the esophageal mucosa [61]. The implications for persuasion of the patient are also important.

Caveat: Definitions of "Normal" and "Abnormal"

One of the key points the development of any test is the actual determination was what is "normal" and what is "abnormal." This, of course, varies from test to test, and with some tests, there is some nuance. Broadly speaking, the patient first, then the physician must determine if the information and/or data being received is just the "normal variation" that the patient experiences within themselves or the physician would expect to see among humans, or is it "abnormal" in the sense that it indicates the possible presence of disease. As previously mentioned, much a what is considered normal or abnormal not only has a biological basis but also a social and cultural basis (see Chap. 6). I am only going to discuss the biological basis, as the social and cultural basis of what is considered abnormal, especially in behavior, is far beyond the scope of this book. There are four basic categories of data types the physician must determine whether there is simply normal variation or whether what is observed is abnormal: the patient's symptoms, the physician's physical examination, quantitative objective testing, and qualitative images.

It goes without saying, people have a broad array of physical and psychological experiences. People are aware of varying degrees of their own bodies and psyches. Everybody experiences sensations in different regions of their bodies from time to time. Determining was is a normal from an abnormal sensation is a matter of degree and perception. Consider the experience of "pain." Nearly everyone would consider pain abnormal; however, when does exactly a sensation go from being "no pain" to "pain"? Consider the degrees of nuance of pain descriptions: ache, discomfort, irritation, sore(ness), tender(ness), twinge, hurt, pang, sting, throb, cramp, agony, misery, torment, etc. Additionally, consider the "visual analog scale" of pain from 0 to 10 [80], where 0 is no pain and 10 is the worst pain ever. How an individual patient interprets the scale is obviously subjective and has a great deal of interobserver variability (although that would be nearly impossible to test because there is no gold standard for pain measurement).

It is not just pain, but every physiological activity that has some conscious recognition is perceived on a spectrum by people, such as breathing, talking, urinating, defecating, seeing, hearing, and on and on. The unifying theme, however, is that all of these are patient-perceived sensations, and the individual is the one deciding on what is abnormal for them. There are no "objective" tests to confirm the sensation that the individual is feeling, assuming that the individual is being honest in their report. Although there are objective tests of the corresponding physiological function, e.g., pulmonary function tests, it is not unusual for these not to correspond to the level of symptoms reported by the patient, e.g., dyspnea or shortness of breath. Although the patient decides if a symptom is "abnormal for me," it is the physician that must interpret whether this corresponds to a disease state, vis-à-vis semiotic interpretations of signs as discussed above.

It is, of course, self-evident that the human form varies from individual to individual. Determining what is an expected normal variation from an abnormal variation in the physical examination is both the task of the patient and physician. It is, naturally, common that a patient will notice a change in their body, such as a lump, a skin rash, or some other deformity. For them, it is the change of their body from what it was that leads to the determination that something is abnormal. The physician skilled in physical examination can determine more, but this requires training and experience to both understand what is abnormal and how to detect it. This determination of abnormality is a qualitative judgment by the physician, which is very difficult, if not impossible, to standardize from physician to physician. This lack of standardization is sometimes referred to as "interobserver variability." This is where the physician's "tacit knowledge" of the human body and their own physical examination skills come into play. The physician, through a focus attention on how they perform an examination, how accurate their examination was in the past, etc., will determine how reliable their examination is; and, therefore, how it is to be used as premises in an argument toward a diagnosis, or for that matter, increasing the probability of the disease being present to more effectively use objective testing.

Unlike symptoms or physical examination signs, the determination of abnormalities on quantitative tests is more formalized. What I mean by "quantitative" is anything that produces a number, whether it is a test on a bodily fluid or a physiological test. The example given above of 24-h pH monitoring is an example of a quantitative test. There are also some aspects of the physical examination that are quantitative, such as temperature, blood pressure, heart rate and respiratory rate. Many of the standard tests used, such as the complete blood count, go back decades. However, standards exist for these tests, which are regulated by governmental agencies. One standard of normalcy, however, is the 95% confidence interval, i.e., a certain number of "normal" individuals, which can be defined in a number of ways (e.g., in the 24-h pH monitoring above, it was those individuals without symptoms of GERD), volunteer to get the test done and the results are determined. This number may range from 120 to 200 individuals, ideally, and depending on the test, other factors may need to be taken into consideration. These results are subject to the usual descriptive statistical analysis, such as means, medians, standard deviations, etc. The range of results that includes 95% of the results is defined as the "normal range" (or "reference range") if the results follow a standard normal distribution. If the results were skewed, nonparametric statistical tests with a range between the 2.5th and 97.5th percentiles can be used [81].

This determination of "normal" is somewhat arbitrary in that 5% of individuals with no sign of disease will be classified as "abnormal." Additionally, there will be individuals with the disease the presence of which is being tested who will have test result values within the normal range. It is rare to find a quantitative test that perfectly discriminates between individuals with and without the disease. This is why laboratory medicine experts caution that a test result outside the normal range may not indicate disease and a result value in the normal range may not indicate an absence of disease. (See the discussion of Bayesian probabilities above).

Last, determination of normal and abnormal in "visual" tests are qualitative as well. What I mean by visual tests are those that require visual interpretation of images obtained through technological means. For example, images obtained through radiological, ultrasound, magnetic resonance, position-emission or any other such technology that produces an image; histologically process samples of tissue or other tissue processing that produces a product that requires viewing to interpret; or technologically assisted viewing of otherwise hidden surfaces of the human body, such as endoscopies of all sorts, which require interpretation. Some "nonvisual" tests can also fit into this category, such as electrocardiograms or manometries, which produce patterns of electrical, pressure, or other bodily activities that generally require a visual interpretation. In these types of tests, a physician trained in "reading" these images provides a judgment as to what is normal and abnormal and, if abnormal, what the possible abnormality is. This is not to say that there is not some quantifiable data from these tests. For example, a radiological image can measure the size of a tumor, and an echocardiogram can measure blood flow across a heart value. Similarly, a pathological slide can measure the size of a tumor or the number of bacteria in a sample. Additionally, in all of these tests, there are some pathologies that can be "graded" into classes of severity based on specific criteria. Nevertheless, as with physical examination, all of these tests require an interpretation by a physician and, therefore, are subject to the foibles of interobserver variability.

The essential point I am making with these descriptions of testing is that the results are not as conclusive in all circumstances as we would like (or, for that matter, how they are viewed both within the professional or popular mind). This is not to say that no tests are conclusive, many provide definitive answers: the physician observing a fungating tumor or a protruding hernia is not in doubt that there is a disease, or even what the disease is, similarly for tests in the other categories. Therefore, when a test is definitive, then the physician can reliably use the results as a true premise in any argument toward a diagnosis. If the tests are not definitive, the level of the "truthfulness" of the premises may affect the confidence the physician or patient has in the diagnosis.

7.4.6 The Diagnostic Task

The next section will discuss a variety of descriptions of the diagnostic task. This mostly has to how this task is organized and the type of logical inferences made. It is interesting to me that there are a variety of proposals, which are not always consistent with each other. Nevertheless, it is worth considering them.

Barosi [82] proposed that the diagnostic task of a physician occurs in three phases: hypothesis generation, hypothesis testing, and hypothesis closure. Hypothesis generation—inferential form of abduction constrained under the criteria of plausibility. Hypothesis testing—deductive inference (from generated hypothesis to expected findings) followed by an eliminative induction, constrained under the criteria of covering, which intends to select the best explanation. Hypothesis closure—deductive-inductive type of inference very similar to the inferences operating in hypothesis testing [82]. Induction matches the consequences of the generated hypotheses against the patient's characteristics or preference under the criterion of utility [82]. Therefore, although Barosi reasonably divides the diagnostic tasks into phases that are recognizable to a physician, his view is that this is an inductive process, as opposed to a deductive process that was averred by Feinstein [28].

Another viewpoint is that of Ridderikhoff [83]. Traditionally, physicians follow their own pathway to diagnosis, and the method is adapted to the nature of the problem, that is, content dependency [83]. In other words, because of their knowledge and experience, physicians will pursue different methods in achieving a diagnosis. For example, for a patient with new complaints of heartburn, one physician may choose a "comprehensive" policy of objective testing prior to prescribing medications, while another may prescribe a PPI and monitor the patient's response as both a diagnostic test and therapeutic maneuver. However, for Ridderikhoff [83] cognitive bias, uncertain or unreliable data, suboptimal data acquisition, early reduction of possible states of affairs, and the communication and interaction of problems between patients and doctors make the thought of strict and rational processes of information handling unrealistic. This is an important point because of the vagaries of information flow and reliability, and it is unlikely that the practicing physician is able to apply the same methods in determining data truthfulness.

Ridderikhoff [83] then asks the question of what type of reasoning physicians use in their diagnostic task. He discusses three presumed models of diagnostic reasoning: (1) deductive, in which the conclusion (i.e., the diagnosis) should be fully explainable from the acquired evidence; (2) induction, in which the argument goes from particular bits of information to general conclusions; and (3) hypotheticodeductive, in which a hypothesis is tested for its probable truthfulness. To test what type of reasoning is used by physicians, Ridderikhoff [83] presented a study to determine the type of problem-solving logic used by physicians at various levels of experience. In a simulated doctor–patient encounter, deductive and hypotheticodeductive strategies were not used. All participants used the inductive method, specifically, the speculative variant. This variant may be described as a process of iterative pattern recognition (e.g., illness scripts as described above). This strategy allowed for flexibility and quick response to the patient's needs [83]. The number of patterns (or scripts, using the terms of Bowen and Abernathy and Hamm) that the physician has stored and is retrievable will determine how well the physician can match his menu of scripts/patterns to the patient's story/narrative. Ridderikhoff [83] describes this as a "treasury of hypotheses" or a "bag of ideas and thoughts" that come to a physician's mind while evaluating a patient. The physician, as they gather more information on a patient, continually revises the possibly matchable patterns to the patient's problem in an iterative fashion [83].

Although Ridderikhoff [83] proposes that this is an inductive process, it seems to me, given that lack of precision and the overall probabilistic nature of most of the data, that the logical process is more informal. I also must point out that many authors who have been referenced in this book appear, at least to me, to us different terms for the same general idea. The fact that several authors have understood the process in a similar manner, at least to me, does give weight to the possibility that this is at least a useful, if not absolutely correct, way to consider how physicians reason during the diagnostic process.

7.4.7 Formal Logical Diagnostic Reasoning Theories

For the stake of providing an alternative view, that is, views that describe the reasoning process of physicians in more formal, rather than informal, terms, I briefly mention the work of Doroszewski [84] and Moore and Hutchins [85], who take a more formal mathematical and model logic approach to diagnosis.

Doroszewski [84] produced a thesis that there are three main stages of medical diagnosis: (1) initial exploration, (2) hypothesis-directed investigation, and (3) final diagnosis making. Similar, but not quite the same, as Ridderikhoff [83] above. Within these stages, the components include the leading hypothesis, working hypothesis, main diagnostic hypotheses, statements accepted as certain, intermediary and reverse hypotheses, and therapeutic suggestions of immediate consequence. Explanation of the observed symptoms, signs and test results of the explaining hypothesis plays a major role in constructing the mental model of the patient's state. He feels that this process corresponds to a "scientific investigation" of the collection and grouping of empirical material, and the tentative formation of hypotheses, formulation of hypotheses by induction, derivation of testable consequences from the hypotheses by deduction, and testing the hypotheses. (Note, again, the references to logical form types.) He further goes on to devise a mathematical model of this theory [84], the technical details of which are not necessary for this book. There are clearly some overlaps with the diagnostic process as described by Bowen [63]. However, I must say that the level of precision in Doroszewski's theory does not correspond to my experience as a practicing physician on how the process actually occurs in routine clinical practice. However, the overall form of the stages of diagnosis the he asserts is similar to others, although he has divided the process into narrower, more detailed stages, once again, adding to the overall weight of evidence of the descriptive, if not the normative, account of the diagnostic process discussed.

Moore and Hutchins [85] also created a very precise theory of medical diagnosis that they hoped would be the basis of computer-assisted diagnostic tools. They use symbolic modal logic (which, unlike formal, symbolic logic in which statements are either true or false, can qualify statements as "possible," "necessary," etc., see Chap. 2 for a discussion) to model medical decisions that sometimes have to be made on the basis of incomplete and/or unsatisfactory information. They use the concepts of "certainty" with which a given unit of information is available, the "demand" for that information based on the patient's circumstances, and the "effort" that has been made to obtain it. These concepts, in their theory, are akin to the operators in modal logic. They also recognize that some desired data may be unobtainable in some patients. Their evaluation is based on the following analysis:

> Given a nonempty set of data, D, and a nonempty set of actions, A, there is a sequence of subsets of A, i.e., $A_1, A_2,\ldots, A_a$ and a sequence of corresponding subsets of D, i.e., $D_1, D_2,\ldots, D_a$, such that $D_1,A_1; D_2A_2; \ldots; D_a,A_a$, which in some sense represents an *effective procedure* for evaluating a particular patient with a particular disease.

From this basis, they go on to develop a very precise theory of medical diagnosis using symbolic modal logic with the constraints of demand of information, effort to obtain such information, and acceptance that some information will be unavailable. As precise and potentially useful as this analysis may be for creation of computer-assisted diagnosis (and I do not know if it was ever used for that purpose), it clearly does not describe how medical practitioners come to a diagnosis, nor, does it seem to be a normative method of assessing the quality of diagnostic reasoning.

Rather than attempting an account of medical reasoning based on formal deduction, my assertion is that for the most part medical reasoning and argumentation is informal *because* of the variety of data (facts, probabilities, social constructs, etc.) and each of these requires an interpretation and abstraction for the mental manipulation by the physician and the patient. Interpretation in the medical encounter will be discussed in the next chapter.

Interpretation of Medical/Patient "Texts" as a Hermeneutical Process

Having obtained a history, physical examination and any tests desired by the physician, Leder [86] argues that the diagnostic process is a hermeneutical enterprise. Hermeneutics is the study of how "texts" are interpreted. The word "texts" in this context is not only words on a page or words spoken but also any communication or observation that functions as a "sign" carrying a "meaning" to be interpreted by the receiver of the sign. Therefore, Leder [86] makes the assertion that the ill person is a "text" and that the physician's task is to interpret this text. This text is a set of elements that constitute a whole and takes on meaning through interpretation [87]. In medicine, this text is the "person-as-ill" [86]. This text has a wide variety of forms: (1) the "experiential text", which is what is what is lived by the patient; (2) the "narrative text", which is what is constituted during history-taking; (3) the "physical text" of the patient's body as objectively examined; and (4) the "instrumental text" constructed by diagnostic testing [86]. Please note how this account dovetails nicely with the semiotic account of medical communications as signs [62].

To go on, with the experiential text, the patient interprets their own signs and symptoms and ultimately must decide if these indicate an illness that requires a physician's evaluation. This text becomes their "medical story." The narrative text is written during the initial medical encounter when the physician takes the patient's history. With this text, the "authors" are the patient's body, the patient's mind, and the physician's mind. There is an exchange between the patient and physician regarding the pertinent content of the text, but ultimately, the physician records this in the customary manner of a professionally acceptable medical history (we will discuss the effect of professional norms on the physician, the professional umwelt, later in the chapter). The physical text is the physical examination. This is directed by the physician as they examine the patient. There is usually some type of additional information from the patient during the examination, for example, "does this hurt when I press here?" However, for the most part, it is the physician using their tactile skills that is identifying and interpreting this text. Last, the instrumental text is any diagnostic testing the physician chooses to obtain, the results of which are interpreted by the physician in the context of the other texts. The instrumental text is different than the other texts in that it is the only one that produces an "artifact" of sorts—the lab result, the X-ray, etc., which is independent of the physician and the patient [86]. One can easily see how "illness scripts" as described above fit into this hermeneutical process. In this process, the physician actually has multiple roles: "scientist, biographer, historian, priest[10] and personal advisor" [88]. Moreover, by acknowledging the interpretative nature of clinical understanding, we leave behind pure objectivity; that is, when there is interpretation, there is subjectivity, ambiguity, and room for disagreement [86].

In addition to the "text" of the patient in the clinical encounter, the physician must also interpret the text of any mode of information they are receiving about medical knowledge, e.g., textbooks, review articles, new medical research, lectures, etc. The "hermeneutic telos" is the set of goals that, throughout the clinical encounter, orient the writing and reading of these texts. These goals are coherence, collaboration, and clinical effectiveness [86]. Coherence implies that the text needs to be interpreted coherently. The medical chart can be considered a "tertiary" text in this regard, with the secondary text the physician's understanding and the primary text the patient's own account of their illness. On a conceptual level, the nosology of diseases and syndromes provides the primary integrative tools. Diagnostic coherence does not come only at the end of the evaluation but guides the evaluation throughout [86]. Leder [86] quotes Heidegger: "any confrontation with meaning presupposes a certain 'fore-structure' of understanding." Collaboration implies that the physician and the patient collaborate in understanding these texts [86]. I would further go on to say that this collaboration is vital for both the manifest rationality of the physician's argument on diagnosis and treatment, and the patient's likelihood of being persuaded by this argument. This culminates in the interpretation of the text providing answers leading to therapeutic decisions that will have some level of clinical effectiveness [87]. Coming to an interpretation is important. Any act of interpretation is needed for an application [89]. For the physician, it is the application of knowledge and information in the care of the patient which is the goal.

Language and Communication

Everyday language exists on multiple levels, and this can affect patient–physician communication. This may influence how medical texts are created and the collaboration between the patient and physician. Little [90] acknowledges that much of Karl

---

[10] There are now also 48 and up to 96 hours of pH monitoring, but the essential features are the same.

Popper's view on the scientific method is outdated, but he avers that Popper's ideas may have value in analyzing the clinical process. In Little's [90] analysis, the clinical process consists of inputs, the process itself, and an output. The input is the patient with their problem and underlying beliefs. The output is the "medical achievement" for the patient (i.e., the clinical outcome). The process is the clinical activity from when the patient seeks care to the outcome. He succinctly paraphrases Popper's analysis of the scientific method as follows: P1 → TS1 → EE → P2, where P1 is the initial problem, TS1 is the first trial solution or hypothesis, EE is the phase of error elimination in which the theory is subjected to the process of severe criticism and testing, and P2 is the residual problem remaining after the error elimination process. In clinical terms, P1 is the patient's presenting problem, TS1 is the provisional (or differential) diagnosis, EE is any additional testing, and P2 is the nosological problem of classifying the disease, determining its appropriate treatment and its prognosis. Nevertheless, in this process, there are potential communication problems between patients and physicians, that is, the noise-to-signal ratio, for example, issues with language (as was noted in how effective persuasion methods can be). Little [90] paraphrases Buhler that everyday language exists on a number of levels: the expressive/emotional level, in which words may not be used; the signaling level, which appeals to the receiver for support of joint action; the descriptive level, which communicates the attributes of an object or an experience; and the argumentative level, which requires reciprocity so that discussion and criticism may be exchanged and enhanced [90]. This is consistent with how human language evolution led to communication. With most physicians, the physician's interpretation is not a specific differential diagnosis but a general categorization of seriousness—not serious, sick-not sick, etc.

7.4.8 The Process of Placement of a Patient into a Diagnostic Category

Although I have given examples of various theories of diagnostic reasoning or logic, they all ultimately come to the same point—the diagnosis. This process, in my view, is that of categorization, a nosology of sorts, where the patient is placed into a diagnostic category that (1) best explains the patient's presentation (symptoms, signs, and tests) and (2) allows for matching of that category to a treatment plan. Figure 7.1 presents a schematic of what I call the "funnel" process of continuous smaller, more specific categorization of the patient's condition based on increasing information. The patient, having determined that they have "something medically wrong" with them, seeks the care of a physician. The physician starts the diagnostic process with a history and physical examination. During this stage, the physician starts to develop a differential diagnosis—that is, they draw from their memory potential categories of disease that can be explained by the presentation, as presented in the "physician's cognition" column of Fig. 1.1. At the end of this stage, the number of possible disease categories in which the patient can fit has been greatly reduced.

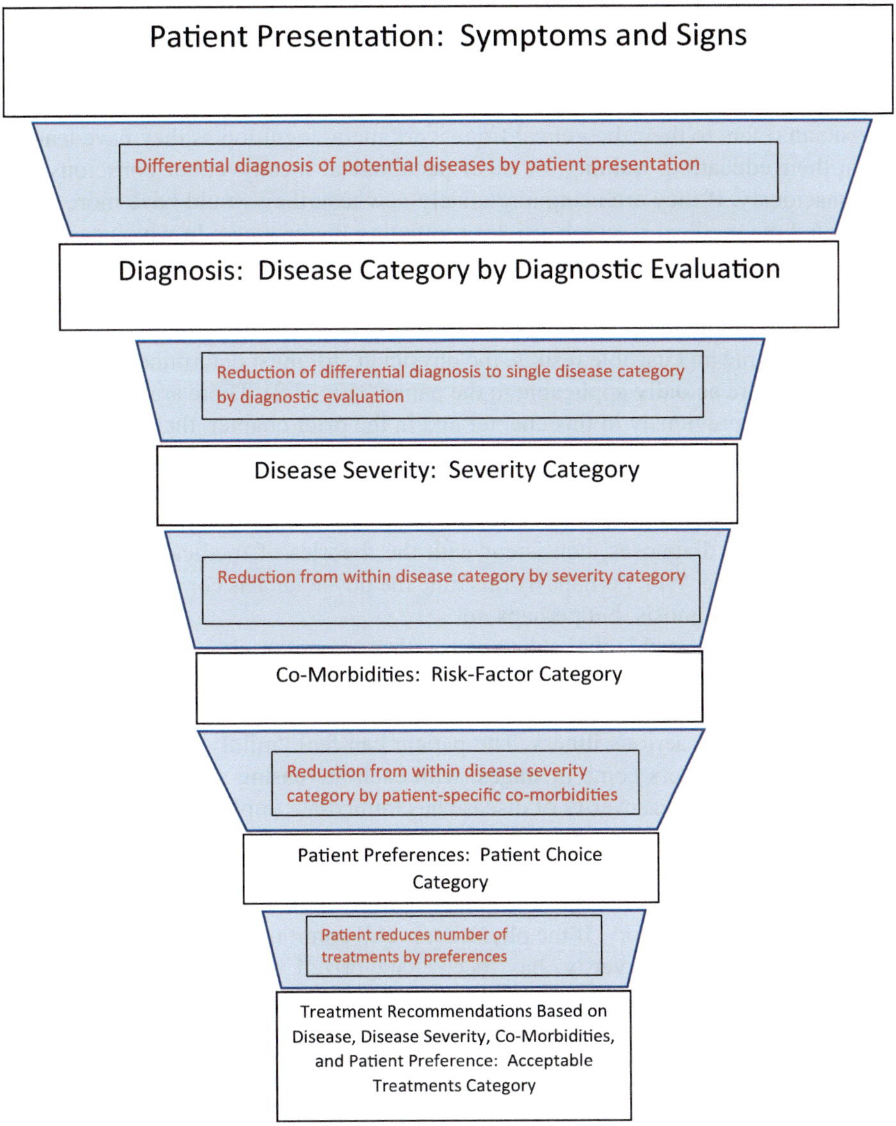

Fig. 7.1 The "Funnel" process of patient categorization to treatment choice. With each step down from the top, certain members of each category set will be eliminated as not being the category to which the patient belongs. The patient starts the process by determining that they are in the category of people who may have a medical problem. The next four sets are determined by the physician. Finally, the last set, the accepted treatment, is accomplished by the patient

Next, the physician orders any objective tests to be later used in their argument development if they feel the need to do so[11] and will eventually review those results. However, this stage requires that the physician make a decision as to which tests will provide reliable and usable information (i.e., premises) in their reasoning. The physician refers to their theoretical framework meta-cognition as they have learned from their education, training, or other pedagogical means, either consciously or unconsciously. If they are using a relatively new test, they would have more likely evaluated the medical research articles promoting the new test. In which case, they would have to assess the reliability of the conclusions of that one, or more, study(ies) through their metacognition processes of evidence for theory and techniques of evidential foundational appraisal (Fig. 1.1). Having been satisfied that the study does provide reliable and useable results, the physician still must determine if the results of the study are actually applicable to the patient (Fig. 7.2). There are many factors, as mentioned previously in this chapter and in the prior chapter, that can affect this applicability. I am not going to reiterate these factors, but the physician will consider them. Nevertheless, once the appropriate test results are returned and interpreted, the physician will further revise their differential diagnosis, eliminating nonexplanatory diagnoses, consistent with the theories of medical reasoning discussed above (Fig. 7.1). Perhaps by this time the physician has come to a conclusion of a definitive diagnosis, but perhaps not.

Although it is possible that a disease is either present or absent, it is more likely that any category of disease has a spectrum of severity. For example, in appendicitis, the appendix can be inflamed, gangrenous or perforated, with each level having the potential for more serious illness. The patient can feel "mildly ill" or they can be incapacitated. Cancers come in stages, with each increasing stage reflecting more advanced disease. The severity of disease has immediate implications for the physician, namely, how quickly and to what extent they need to act. Therefore, disease severity further reduces the number of diagnostic categories. If the physician has determined that the patient is in the category of a single disease, then the severity further refines the category. If the physician is still entertaining more than one diagnosis, the level of severity has been categorized for each disease under consideration.

Last, from the standpoint of patient categorization of the diagnostic process, is the patient's associated comorbidities (Fig. 7.1). These comorbidities may affect treatment choices. For example, a patient with a particular drug allergy cannot be treated with that drug even if otherwise the drug would be an appropriate treatment. Certain comorbidities may make the patient an unfit candidate for an operation. This last stage of the diagnostic process may not necessarily aid in determining which disease the patient has but may, as some comorbidities can either be exacerbated by a disease or vice versa, while others may mimic other disease symptoms, for example, dyspnea in someone with congestive heart failure and with concern for

[11] Often, the physician can make a confident diagnosis based on history and physical examination and will not need to obtain any objective tests. In such instances, this stage is essentially skipped.

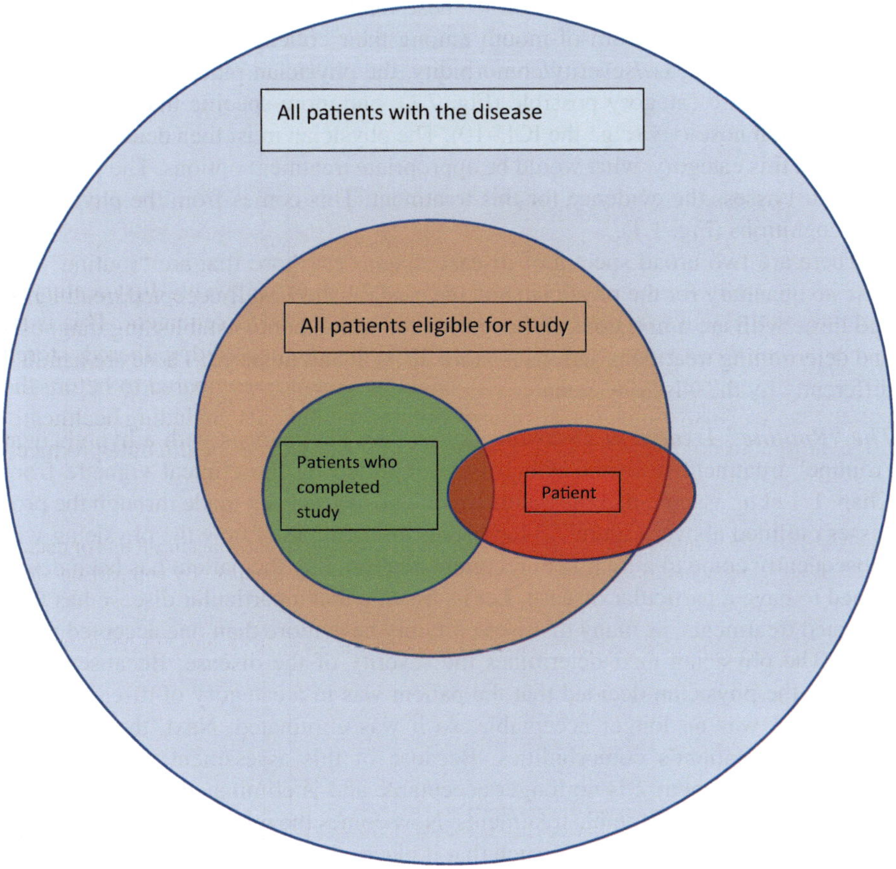

Fig. 7.2 Determination if the conclusions of a medical research article are applicable to an individual patient. This is applicable to both new diagnostic tests and new treatments. With each subsequent smaller circle, fewer patients are in that category. Finally, the patient, represented by the red oval, can be in any of the three categories, depending on their characteristics, but at the exclusion of the other two categories

pneumonia. This final reduction to this category starts the process for treatment decisions (Fig. 7.1), which also begins the process of persuading the patient as to the truth of their diagnostic category (Fig. 1.1).

7.5 Application of Medical Knowledge in Treatment Choices

Ultimately, the purpose of coming to a diagnosis is to recommend treatment. In general, for each diagnostic category, there will be a menu of accepted treatments that meet the "standard of care." Physicians learn of these treatments in their medical education and any revision to these treatment recommendations through journals, conferences, word-of-mouth among their colleagues, etc. By narrowing the category of disease/severity/comorbidity, the physician placed the patient into the most specific category possible (Fig. 7.1), one more specific than any disease classification nosology (e.g., the ICD-10). The physician must then determine, for a patient in this category, what would be appropriate treatment options. The physician then must assess the evidence for this treatment. This comes from the physician's metacognitions (Fig. 1.1).

There are two broad spectra of disease diagnoses: those that are "routine" that pose no quandary for the physician and have established, well-accepted treatments; and those with are ambiguous and complex for which booth establishing diagnosis and determining treatment options is more difficult and nuanced. These are handled differently by the wise physician.

The "Routine" Treatment Decision Let us start the analysis with a hypothetical "routine" treatment decision, which is exemplified by the clinical vignette from Chap. 1. Let us assume that the definitive diagnosis has been made through the processes outlined above. Figure 7.3 represents a schematic of how the physician will subsequently come to a treatment recommendation. Say the patient has been determined to have a particular disease. Let us assume that a particular disease has four accepted treatments, as many diseases certainly have more than one accepted treatment. The physician next determines the severity of the disease. Because of the severity, the physician decided that the patient was in a category of disease where treatment 1 was no longer acceptable, so it was eliminated. Next, the physician assesses the patient's comorbidities. Because of this assessment, the physician decides that treatment 2 is no longer acceptable and is eliminated. This leaves the physician with two acceptable treatments. Now comes the process of persuading the patient who their presentation is such that it places them in this particular category. Because the patient is in this particular category, only treatments 3 and 4 are acceptable treatments, and the physician may very well provide an argument as to how this is the case. The patient will then have an exchange with the physician to ensure that any opaque points are clarified. This exchange leads to the manifest rationality of Johnson [1] such that both the physician and the patient have agreed to the conclusion(s) of the physician's argument, perhaps after some revisions by the physician based on the patient's input/critiques. Ultimately, the patient makes the choice to proceed with treatment 4, which is acceptable to the physician. This completes the flow of the medical encounter in Fig. 1.1. Even though this was presented in a linear fashion, it is most likely this reasoning by the patient is an iterative, nonlinear, parallel process where treatments are considered while the additional information is being obtained and often "low-risk" treatments for the most common likely disease may have been initiated as both a treatment *and* a diagnostic test, as the example of using a PPI for a patient with heartburn presented above.

When I say that this represents a "routine" case, I mean that the medical knowledge with which the physician uses in their metacognitions is generally well accepted by the physician and the medical community. The physician does not have

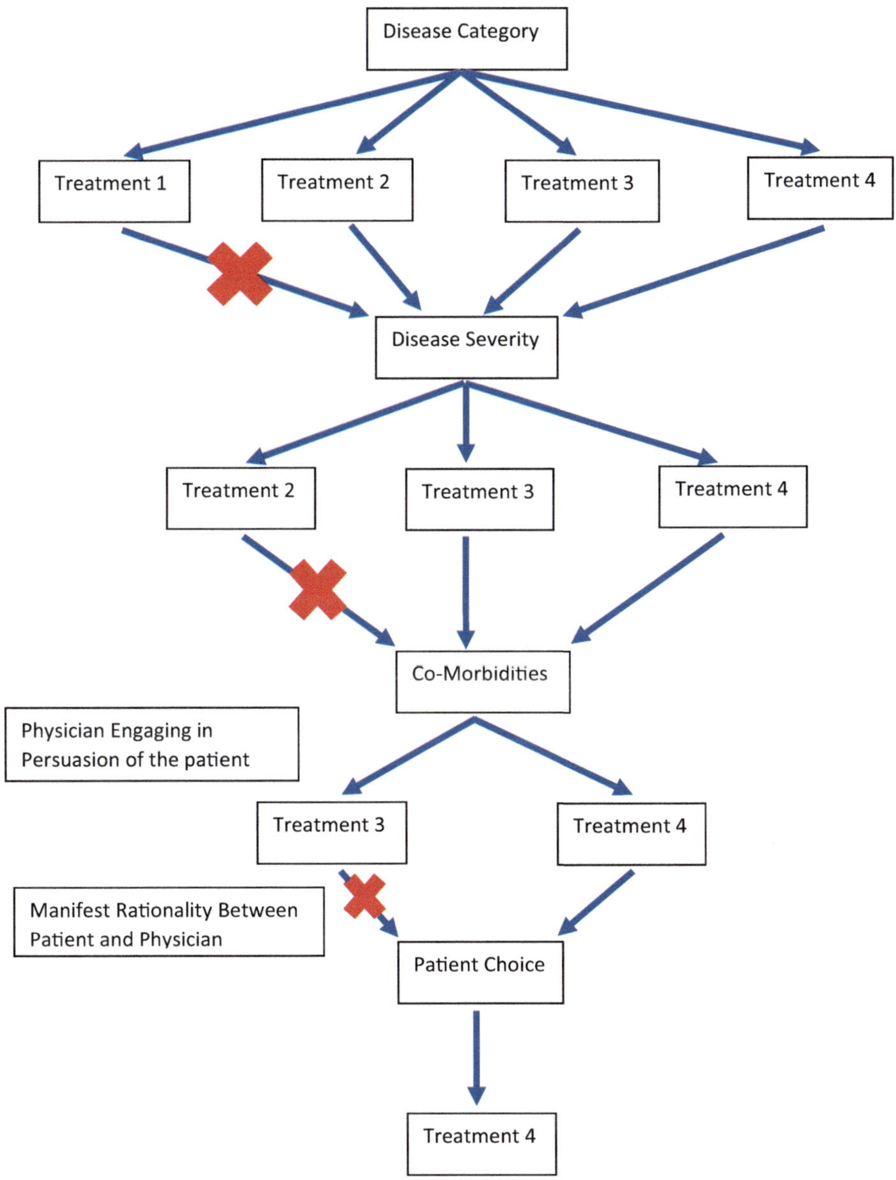

Fig. 7.3 Schematic of treatment recommendation decisions. This is for "routine" treatment decisions for an uncomplicated medical disease with well-accepted treatment options. The physician will go through the process of eliminating treatment options as they obtain more information pertaining to the patient; essentially, as they funnel the patient into an increasingly specific category, the previous treatment that may have been appropriate for the broader category is eliminated until the patient is left either making a choice of the acceptable treatments or agreeing to the only acceptable treatment

to judge the voracity of any new medical knowledge. The only things that they have to determine are which specific category the patient is in and which treatments are acceptable by the medical community for that category.

Potential Pitfalls The hypothetical example above produced an argument with an illative core that was structurally sound logically and produced a valid conclusion. Nevertheless, there are still potential pitfalls that may produce a materially false conclusion, by which I mean that the patient did not have the anticipated outcome.

The first issue is that of knowledge. Physicians do not know all the diseases that can potentially afflict our species. It is truism that you cannot know what you are dealing with if you do not know that what you are dealing with exists. It is not uncommon, and I am confident to say that most physicians have experienced this, that a patient will go some time without a diagnosis being established, because their physician(s) did not even realize that there was such a diagnosis. One cannot come to a conclusion that one cannot imagine. This speaks to a larger issue of diagnoses as conclusions to medical arguments—it is exceptionally rare for a physician to come to a "brand new" disease as a diagnosis (e.g., the AIDS history as recounted in Chap. 6); nearly universally, the physician is trying to "match" the conclusions that they already have to the argument they have constructed. Therefore, if that conclusion is something unknown to the physician, they cannot match it to the premises of their argument.

The second issue is that of probabilities. It is uncommon for any one treatment to be an absolute cure for a disease. Some have very high probabilities, say appendectomy for appendicitis (albeit with the caveat that surgical complications can occur). However, in the vast majority, there are no guarantees. Therefore, even logically sound arguments with valid conclusions may not produce the desired results. This is due to the fact that the probability of a "no cure" happening is stochastic and measurable. See discussion of probabilistic causation in Chap. 5.

The third issue is the pitfall of induction (see Chap. 2). To reiterate, induction is the logical form using probability propositions and/or the logical form where a set of particular observations are used to make a generalization. The probability issue was presented in the preceding paragraph, what I want to address here is the generalization. All medical knowledge addressing prediction, which, as I have mentioned, is the most important aspect of medical knowledge, is based on information about what has happened to patients in the past. The foundational assumption is that those past patients will be the same (or similar enough) as future patients so that the results recorded in the patient patients can be the results anticipated in future patients. In fact, this is the entire foundation of all science; we can only know what has happened in the past and believe that under the same circumstances, it will happen again in the future. However, is this truly so with respect to patients? For the most basic aspects of human biology, probably so. However, there are serious potential differences with past patients which may lead to different results. That is, the sample of patients used in past studies, or even in the experience of a single physician, may not be representative of future patients. For example, as overall medical progress has continued, the severity of comorbid diseases may have lessened or worsened. For example, the patient with congestive heart disease 30 years ago may not be similar to the patient with congestive heart disease now. That is, even though the disease conception of "congestive heart disease" is the same as a description of the disease, the impact on health may be different. Therefore, this affects the estimated predictability of any one decision.

Another reason that past patients may be different from present-day patients is that disease processes may have changed. For example, it is well documented that microorganisms evolve quite rapidly. Many have become resistant to several antimicrobial drugs. Therefore, an infection with one of these microorganisms, even though sharing the same name as pneumonia, is truly a different disease. This is probably true for some malignancies as well. Therefore, decisions based on past information that is not applicable to today's disease may result in poorer predictability.

The environment in which humans live is different. In addition to changes in living standards and habits, humans are also exposed to different environmental factors. Housing has changed, food has changed, and sanitation has changed. In addition, the ease of travel has allowed for the rapid transmission of infectious organisms in a way that was not possible decades ago.

Treatments may have changed. In addition to improved treatments of an index disease, treatments of comorbidities have improved. It is certainly more likely that a patient in need of a cancer operation is more likely to survive their operation if their coronary artery disease is effectively addressed. Therefore, these additional treatments may be such that using past information reduces their predictability.

Last, it is difficult to determine what new treatments are on the horizon. Therapeutic agents and procedures are constantly being innovated. Therefore, what was an untreatable disease a decade or even a few years ago can be successfully treated today. The example given in the last chapter of AIDS going from a near-universal death sentence to a manageable chronic condition is an exemplar of this.

In summary, all these considerations should give the physician pause to consider whether the data from past patients are truly applicable to their present patients. This difference could be for the better or worse, but still is a difference. On the other hand, I do not want to imply total nihilism about past data. We have no other guideposts to help us on this journey with the patient. Only that the *wise* physician will have to decide what information is applicable to their patient.

Patient Categorization into Treatment Groups Based on New Knowledge In the preceding section, I discussed the application of medical knowledge, which is well accepted by the medical community. In this section, I will address the application of new medical knowledge.

As discussed in the prior chapter, healthcare professionals are inundated with "new information" and have to determine if such new medical knowledge meets their criteria for acceptability and then incorporate that knowledge into their body of medical knowledge. Once they have incorporated that knowledge, then they must determine if that knowledge is applicable to an individual patient. This process is somewhat different from the process of established medical knowledge of treatment options illustrated in Fig. 7.3 and more similar to what is illustrated in Fig. 7.2, which was introduced during the discussion of diagnostic testing.

We previously discussed "disease" as a conceptualization for the physician's mental manipulation during the reasoning process of a healthcare professional. A disease is also a material pathological process leading to altered homeostasis in a patient. That "pathological process leading to altered homeostasis" occurs in a certain number of individuals, leading to an incidence (number of new cases per given time period) and prevalence (number of cases in existence at a given time period). Therefore, at any given time period, there exists a set of patients with the disease. This is schematically represented by the large, blue outer circle in Fig. 7.2. However, in any given study, only a subset of this entire class may be eligible for study (the next inner brown circle in Fig. 7.2). For example, in the article by Spechler et al. [9] in the prior chapter, the eligible patients were patients with medical-refractory GERD who were seen in Veterans Affairs gastroenterology medical clinics. Of these eligible patients, only a portion agreed to participate in the study, and a somewhat smaller proportion completed the study (the inner green circle in Fig. 7.2). Therefore, of the entire set of patients with the disease, only a small subset of patients is the group from which the data are generated.

In this sense, the data, argument and conclusions of a particular study are what I refer to as bounded. As mentioned previously, what I mean by "bounded" is that any about the effects of the treatment only logically apply to that group in the study. That is, this group of patients is now a very defined category of patients. Inferences beyond this group require the data to be extrapolated to other patients who were never in the tested group of the study. Therefore, whether any one patient fits within this boundary (or, rather, category) will determine if the results of the study will be applicable to a particular patient. For the results to be applicable to an individual patient, that patient must have the *same characteristics as the study completed patients* (or, at least, similar enough). For an individual patient, that patient may fit into the completed study category, in the eligible but not completed category, or in all patients with the disease category. From a strictly rational point of view, a patient who has a set of characteristics not meeting the category of patients completely the study cannot have the results of that study applied to them.

This observation that medical studies, especially randomized, controlled trials, omit a large swath of patients was also made by others. Feinstein [21] was critical of randomized, controlled trials because they do not include many types of patients seen in clinical practice, such that the "average" randomized, controlled patient may not reflect the actual patient who the physician is treating. This is the problem of if the patient is actually in the category of patients whom the trial included. Trials are designed to have as a homogenous group of patients as possible to reduce confounding variables, that is, treatment efficacy. This reduces the size of the category for which the data are then relevant, that is, treatment effectiveness. Randomized, controlled trials do not include "soft data", which may be very important for an individual patient [21] that the wise physician will know is relevant in treatment decisions. Others have also criticized the unthinking reliance on randomized, controlled trials [91–94].

Although all of these concerns are true and should be addressed by the physician, it is nevertheless true that even imperfect data may be useful on a practical level. That is, are the conclusions, although not strictly applicable, "good enough" for the physician to use as premises in a treatment argument, especially if there is only even less reliable information available? What this question truly asks is: Are there any characteristics of my patient which would otherwise qualify them NOT to be in the category of patients for whom the study is applicable that I can ignore? That is, what patient-specific information should and should not be included? For example, in the study by Spechler et al. [9], patients came from Veterans Affairs medical clinics. They acknowledged that this is a selected group of patients: "...a predominance of white men reflecting the veteran patient population." A physician may decide that this particular characteristic is not relevant in determining the applicability of the data to their patient, for example. Another physician may decide that it is relevant, for example, if that physician has a female patient. In either circumstance, the physician, however, needs to make a conscious judgment to either believe what would other be an exclusionary characteristic is not relevant in their reasoning.

On the other hand, errors can occur if the physician simply accepts the conclusion of a study and ignores the inclusion/exclusion criteria. This can lead to potential miscategorization if the physician does not subcategorize patients appropriately. For example, applying the results of a randomized, controlled trial to a patient with the disease tested, but having an exclusion criterion. Once again, let us look at the study of Spechler et al. [9]. One of the specific inclusion criteria was the use of MII-pH monitoring to diagnostically confirm refractory reflux. If a physician has a patient with what they consider refractory GERD but does not confirm the diagnosis with MII-pH monitoring, this would not be a trivial exclusion. This could produce a critical miscategorization of a patient into a category in which they should not be.

Both the process of ignoring irrelevant criteria and not ignoring important criteria is a matter of practical wisdom, to be discussed more below.

7.5.1 *Operative Decisions*

Much of what was discussed is in relation to physician decisions in a clinical setting with a conscious, participatory patient. However, there is a special class of decisions that healthcare professionals may need to make as the treatment is happening. The "procedural" specialties have such additional components to medical treatment decisions. These include a proceduralist's manual handicraft, which is an essential feature of treatment decisions and intraoperative decisions.

With respect to surgical or procedural handicraft compared to dispensing of a drug, it matters not who is prescribing or dispensing a medication for the drug will have the same effect on the patient; however, it may matter a great deal who performs the operation or procedure.[12] In these procedures, manual skill and anatomic recognition are essential in performing the procedure, especially if complex or with

[12] In the surgical community, there is no more a derogatory term for a surgeon that to say that they have "hands of stone" or "stone-hands," implying that they have little manual dexterity in the execution of an operation.

altered anatomy. For example, in a study of operative skill in the conduct of bariatric operations, Birkmeyer et al. [95] demonstrated through video review of actual operations that those operations judged by other expert bariatric surgeons to be done with a higher skill level were the operations that led to better results. Essentially, the skill of the surgeon, or, for that matter, other proceduralists such as interventional radiologists, cardiologists, gastroenterologists, etc., matters a great deal.

The other issue in procedural interventions is stumbling across the unexpected in the course of an operation. Most elective operations are routine and preplanned. In the vast majority of times, the operation is chosen based on the known efficacy of the operation for the particular problem and proceeds as planned. However, there are times when the surgeon is confronted with an intraoperative situation that is unexpected [96]. In these circumstances, not all decisions will have solid evidence, certainly not in the sense of evidence-based medicine. Evidence-based medicine cannot be a good guide in these situations because it is skeptical of explanations from basic biological sciences and views disease only from a population level [16]. However, to simply say that since there is no good evidence for this situation, I will make no decision at all, is just not an option available to the surgeon, or other proceduralist. They *must* make a decision; there is no alternative but to act. This is the essence of practical wisdom or *phronesis*, making the right decision with the information at hand. The surgeon, in the midst of an operation, when confronted with a situation for which there is no good evidence, must reason from first principles. These principles are based on anatomic, physiologic and pathologic knowledge, in conjunction with the knowledge of the patient. This may require creating solutions that are *ad hoc*, which the surgeon may never again do. It may also require seeking an opinion from a trusted colleague. Moreover, it is not just making a decision; the proceduralist must be able to *execute* the decision. In an intraoperative setting, having come up (most likely through abduction) with a satisfactory solution is useless unless the surgeon has the manual dexterity to actually perform the physical task.

What I have described is an individual doctor reasoning about an individual patient under time constraints (and perhaps other pressures). This, at least in my opinion, is a form of "precision medicine." It is worth discussing the difference between precision medicine and evidence-based medicine.

7.5.2 Tension Between "Precision Medicine" and "Evidence-Based Medicine"

I have discussed at length the tenets of evidence-based medicine. This means that the physician uses the "best available" data in decisions pertaining to patient care. It also implies that the data come from populations of patients that were analyzed with the most applicable statistical techniques. I have been critical of the assertion that it provides the "best" evidence exclusively, although I will concede that it can provide appropriate evidence when applied with wisdom and understanding. My general assertion is that the physician desires the "most appropriate" information and that this information may not necessarily be from the methods to generate the "best evidence" or, at least, such information has not been generated by these methods.

Recent developments in medical technologies have spawned the movement of "precision medicine." In 2011, the National Research Council [97] produced the following definition of precision medicine:

> The tailoring of medical treatment to the individual characteristics of each patient…to classify individuals into subpopulations that differ in their susceptibility to a particular disease or their response to a specific treatment. Preventative or therapeutic interventions can then be concentrated on those who will benefit, sparing expense and side effects for those who will not.

Quite frankly, this sounds very much like ensuring that the patient is in the right category of patients for which the treatment is effective. A more colloquial rendering of precision medicine is "the right medicine, for the right patient, at the right dose, at the right time," acknowledging that a "one size fits all" approach is not ideal [98]. I would further go on to say that a one-size-fits-all has led to overtreatment of some patients (with possible adverse effects) and undertreatment of others (leaving them at the mercy of the natural history of the disease).

The right treatment involves discovering an individual patient treatment effect [99]. That is, what will work for this particular patient. On the other hand, the presently accepted gold standard of evidence-based medicine, the randomized, controlled trial, produces an "average" treatment effect [99]. It is a truism that all practicing physicians will acknowledge that the response to a specific treatment will vary across the heterogeneity of a population, with some individuals having a good response and others having a poor response for a variety of biological reasons [98], often unknown. Please recall the hypothetical randomized trial presented in Chap. 5 (Fig. 5.2). The results of the trial showed an odds ratio of 1.5 "cure" with treatment compared to placebo. However, 40% of placebo patients were "cure," while 40% of treatment patients were not. Precision medicine aims to determine the different characteristics of the patients in these groups. In fact, randomized, controlled trials hide the heterogeneity of individual patient responses by focusing on the "average" treatment effect [99]. That is, we are learning about the characteristics of the treatment in a group of patients, rather than the characteristics of the patients responding or not responding to the treatment.

Precision medicine avers to harness improved knowledge of the pathogenesis of disease in an individual patient's disease [98] as well as large datasets [100]. That is, improved knowledge of pathogenesis in an individual patient can identify the causal attribution sequence that will yield knowledge of specific therapeutic targets for the individual's disease. I must say, as a surgeon, this has great appeal; I surgically treat the patient's disease *as the disease is in that patient*, not the populations "average" disease. The use of large, granular, accurate, individual-patient oriented datasets are simply necessary to better classify and categorize patients. Although the exact details of these techniques are beyond the scope of this book, I will end this section with the following quote from Tonelli and Shirts [101]:

> Precision medicine explicitly prioritizes the individualization of care and focuses attention on unique characteristics of a particular patient. In this fashion, [it] differs greatly from [evidence-based medicine], which seeks to determine the best course of action for a patient with an appeal to generalizable knowledge gained from population studies...To realize the goals of [precision medicine], the hierarchy of evidence pyramid must yield to a more horizontal conception of medical knowledge.

In other words, as previously discussed, "best" evidence may not be the most appropriate evidence for an individual patient. These are the judgments that the physician must make when constructing their diagnostic and therapeutic arguments in the process of persuading themselves and their patients.

7.5.3 *Outside Pressures That May Affect Physician Decision-Making*

I will now discuss aspects of physician decision-making that will make some practicing physicians (and, for the record, I was a practicing general surgeon for over 30 years) uncomfortable. To state this clearly, pressures outside of what the physician believes is best for the patient may influence their decisions. This may come as a shock or a surprise to some layman, although others may say this is stating the obvious. It starts with the fact that the practice of medicine is a business. This is true not only for physicians in private practice but also for academic physicians.[13] In fact, there are journals, such a *Medical Economics, Managed Healthcare Executive, Physician's Practice,* among others, courses at any number of medical society meetings on "coding and billing," as well as casual conversations in doctors' lounges all having to do with physicians' business concerns. Because it is a business, physicians find themselves under financial pressure.

Because physicians can find themselves under financial pressure, they may make medical choices based on these financial pressures. Although outright fraud is rare in medical practice, it does occur. In fact, the United States Department of Justice has 80 prosecutors in their Health Care Fraud Unit [102], which have been quite successful in identifying and prosecuting health care fraud cases, including cases against physicians and their practices. Although it is difficult to know how many patients were medically harmed, as opposed to "just" financially harmed, it is very likely that some physicians will recommend an appropriate, more lucrative treatment while demurring an equally appropriate, less expensive treatment. Even

---

[13] It has also been curious to me that doctors teaching in medical schools are generally required to have a medical practice that generates revenue for the medical school. In fact, in many medical schools, clinical revenue is the primary source of funding, not state government (for public medical schools) or tuition. As far as I know, no other "professional" schools, such as law schools or business schools, require their faculty to practice law or manage a business as a means of generating revenue for their particular schools.

supposedly nonprofit institutions will aggressively bill patients for services.[14] There is a reason why there are so many billboards and commercials for health care—it is about generating revenue.

One of the other main influences on physician treatment recommendations and patient acceptance of medical recommendations is medical insurance coverage. Medical insurance companies vary for what type of medical care they will pay healthcare providers. The majority of policies will also have some type of deductable. Physicians and hospitals generally have to submit for "preapproval" prior to the initiation of healthcare procedures. Even if a procedure or consultation is preapproved, this does not insure payment from the insurance company. The result of all of this is that some recommendations that the physician would like to make or the patient would like to accept are simply not considered due to insurance company denial policies. These policies have nothing to do with optimal care; however, they do pervert medical persuasion and argumentation and limit the possible premises and conclusions drawn.

The last effect of physician medical decisions that I would like to discuss are choices based on "defensive" medicine. For those who may not be aware of this phrase, defensive medicine is the practice of ordering tests or other procedures not necessarily because the doctor thinks it is necessary for the best care of the patient, but for the fear that if they did not and the patient had a poor outcome, they would be sued for malpractice [103]. The general assumption is that this practice, which is quite prevalent [103], increases the costs of care without improving outcomes. Whether this is true or not is not the point of me presenting this information but only to add to the list of "nonpatient care" influencing physician decisions.

We published an analysis of the surgical treatment options for GERD with respect to stakeholder valuation of the varying procedures [104]. What we determined is that each stakeholder has a different calculus in determining the value of the procedure for them. Again, this is only to acknowledge the obvious—not all the decisions are purely about the well-being of the patient.

7.6 Intuition in Clinical Practice

7.6.1 Practical Wisdom

There is knowledge, and then there is the use of that knowledge. Being able to assess when and how to use knowledge is wisdom. I spent the last two chapters on how medical knowledge is generated and how physicians incorporate this knowledge into patient care. However, this is an incomplete account. As discussed in

[14] The *New York Times* published a piece on patients who were entitled to free care but were billed and hounded by a hospital for payment. Jessica Silver-Greenberg and Katie Thomas, "They Were Entitled to Free Care. Hospitals Hounded Them to Pay." *New York Times*, September 24, 2022.

Chap. 6, contemporary epistemology focuses on justified true beliefs as independent propositions. This is far from a uniform opinion about knowledge. For instance, Kvanvig [105] objects both to the focus on a single belief of a single person at a single time and the object of a belief is presumed to be a discrete proposition. Instead, he asserts that a particular belief cannot be separated from other beliefs of the person or beliefs of other people. This is an important concept in that when physicians take in information about a patient, what and how they hear it is in relation to their existing medical knowledge, as well as their social umwelt.[15]

Just accumulating knowledge is not enough to lead to wisdom. An aggregation of facts does not lead to understanding. Zagzebski [33] quotes Julius Moravcisk that *understanding* is more than just the reproduction of facts; it possesses the right concepts and intuitive insights into the connection of the proper parts of a sequence. She further goes on to quote Gail Fine: Understanding, but not knowledge, requires explanation and interrelated accounts of knowledge. On the other hand, knowledge, but not understanding, requires certainty and allows one to know propositions individually, just not collectively. One understands a proposition as part of and because of one's understanding of a system or network of truths, that is, as a pattern of a whole chunk of reality [33]. To Zagaebski's "system or network," I would add "frameworks and theories." Understanding involves the comprehension of structures of reality other than its propositional structure.

Wisdom has certain properties that make it both useful and valuable but also acquired through the course of life, rather than a course of study. Wisdom is an epistemic value qualitatively different from the piling up of beliefs that have the property of justification, warrant or certainty [33]. Wisdom is a matter of grasping the whole of reality. Wisdom takes a different form in each individual case and resists any analysis that does not make essential reference to the standpoint of the individual. Human knowledge has increased, but the totality of human wisdom has not [33]. The experience needed for wisdom requires a certain amount of time, whereas the growth of knowledge can be accelerated by teaching [33]. Wisdom cannot be misused, but knowledge can. Wisdom unifies knowledge, desires and values [33]. There is no manual of "how to" acquire wisdom. However, the wise person has an understanding of the foibles of the human condition, what is good for this condition, and the right way to strive for it (even though it may never be obtained).

On the other hand, evidence-based medicine is not understanding or wisdom because it is entirely related to "disease" as a concept, not the entirety of disease as manifested in a patient (Fig. 6.1). It places research design methodology at the pinnacle of knowledge. This knowledge (or, rather, the "data" in "data-driven") will "decide" what is right for the patient, almost as if the physician is irrelevant in the process. However, data never speak for themselves and certainly cannot persuade without an interpretation. Simply put, the human mind has not evolved in this manner.

---

[15] There is a quote attributed to Einstein: "Not everything that can be measured is important, and not everything important can be measured."

Professional Wisdom

I have introduced and discussed the concept of practical wisdom, but this also applies specifically to professionals. Edmondson et al. [106] introduce the concept of "professional wisdom." They first start with referencing their assertion that "wisdom" combines experiential, intellectual, ethical, emotional, and practical capacities [107, 108], as was also noted above. They also assert that wisdom is more strongly social in nature than is usually appreciated [106]. Edmondson and colleagues [106] point out that the social nature of wisdom is quite insightful. This also has explanatory power. One of the core tenets of evidence-based medicine is that there is variation in care rendered and the medical outcomes produced. This, they consider, is a net negative. Proponents of evidence-based medicine, furthermore, assert that this variation is due to the uneven application of the "best evidence," while those advocating "tacit knowledge," "wisdom,", etc., feel that the variation is required due to variation in patients. On a practical matter, it could be that both are at odds with a physician's other motivations (discussed above) and, perhaps, their knowledge base, which is why we have variation.

Wisdom is a form of informal reasoning [106]. In clinical reasoning, deductions are rarely strict, premises rarely lawlike, and evidence rarely conclusive, but clinicians still must make adequate decisions [106]. Wise decisions are called for at points between knowledge and uncertainty where action or insight is vital, but neither everyday nor expert knowledge provides solutions [106]. To me, this is consistent with Kahneman and Tversky's judgment under uncertainty, discussed in chapter [109].

The "extracognitive" aspects of argumentation can play a role [106]. For example, there may be limitations in information that can affect the ability to decide [106]. At other times, there may be more than one available solution from which to choose [110]. How is such a decision made? Professionals are heavily influenced by the contexts of their choices. These individuals take some of their decision-making cues from their professional or institutional setting [106]. This is consistent with a professional social umwelt that I previously stated exists. In this setting, professionals become accustomed to knowing what sorts of responses their peers regard as adequate and possibly adapt their expectations to response they know to be likely acceptable [106]. This is not always a good thing: Theories and ideologies can persist over long periods even when they have been largely falsified [111]. I have previously given the example of the persistence of the belief that the primary causative agent in peptic ulcer disease was gastric acid long after it was shown that the primary agent was *Helicobacter pylori*. It takes a certain amount of wisdom, humility and courage to escape the trap of just doing something because everyone else does.

At times, for both the professional and the patient, overcoming their social or professional umwelt is required to make good decisions. Reasoning well may demand facets of character and political judgment that make radical demands of the reasoner [106]. This is consistent with the prior discussion in Chap. 4 that accepting conclusions of arguments that are contradictory to one's social (or professional) umwelt requires exceptional integrity. Another extracognitive feature that may be particular to experts is that they tend to be less certain in their judgments than non-experts, as though expertise develops *humility* (an intellectual virtue [33]) that allows for continuous critical assessment.[16] According to Aristotle in *Rhetoric*, other important virtues of the wise person also include devotion to the common good, courage, responsiveness to listener's problems with the argument presented, as was discussion in Chap. 4 and in *Virtues of the Mind* [33]. This constant self-assessment leads to more perfected solutions [112].

The Non-Routine, Complex, Ambiguous Decision

I gave an account of the routine decision above. Now is time to give an account of the more uncommon but more vexing complex or ambiguous case. Every physician has had these cases. Cases that simply "don't make sense." The symptoms do not follow a recognizable pattern, treatments that should have worked, have failed, treatment reactions are unexplained by the pharmacology of the drug, etc. These are the cases that weigh on a physician.

These are exactly the types of cases for which there is no "best-evidence." These are the cases where numerous tests are ordered and several specialists consulted. These are exactly the type of cases that require wisdom, understanding, humility and intuition. I can offer no normative account of how a physician should approach cases such as these, as they are all unique. My point is that approaching these cases requires more than knowledge and facts. In addition, much cannot be standardized in the approaches.

Intuition: The Counter-Argument

In Chap. 2 and in this chapter, I have acknowledged that intuition as a method of medical decision-making exists among most, and especially experienced, physicians. My view is that intuition is a form of subconscious recognition of atypical situations and that the solutions it produces are akin to abduction. However, I will concede that not all share my view. Some are more confident in intuition. Broude's view [19] of intuition is that by itself, intuition is insufficient as explicit knowledge but is an inherent part of the process of linking tacit knowing with explicit knowledge [19]. Intuition is a cognitive element of clinical reasoning that incorporates tacit elements of clinical reasoning in a rational manner, albeit one that resists explicit formulation [19].

On the other hand, others have less sanguine views. Feinstein [28] opposes "intuition" based on "hunches" or "nebulously defined" clinical experience. Nevertheless, he acknowledges that intuition is a part of medical practice but implored it to be

[16] One can recall my "Lego Theory" of knowledge accumulation—that is, the more you know about a topic, the easier it is to know more, because your existing knowledge acts as places for new knowledge to anchor, just as the prongs of Lego bricks.

more explicit: "without intuition, imagination or esthetics, the 'scientist' is a dullard. Without rationality, discipline or logic, the 'artist' is a dawdler" [28]. Dudley's [113] view is unequivocally negative. For him, he asserts that we are bounded by unprovable axioms or conventions that must be the starting point of any system of reasoning we care to adopt. This is the commonly accepted knowledge that all humans have in general, and medical professionals have through there education which has gone unchallenged (i.e., the physician's theoretical framework meta-cognition of Fig. 1.1) and the bootstrapped knowledge that was discussed in Chaps. 4 and 6. Therefore, for Dudley [113], any particular method or technique of reasoning in order to solve a problem must be based on pragmatics—that is, does it work in the world as we experience it. Therefore, if we are to accept "intuitive reasoning" as a legitimate method of clinical reasoning, it must consistently give good results [113]. In addition, this is the rub—it is impossible to replicate an individual's intuitive reasoning and, as a general technique, it has not been proven to yield consistently good results. Dudley [113] does concede that it is possible that prolonged contemplation of a group of facts and concepts can result, through "cerebral processes that are subliminal," in a new synthesis or provides a breakthrough. This is how Abernathy and Hamm [24] view intuition and sounds similar to abduction. However, Dudley's most pointed criticism is that appealing to one's intuition as a defense of one's clinical decision-making is truly an appeal to protect the clinician from engaging in the difficult task of analyzing a "complex matrix of patient information" [113]. In this, he is right. Intuition occurs *because* a physician has focused their attention on a patient with a perplexing presentation, not just because they want to produce a quick decision and move on to something else.

7.7 How a Patient Accepts a Physician's Recommendations

Once a physician comes to a decision as to the patient's diagnosis and which would be the appropriate treatments, this is presented to the patient. The physician may be blunt and authoritarian by saying "this is what you have and this is what we need to do." Or, more commonly, they will report on the findings of the various tests ordered and how the diagnosis explains the patient's symptoms (Fig. 1.1). Whether one wants to call this an explanation or an argument, it still is a matter of persuasion. The patient needs to be convinced that the diagnosis offered is from what they are suffering. Patient participation in this process and ultimately any therapeutic decisions is a form of manifest rationality, as discussed by Johnson [1].

In presenting the treatment options, the physician will have to convince the patient how the varying treatments will affect their condition. This may include discussion of how a medication targets the causal sequence leading to the disease or how an operation will correct the anatomic defect. Usually, during this process, the physician will discuss the various "risks and benefits." The benefits are how the recommended treatment will likely improve the patient's condition, while the risks are the possible adverse outcomes. Such relevant issues may include survival (e.g., after a cancer diagnosis) or quality of life. Sometimes, this is accompanied by actual probabilities of this happening, such as "for a patient like you, this operation as a 1 in 100 chance of death," while others may simply say, "you could die from this operation." The physician may have to "translate" the probabilistic nature of prognosis into laymen's terms. For example, if a disease has a median survival of 12 months, half of the patients with the disease died before 12 months, while the other half died after 12 months. Not that this particular patient will live 12 months. Similarly, if a disease has a 25% 5-year survival, it means that three-quarters of the patients died before 5 years, while the remainder died after 5 years, not that this particular patient as a 25% chance of living 5 years.

In this process, the entire persuasive enterprise can be an explicit illative core of the argument, or much can be implicit and assumed, by the physician, patient and patient's loved ones who may be present for this discussion. When there are unsaid assumptions in an argument that are assumed, this is an enthymeme. Aristotle defined an enthymeme as a syllogism from what is likely to be the case or from signs, whether the inference is expressed completely or not. These can be "distributed" among several different contributors, augmenting the "sociality" of how conclusions evolve [106]. In the medical context, the appropriate use of tests and consultants can function as these additional contributors. These tests and consultants provide the premises for the illative core of the physician's argument. This process, hopefully, leads to a "reasonable conviction" by both the physician and the patient as to the validity of the conclusion.

Such judgments take place in situations that are markedly personal and interpersonal. These reasonable convictions are generally constituted partly of emotional, ethical, social and even political elements [106]. This occurs in the background of the patient and physician's social/cultural or professional umwelt (see Chap. 3). To me, this appears to be a very good description of how a wise, thoughtful clinician will approach a patient with complex medical issues. In addition to coming to a diagnosis, it is coming to a diagnosis in the context of the patient's entire mental and social environment. The interplay of argument, the listener's reactions, and the arguer's ethos forms the basic condition under which human communication takes place [106]. This is the essence of manifest rationality and persuasion in the context of what the human mind can accept (Fig. 4.2). The speaker's trustworthiness is an essential feature of enthymematic reasoning.

The physician will generally give the patient an opportunity to ask any questions. After this back and forth, the patient may reach a decision (Figs. 1.1, and 7.1 and 7.3).

7.8 Conclusions

What I have attempted in this chapter is to give a descriptive account of how a rational physician will incorporate medical knowledge into their corpus of medical knowledge and how they will use this knowledge for diagnosis and treatment decisions. I have not attempted to deliver any normative rules for this process as I am not sure there are uniform and/or comprehensive rules, certainly not ones that are universally accepted. The incorporation of medical knowledge requires the physician to have confidence that the information given is both true and useful. I have given accounts of various methods of reasoning to achieve this. It still appears to me that physicians use informal logic for this purpose. I have tried to give an account of diagnostic medical reasoning. Rather than being a formal process, it appears that it is an informal, iterative process that relies both on using patient data in a manner that is both semiotic and hermeneutical, leading to recognition of patterns or scripts. The physician then interprets these scripts in a manner that continually refines the possible categories that the patient is in, with the ultimate goal of matching the patient diagnostic category to the appropriate treatment. How physicians accept treatments that are appropriate for a patient category was also discussed and is similar to how diagnostic tests are adopted. I have discussed the strengths and weaknesses of evidence-based medicine, which is best applied in routine cases for which there is evidence. I have also discussed precision medicine, which incorporates patient-specific rather than population-based data. Last, I discussed *phronesis*, intuition, and practical and professional wisdom and understanding, and how these are used by the physician is complex and ambiguous. This process then leads to creation of an illative core argument which is presented to the patient. The patient will then engage in this process to achieve manifest rationality with the physician, and, thereby, be persuaded to accept the diagnosis and the agreed upon treatment.

References

1. Johnson RH. Manifest rationality: a pragmatic theory of argument. New York: Routledge; 2012.
2. Sackett DL, Rosenberg WW, Gray JA, et al. Evidence-based medicine: what it is and what it isn't. BMJ. 1996;312:71–2.
3. Zarkovich E, Upshaw REG. The virtues of evidence. Theor Med. 2002;23:403–13.
4. Evidence-Based Medicine Working Group. Evidence-based medicine. A new approach to teaching the practice of medicine. JAMA. 1992;268:2420–5.
5. Sackett D, Haynes R, Tugwell P, Guyatt G. Clinical epidemiology: a basic science. 2nd ed. Boston: Little, Brown; 1991.
6. Mike V. Outcomes research and the quality of health care: the beacon of an ethics of evidence. Eval Health Prof. 1999;22:3–32.
7. Mittinen OS. Evidence in medicine: invited commentary. CMAJ. 1998;158:215–21.
8. Peters JH, DeMeester TR, Crookes P, et al. The treatment of gastroesophageal reflux disease with laparoscopic Nissen fundoplication: prospective evaluation of 100 patients with "typical" symptoms. Ann Surg. 1998;228:40–50.
9. Spechler SJ, Hunter JG, Jones KM, et al. Randomized trial of medical versus surgical treatment for refractory heartburn. N Engl J Med. 2019;381:1513–23.
10. Rogers EM. Diffusion of innovations. 5th ed. New York: The Free Press; 2003.
11. Silverstein FE, Faich G, Goldstein JL, et al. Gastrointestinal toxicity with celecoxib vs nonsteroidal anti-inflammatory drugs for osteoarthritis and rheumatoid arthritis: the CLASS study: a randomized controlled trial. JAMA. 2000;284:1247–55.
12. Cotter J, Wooltorton E. New restrictions on celecoxib (Celebrex) use and the withdrawal of valdecoxib (Bextra). Can Med Assoc J. 2005;172:1299.

13. COX-2 selective (includes Bextra, Celebrex, and Vioxx) and nonselective nonsteroidal anti-inflammatory drugs (NSAIDS). https://fda.gov. Posted 7 Apr 2005, last accessed 26 Sept 2022.
14. Gartlehner G, Hansen RA, Nissman D, et al. Efficacy trials in systematic reviews. Rockville, MD: Agency for Healthcare Research and Quality; 2006. (Technical Reviews, No. 12).
15. Center for Evidence-Based Management. What is a systematic review? https://cebma.org. Last accessed 27 Sept 2022.
16. Chin-Yee BH. Underdetermination in evidence-based medicine. J Eval Clin Pract. 2014;20:921–7.
17. Stanford K. Underdetermination of scientific theory. In: Zalta EN, editor. The Stanford encyclopedia of philosophy. Stanford, CA: Stanford University; 2021. https://stanford.edu/archives/win2021/entries/scientific-underdetermination.
18. Polanyi M. The tacit dimension. Gloucester, MA: Peter Smith; 1983.
19. Braude HD. Clinical intuition versus statistics: different modes of tacit knowledge in clinical epidemiology and evidence-based medicine. Theor Med Bioeth. 2009;30:181–98.
20. Polychronis A, Miles A, Bentley P. Evidence-based medicine: reference? Dogma? Neologism? New orthodoxy? J Eval Clin Pract. 1996;2:1–3.
21. Feinstein AR, Horwitz R. Problems in the 'evidence' of evidence-based medicine. Am J Med. 1997;103:529–35.
22. Malterud K. Reflexivity and metapositions: strategies for appraisal of clinical evidence. J Eval Clin Pract. 2002;8:121–6.
23. Henry S. Recognizing tacit knowledge in medical epistemology. Theor Med Bioeth. 2006;27:187–213.
24. Abernathy CM, Hamm RM. Surgical intuition: what it is and how to get it. Philadelphia: Hanley & Belfus, Inc.; 1995.
25. Elstein AS. Clinical problem solving and decision psychology. Acad Med. 2000;75(Suppl 10):S134–6.
26. Sackett DL, Richardson WS, Rosenberg W, Haynes RB. Evidence-based medicine: how to practice and teach EBM. Churchill: Livingstone; 1997.
27. Feinstein AR. An analysis of diagnostic reasoning: II. The strategy of intermediate decisions. Yale J Biol Med. 1973;46:264–83.
28. Feinstein AR. Clinical judgment. Baltimore, MD: Williams & Wilkins; 1968.
29. Feinstein AR. Scientific methodology in clinical medicine. I. Introduction, principles, and concepts. Ann Intern Med. 1964;61:564–79.
30. Feinstein AR. Scientific methodology in clinical medicine. II. Classification of human disease by clinical behavior. Ann Intern Med. 1964;61:757–81.
31. Feinstein AR. Scientific methodology in clinical medicine. III. The evaluation of therapeutic response. Ann Intern Med. 1964;61:1162–93.
32. Feinstein AR. "Clinical Judgment" revisited: the distraction of quantitative models. Ann Intern Med. 1994;120:799–805.
33. Zagzebski LT. Virtues of the mind: an inquiry into the nature of virtue and the ethical foundations of knowledge. Cambridge: Cambridge University Press; 1996.
34. Malik A, Conroy M, Turner C. *Phronesis* in medical ethics: courage and motivation to keep on the track of rightness in decision-making. Health Care Anal. 2020;28:158–75.
35. Tyreman S. Promoting critical thinking in health care: phronesis and criticality. Med Health Care Philos. 2000;3:117–24.
36. Kaljian LC. Patient care and population health: goals, roles and costs. J Pub Health Res. 2014;3:81–2.
37. Kaljian LC. Teaching practical wisdom in medicine through clinical judgment, goals of care, and ethical reasoning. J Med Ethics. 2010;36:558–62.
38. Healy MJR. Formal reasoning and the surgeon. Theor Surg. 1991;6:87–8.
39. Montgomery EB. Medical reasoning: the nature and use of medical knowledge. New York: Oxford University Press; 2019.

40. Marcum JA. The role of emotions in clinical reasoning and decision-making. J Med Philos. 2013;38:501–19.
41. Marcum JA. An integrated model of clinical reasoning: dual-process theory of cognition and metacognition. J Eval Clin Pract. 2012;18:954–61.
42. Kassirer JP. Our stubborn quest for diagnostic certainty: a cause of excessive testing. N Engl J Med. 1989;320:1489–91.
43. Riffenburgh RH. Using the reference guide. In: Riffenburgh RH, editor. Statistics in medicine. 2nd ed. New York: Academic; 2006.
44. Maung HH. The causal explanatory functions of medical diagnoses. Theor Med Bioeth. 2017;38:41–59.
45. Benzi M. Medical diagnoses and actual causation. L+PS—Logic. Philos Sci. 2011;9:365–72.
46. Blaxter M. Diagnosis as a category and process: the case of alcoholism. Soc Sci Med. 1978;12:9–17.
47. Salmon WC. Causal and theoretical explanation. In: Salmon WC, editor. Causality and explanation. Oxford: Oxford University Press; 1998.
48. Scriven M. Causation as explanation. Nous. 1975;9:3–16.
49. Lewis DK. Causal explanation. In: Lewis DK, editor. Philosophical papers, vol. 2. Oxford: Oxford University Press; 1986.
50. Woodward J. Making things happen: a theory of causal explanation. Oxford: Oxford University Press; 2003.
51. Lipton P. Inference to the best explanation. 2nd ed. New York: Routledge; 2003.
52. Hempel CG. Aspects of scientific explanation. New York: The Fress Press; 1965.
53. Gorovitz S, MacIntyre A. Toward a theory of medical fallibility. Hastings Center Rep. 1975;5:13–23.
54. Cartwright N. How can we know what made the ratman sick? Singular causes and population probabilities. In: Jokic A, editor. Philosophy of religion, physics, and psychology: essays in honor of Adolf Grunbaum. Amherst, NY: Prometheus Books; 2005.
55. Dragulinescu S. On anti-Humeanism and medical singular causation. Acta Anal. 2012;27:265–92.
56. Darden L. Mechanisms versus causes in biology and medicine. In: Chao H, Chen S, Millstein RL, editors. Mechanism and causality in biology and economics. Dordrecht: Springer; 2013.
57. Russo F, Williamson J. Interpreting causality in the health sciences. Int Stud Philos Sci. 2007;21:157–70.
58. Nervi M. Mechanisms, malfunctions and explanation in medicine. Biol Philos. 2010;25:215–28.
59. Anderson H. Mechanisms: what are they evidence for in evidence-based medicine? J Eval Clin Pract. 2012;18:992–9.
60. Whitbeck C. What is a diagnosis? Some critical reflections. Metamedicine. 1981;2:319–29.
61. Bennett RD, Straughn DM, Velanovich V. Gastroesophageal reflux disease, hiatal hernia, and Barrett esophagus. In: Zinner MJ, Ashley SW, Hines OJ, editors. Maingot's abdominal operations. 13th ed. New York: McGraw-Hill Education; 2019. p. 393–422.
62. Nessa J. About signs and symptoms: can semiotics expand the view of clinical medicine? Theor Med. 1996;17:363–71.
63. Bowen JL. Educational strategies to promote clinical diagnostic reasoning. N Engl J Med. 2006;355:2217–25.
64. Koens F, Mann KV, Custers E, Ten Cate OT. Analyzing the concept of context in medical education. Med Educ. 2005;39:1243–9.
65. Schmidt HG, Norman GR, Bohuizen HP. A cognitive perspective on medical expertise theory and implications. Acad Med. 1990;65:611–21. (Erratum, Acad Med 1992;67:287).
66. Nendaz MR, Bordage G. Promoting diagnostic problem representation. Med Educ. 2002;36:760–6.
67. Bordage G, Lemieux M. Semantic structures and diagnostic thinking of experts and novices. Acad Med. 1991;66(Suppl):S70–2.

68. Bordage G. Why did I miss the diagnosis? Some cognitive explanations and educational implications. Acad Med. 1999;74(Suppl):S138–43.
69. Norman G. Research in clinical reasoning: past history and current trends. Med Educ. 2005;39:418–27.
70. Elstein AS, Schwarz A. Clinical problem solving and diagnostic decision-making: selective review of the cognitive literature. BMJ. 2002;324:729–32.
71. Custers EJ, Regehr G, Norman GR. Mental representations of medical diagnostic knowledge: a review. Acad Med. 1996;71(Suppl):S55–61.
72. Eva KW. What every teacher needs to know about clinical reasoning. Med Educ. 2005;39:98–106. (Erratum, Med Educ 2005;39:753).
73. Trevethan R. Sensitivity, specificity, and predictive values: foundations, pliabilities, and pitfalls in research and practice. Front Public Health. 2017;5:307.
74. Velanovich V. Bayesian analysis is the diagnostic process. Am J Med Qual. 1994;9:158–61.
75. Ivanov A. Barriers to the introduction of new medical diagnostic tests. Lab Med. 2013;44:e132–6.
76. Johnson LF, DeMeester TR. Development of the 24-hour intraesophageal pH monitoring composite score. J Clin Gastroenterol. 1986;8(Suppl 1):52–8.
77. Dent J. Review article: from 1906 to 2006—a century of major evolution of understanding of gastro-esophageal reflux disease. Aliment Pharm Ther. 2006;24:1269–81.
78. Velanovich V. Practice-changing milestones in anti-reflux and hiatal hernia surgery: a single surgeon perspective over 27 years and 1,200 operations. J Gastrointest Surg. 2021;25:2757–69.
79. Johnsson F, Joelsson B, Isberg P-E. Ambulatory 24 hour intraesophageal pH-monitoring in the diagnosis of gastroesophageal reflux disease. Gut. 1987;28:1145–50.
80. Kelly A-M. The minimum clinically significant difference in the visual analog scale pain score does not differ with the severity of pain. Emerg Med J. 2001;18:205–7.
81. Reference Ranges. https://labortorynavigator.com. Last accessed 29 Sept 2022.
82. Barosi G, Magnani L, Stefanelli M. Medical diagnostic reasoning: epistemological modeling as a strategy for the design of computer-based consultation programs. Theor Med. 1993;14:43–55.
83. Ridderikhoff J. Problem-solving in general practice. Theor Med. 1993;14:343–63.
84. Doroszewski J. Hypothetico-nomological aspects of medical diagnosis. Part I: general structure of the diagnostic process and its hypothesis-directed stage. Metamedicine. 1980;1:177–94.
85. Moore GW, Hutchins GM. Effort and demand logic in medical decision making. Metamedicine. 1980;1:277–303.
86. Leder D. Clinical interpretation: the hermeneutics of medicine. Theor Med. 1990;11:9–24.
87. Daniel S. The patient as text: a model of clinical hermeneutics. Theor Med. 1986;7:195–210.
88. Toulmin S. On the nature of the physician's understanding. J Med Philos. 1976;1:32–50.
89. Gadamer H-G. Truth and method. New York: Crossroad; 1984.
90. Little JM. The problem of clinical process—a Popperian analysis. Theor Surg. 1993;8:146–50.
91. Sleigh JW. Logical limits of randomized, controlled trials. J Eval Clin Pract. 1997;3:145–8.
92. Kaptchuk T. The double-blind, randomized, placebo-controlled trial: gold standard or golden calf. J Clin Epidemiol. 2001;54:541–9.
93. Altman DG. Statistics in medical journals: some recent trends. Stat Med. 2000;19:3281–4.
94. Grossman J, Mackenzie F. The randomized, controlled trial: gold standard or merely standard. Perspect Biol Med. 2005;48:516–34.
95. Birkmeyer JD, Finks JF, O'Reilly A, et al. Surgical skill and complication rates after bariatric surgery. N Engl J Med. 2013;369:1434–42.
96. Velanovich V. Operative decisions. Theor Surg. 1991;6:38–40.
97. National Research Council. Toward precision medicine: building a knowledge network for biomedical research and a new taxonomy of disease. Washington, DC: National Academic Press; 2011.

98. Seyhan AA, Carini C. Are innovation and new technologies in precision medicine paving a new era in patient centric care? J Transl Med. 2019;17:114.
99. Blackstone EH. Precision medicine versus evidence-based medicine: individual treatment effect versus average treatment effect. Circulation. 2019;140:1236–8.
100. Ginsburg GS, Phillips KA. Precision medicine from science to value. Health Aff. 2018;37:694–701.
101. Tonelli MR, Shirts BH. Knowledge for precision medicine: mechanistic reasoning and methodological pluralism. JAMA. 2017;318:1649–50.
102. Health Care Fraud Unit, the United States Department of Justice. https://justice.gov. Last accessed 30 Sept 2022.
103. Studdert DM, Mello MM, Sage WM, et al. Defensive medicine among high-risk specialist physicians in a volatile malpractice environment. JAMA. 2005;293:2609–17.
104. Zheng QV, Velanovich V. Modeling stakeholder valuation: an example using surgical treatments for gastroesophageal reflux disease. Cureus. 2021;13(11):e19559.
105. Kvanvig J. The intellectual virtues and the life of the mind. Lanham, MD: Rowmen and Littlefield; 1992.
106. Edmondson R, Pearce J, Woerner MH. Wisdom in clinical reasoning and medical practice. Theor Med Bioeth. 2009;30:231–47.
107. Edmondson R. Wisdom in later life: ethnographic approaches. Age Soc. 2005;25:339–56.
108. Edmondson R, Pearce J. The practice of health care: wisdom as a model. Med Health Care Philos. 2007;10:233–44.
109. Kahneman D, Slovic P, Tversky A. Judgment under uncertainty: heuristics and biases. Cambridge: Cambridge University Press; 1982.
110. Norman GR, Schmidt HG. The psychological basis of problem-based learning: a review of the evidence. Acad Med. 1992;67:557–65.
111. Egidi M. Discrepancies: competing theories and ideologies as cultural traps. In: Rizzello S, editor. Cognitive developments in economics. London: Routledge; 2003.
112. Gera-May I. "We seem to have always spoken in pross…" policy analysis as a clinical profession: implications for policy analysis practice and instruction. Policy Stud J. 2007;35:135–64.
113. Dudley HAF. Intuition: intellectually effete, and a nonthinker's picket fence. Theor Surg. 1991;6:78–80.

Chapter 8
Correlations with "Non-Western" Medical Theory and Practice: Traditional Chinese Medicine, Traditional Indigenous Medicine, Faith Healing, and Homeopathy

8.1 Non-Western Medicine Has a Theoretical Foundation Too

The purpose of this chapter is to apply the concepts developed in this book about argumentation and persuasion to non-Western allopathic medical practices. The prior chapters almost exclusively used allopathic medicine as practiced originally in Europe and then eventually exported around the world as the basis for analysis. However, prior to this social and political development, all cultures and communities probably had some form of medical care. Prior to modern times, with its increasing ease of communication, humans in their communities developed their own medical practices. My assertion is that these practices were based on a theoretical foundation, consistent with their cultures. Therefore, each people's culture and social umwelt, how they view their world and how knowledge was derived from the world, is how they developed their theoretical foundation medicine, which became the *raison d'etre* for subsequent practice.

I will further assert that the same evolution of the human brain and mind that led to the development of allopathic Western medicine also led to these other medical traditions. I will reiterate what was said in Chap. 1: the human mind evolved to survive, not to discern truth. Therefore, these practices developed in the milieu of their respective cultures and societies not only to promote health and alleviate the suffering of individuals but also to foster group cohesion. These medical traditions, like Western allopathic medicine, exist within a social/cultural umwelt of the people within that culture and a professional umwelt of the practitioners of the tradition. My goal is not to be critical of any medical tradition but, rather, to demonstrate the universality of the illative core of argumentation in human persuasion and how the individual social and cultural umwelt can determine whether the argument is accepted. All of these traditions have a rational basis in a network of self-supporting

V. Velanovich, *Medical Persuasion*, https://doi.org/10.1007/978-3-031-30371-5_8

justified true beliefs that do have an epistemic basis, even if these beliefs differ from culture to culture.

Toward this end, I will take examples of non-Western allopathic medicine. These will include traditional medical practices as well as an example of alternative and complementary medical practice. I will fully acknowledge that I am not an expert or a practitioner of any of these traditions. I will accept as a criticism that since I am not a member of a particular tradition's culture, other than my own, I may be prone to error in interpretation. As true as this is, my other option is simply to make no attempt at understanding these other medical paradigms. This, I believe, would be an even greater failure on my part. Moreover, my intention is to give just enough of an account to illustrate their underlying theory, which may or may not be overtly considered a theory by their practitioners, and how that theory results in the tradition's medical practice. This will be the same approach that I took with Western allopathic medicine. I will strive in my account to be respectful to these traditions and in no way to imply superiority of one over any other, including Western allopathic medicine.

Toward this end, I will not directly compare any one tradition with any other, as I believe that each is its own independent, stand-alone theory, not requiring justification by comparison. I also have no intention on discussing or analyzing actual efficacy or effectiveness of treatments. I am not endorsing or dismissing any of these traditions. This is not relevant for the discussion of theory, nor do I feel I am qualified in any way to address such an analysis. This is for each tradition's practitioners to do, or, possibly, regulatory agencies. There will be no comparisons to Western medicine as a "gold standard" of what should be optimal medical care because one can argue effectively that Western medicine misses much pertaining to the well-being, especially spiritual well-being, of its patients. I may acknowledge different theoretical concepts, such as what "disease" will mean different things in these traditions. Additionally, it must be acknowledged that there may be concepts that are not directly translatable from the native language into English. Therefore, I am sensitive to the issue that important nuance and understanding may be lost or misunderstood. Hence, my approach is not to claim understanding but make a sincere attempt to understand with humility. For any errors I have made, I humbly apologize.

The examples I have chosen are traditional Chinese medicine, traditional North American indigenous medicine, traditional African medicine, American faith healing, and homeopathy. This is not to say that other medical paradigms are not worthy of study or inclusion, only that these were accessible, illustrative, and of interest to me.

8.2 Traditional Chinese Medicine

8.2.1 Brief History of Traditional Chinese Medicine

What is now known as "traditional Chinese medicine" had its origin more than 4000 years ago [1]. The main concept of *qi*, or vital force, has its roots in a Confucian philosophical theory described in *The Analects of Confucius* some 3500 years ago [2]. The first known text of traditional Chinese medicine was written approximately 2600 BCE, the *Huangdi Neijing*, translated into English variously as *The Yellow Emperor's Inner Classic* [1], *The Yellow Emperor's Canon of Medicine* [3], among others. At the time of its development, traditional Chinese medicine was a canon of Chinese philosophy, astronomy and literature, coupled with the common experience of dealing with medical disorders using puncture, mind control (*qipong*), and plant-based therapies [4]. Anatomical and surgical operations are relatively uncommon in traditional Chinese medicine because of the Confucian tenets of the sacred body [1]. Therefore, traditional Chinese medicine was developed, for the most part, along nonsurgical lines.

Traditional Chinese medicine continued to evolve over the next thousands of years. During the Eastern Han Dynasty (first to the third century CE), Zhang Zhongjing wrote the *Shanghan Lun* (translated into *Treatise on Cold Damage and Miscellaneous Disease* [3], among others), emphasizing the patient's physique in relation to disease susceptibility [3]. The *Bencao gang mu* (translated into *Guidelines and Details of Materia Medica* [1] or *Compendium of Materia Medica* [5]) was written by Shizhen Li in the sixteenth century during the Ming Dynasty, containing approximately 11,000 herbal medical preparations from some 1892 medical materials derived from plants, minerals and animal products, many imported from outside China through the Silk Road [1, 5]. Even recently since the 1970s, there has been additional writing on the patient's "constitution" and its relationship to health and disease [3]. The *Chinese Pharmacopoeia* was most recently updated in 2015 [6], containing 5608 medical products, including herbal medicines, animal-derived products, minerals, food and conventional drugs. This was added to the *Index of Pharmacopoeias* by the World Health Organization in 2002 [7].

Because of this long history of thought and practice in traditional Chinese medicine, this history is sometimes referred to by its practitioners as a "Seal of Trust," that is, evidence of its effectiveness and value. Certainly, the practice of traditional Chinese medicine is quite active not only in China but also in North America and Europe, as well as other parts of the world.

8.2.2 Theoretical Foundation of Normal Human Functioning

This will be a very rudimentary account due to both my lack of expertise and space constraints. Although much detail and nuance will be left out, I hope to provide enough information to support the basis of my thesis. Traditional Chinese medicine recognizes the human body by "system discrimination" and in a "cybernetic way" as a holistic theory with emphasis on the human's relationship to their social and natural environment [4]. What is meant by "system discrimination" is that the human body is a complex with integrated systems, and there is an "external reflection" of "internal activities," such that observed external signs reflect internal function [4], for example, how the parts of the tongue reflect the conditions of some internal organs, discussed below. What is meant by "cybernetics" is that the human body is a "self-controlled network", and this network is connected throughout the body [4], for example, by the meridians, which will be discussed below. Moreover, traditional Chinese medicine attempts to integrate the mind, body, natural and social environments, and health with the fundamental view that is holistic based on harmony among these factors [1, 4].

There are several foundational tenets of traditional Chinese medicine. These include:

1. The vital life force of *qi*.
2. The opposites of *yin* and *yang*.
3. The Five Elements.
4. The *Jing-luo* or meridians.
5. The *Zang-fu* organs.
6. The inclusion of environmental factors [1, 8].

Qi is translated into English as a "vital life force," but this does not truly encompass the concept in classical Chinese philosophy from whence it came. It is an all-encompassing force that binds together all things in the universe—it is both "everything and nothing" [8]. *Qi*, however, "flows" through humans, and its flow and "balance" are essential for human health. There are different types of *qi*. For example, within the human body, there are four types: parental (*yuan qi*) is the *qi* that is inherited from one's parents at conception; pectoral (*zong qi*) is the *qi* that is produced by breathing; nutritional (*ying qi*) is derived from eating foods and is responsible for the circulating nutrition throughout the body; and defensive (*wei qi*) is responsible for protecting the body from illnesses.

Qi is made up of *yin* and *yang* portions, which are opposite of each other [8]. However, it must be understood that *yin* and *yang* do not have independent existences, and these elements are always together. Figure 8.1 shows the very familiar *yin-yang* symbol representing the balance of opposites. The outer circle represents the universe and everything in it, while the two smaller inner circles represent the notion that everything has the "seeds" of its opposite. Table 8.1 lists examples of such opposite for general phenomena and specifically for traditional Chinese medicine [8].

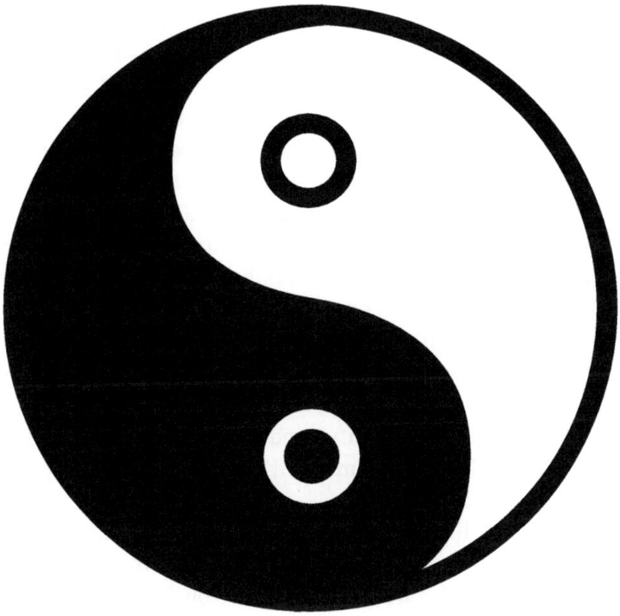

Fig. 8.1 The traditional *yin-yang* symbol. The outer circle represents everything in the universe. The white section is the *yang*, and the black section the *yin*. The two smaller circles represent the concept that everything has the seeds of its opposite

Table 8.1 Examples of *Yin-Yang* opposites

General examples		Traditional Chinese medicine examples	
Yin	*Yang*	*Yin*	*Yang*
Structure	Function	Dark	Light
Night	Day	Cold	Warm
Cold	Hot	Negative	Positive
Earth	Sky	Passive	Active
Moon	Sun	Female	Male
Slow	Fast	Solid	Hollow
Humidity	Dryness	Liver	Gallbladder
Ascends energy	Descends energy	Heart	Small intestine
Fluids	Energy	Spleen	Stomach
Calm	Expressive	Lungs	Large intestine
Death	Birth	Kidneys	Urinary bladder

In Chinese philosophy, the five-element theory describes the interaction and relationship between things. These elements are wood, fire, earth, metal and water [4]. They divide the human body into five systems. Movement and interchange among the five elements are used to explain the human body and its physiology.

The *jing-lua*, or meridians, are the "channels" through which *qi* and other fundamental substances flow in the body [1, 8]. Historically, meridians have been described as following "vascular nerve bundles" [1]. However, no "scientifically" viable explanation for the existence of the meridians in a "non-philosophical" context has been established [1]. On the other hand, traditional Chinese practitioners believe that the meridians are "nonphysical" [8]; therefore, it is not surprising that no anatomic correlations are identified. The *jingmai* are the main meridian channels, while the *luomai* are the collateral channels. There are 12 major or primary meridians that connect the *Zang-fu* organs (discussed below) and are the main pathways that transport *qi* and *xue* throughout the body. There are eight extraordinary meridians that connect the 12 primary meridians. There are 12 divergent or distinct meridians that are responsible for connecting the *wei* (defensive) and *yuan* (parental) *qi*. There are six *yin* meridians, three in the arm (associated with the heart, lung and pericardium) and three in the leg (associated with the liver, kidney and spleen). There are six *yang* meridians, three in the arm (associated with the small intestine, large intestine and the coelomic cavity) and three in the leg (associated with the urinary bladder, gallbladder and stomach) [8]. This leads to a complex network throughout the body (Fig. 8.2).

Zang-fu organs are a collection of organs that produce and regulate *qi* within the human body [8]. They should not be thought of anatomically but rather as their interconnective functions [8]. Each organ's function is its *qi*. There are five *Zang*

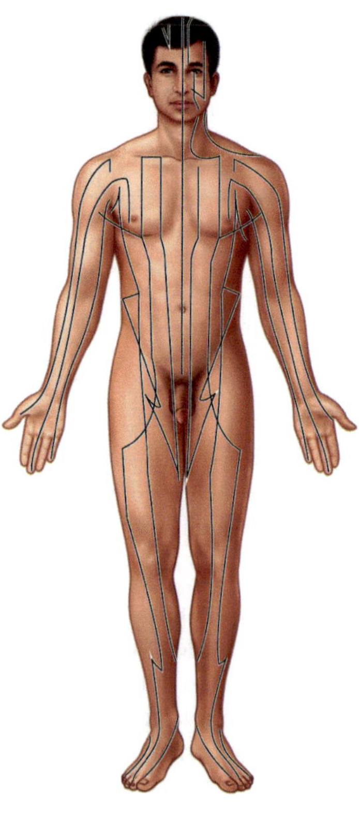

Fig. 8.2 A traditional illustration of the surface location of the meridians

organs that are *yin* and six *fu* organs that are *yang*. *Zang* organs produce and store five fundamental substances: *qi, xue* (blood), *jinye* (body fluids), *jing* (essence), and *shen* (spirit) [8]. The heart stores *shen*; it governs blood and the meridians and emotionally controls joy. The spleen is responsible for the transportation of *qi* and *xue* from nutrition and water and actuating them to the other *Zang* organs and contains *xue* within the meridians. It governs the limbs and controls deliberation. The lung actuates the pectoral *qi*. It governs the skin and hair and emotionally controls grief. The kidney is responsible for the containment of *shi*, which guides conception, development, birth and growth, as well as the production of marrow. Last, the liver ensures that *qi* can flow and be stored and maintains the tendons [8].

The primary function of the six *fu* organs is to transmit and digest nutrients without storing them and to excrete waste. The stomach first digests and extracts nutritional *qi*. The small intestine further purifies the partially digested nutrition from the stomach from a turbid to clear substance. It then transports this substance throughout the body while expelling the turbid substance. The large intestine receives waste from the small intestine, absorbs any remaining good fluids, and then turns the remaining waste into feces. The urinary bladder also receives turbid fluid from the small intestine, which stores and eliminates urine. The gallbladder transforms any of the liver's remaining *qi* into bile. The coelomic cavity (the *sanjiao*) holds the organs in place [8].

The *Zang-fu* organs follow the *Wu Xing* cycle, corresponding to the five elements and having "generating" and "restraining" interactions (Fig. 8.3) [8]. This corresponds to the notion that change in the universe occurs in a cyclical pattern of five stages. This cycle can relate to each element in different ways. The three major *yin-yang* systems (the five fundamental substances, *Zang-fu,* and meridians) are collectively known as the functional entities. These functional entities are responsible for the five cardinal functions: actuation, warming, defense, containment and transformation. The environmental factors of wind, damp, hot and cold can affect this process.

I will reiterate that this is just the barest of outlines of the basis of traditional Chinese medicine. A competent understanding would require years of study and instruction. Nevertheless, it is easy to see that there is a theory structure here that meets the criteria for biomedical theories, especially the interlevel, interfield theory of Schaffner [9], although what constitutes the "levels" and "fields" is different than what Schaffner used as examples. Nevertheless, there is a conceptual framework in place that provides a way to understand causal attribution (as defined in Chap. 5), a method of predictability, and a way to identify therapeutic targets.

8.2.3 Concept of "Disease"

I previously defined a disease as "an abnormal deviation of the homeostatically operational structure and function of a specific human body or mind, such that the individual will perceive adverse well-being or will have shortened survival, with or

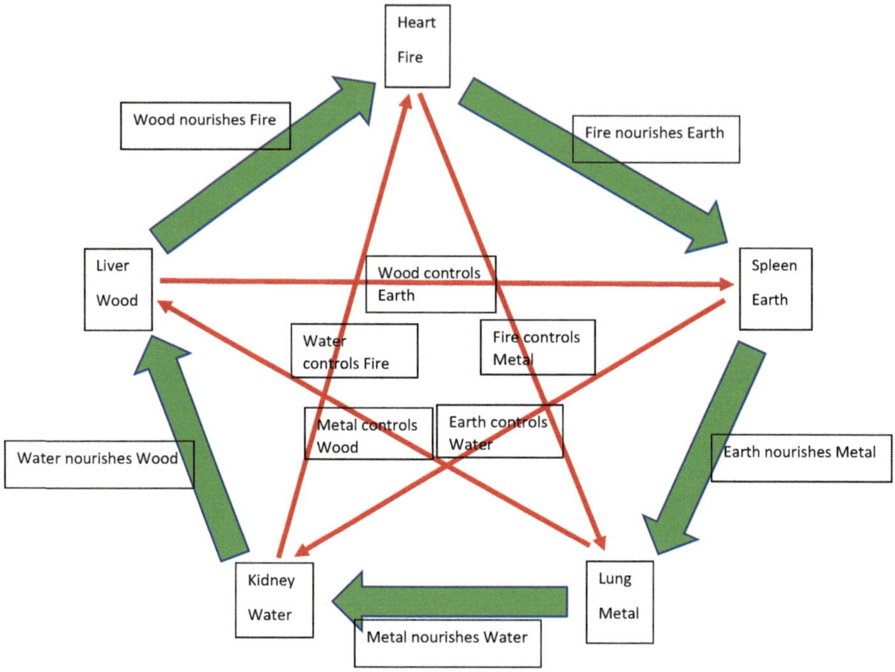

Fig. 8.3 A stylized representation of the *Wu Xing* cycle of the *Zhang-fu* organs

without intervention." This leads to a specific approach in the identification of disease manifestations and causes, with the goal of identifying therapeutic targets within Western allopathic medicine. Because of its theoretical foundations, the traditional Chinese concept of disease is somewhat different.

What Is a "Disease" in Traditional Chinese Medicine?

The traditional Chinese concept of health is that all of the *yin-yang* factors described above must remain in balance. When there is an imbalance or disturbance in these self-controlled systems, a "disease" occurs [4, 8]. However, rather than conceptualize a disease as specific disturbances in *qi* or *yin-yang* in a way that would identify a pathogen or pathogenesis, when a person is ill, they manifest different symptoms, and since everything has a *Wu Xing* (i.e., normal cycle), a pattern of disharmony can be identified. Rather than having a "disease" defined by anatomic pathology or pathophysiology, in traditional Chinese medicine, there is a unique imbalance of *qi* and *yin-yang* that is unique to that patient's functional entities related to *Wu Xing* and their constitution [3, 8]. This will produce a symptom pattern, a *zheng*, which is a result of the disharmony of the functional entities. *Bing* can be considered a "disease category" or "diagnosis" but is not independent of *zheng*. People may have the same *bing* but different *zheng,* so this will lead to different treatments.

Causal Attribution of Diseases

In traditional Chinese medicine, illness can be identified as to how the functional entities are imbalanced as measured by excesses or deficiencies, although traditional Chinese medicine does not strongly differentiate between causes and effects of disease [8]. The three major categories (*bing*) of disease are as follows:

1. External—disease caused by one of the six "excesses" (wind, cold, dampness, dryness, heat/fire, and summer heat) and "bad *qi*."
2. Internal—disease caused by the seven emotions or affects (anger, fear, anxiety, fright, grief, pensiveness, and joy, which affect the *Zhang-fu* organs).
3. Other irregularities—disease caused by something that is neither external nor internal, such as having an imbalance in the diet [8].

Theoretical Foundation of Diagnosis and Diagnostics

It is the traditional Chinese practitioner's task to thoroughly account for a patient's *zheng* to explain all of the patient's symptoms. The method for identifying the patterns of imbalance is a complex process of eight principles known as the *bian zheng* [8]:

1. *Yin*. Yin, with yang, is the most general classification for pattern diagnosis and describes the relationship between three pairs of principles. Generally, yin means cold.
2. *Yang*. This describes the relationship between the other three pairs of the principles. Yang, in general, means heat.
3. *Interior*. This describes diseases that manifest themselves in the *Zhang-fu* organs or deep inside the body, such as in *qi*, blood or bone marrow. More broadly, it is used to describe disease *not* classified as exterior.
4. *Exterior*. This describes diseases that manifest themselves on the surface of the body, such as hair, nails, and meridians. Its clinical features include body chills, fever, aversion to cold temperatures and winds, a weak pulse and headaches.
5. *Heat*. Heat describes an absence of an aversion to cold. If paired with an exterior pattern, its symptoms can include a rapid pulse, fever, body chills, dehydration and sore throat. If paired with an interior pattern, symptoms are a preference for cold drinks, clear urine and a slow pulse.
6. *Cold*. Cold describes an aversion to cold. If paired with an exterior pattern, symptoms are body aches, a tense pulse, body chills, and headaches. If paired with an interior pattern, symptoms include nausea, stomach pain, vomiting, and diarrhea.

7. *Deficiency*. This is a vacuity in *qi*, blood (*xue*) or body fluids (*jingye*). Depending on how it is related to interior/exterior and cold/heat, symptoms can include constipation, anorexia, dizziness and slow pulse.
8. *Excess*. Any disease that cannot be identified as a deficiency pattern is considered an excess pattern. One the six excesses can be present. Depending on how it is related to interior/exterior and cold/heat patterns, symptoms can include a quick pulse, sweaty palms and sharp stomach pains [8].

Having established the basic patterns of imbalances, the traditional Chinese medicine practitioner will use this knowledge in conjunction with the "four pillars of diagnosis" [8]:

1. Inspection—a visual analysis of the face, skin and tongue. The inspection of the tongue is especially important in traditional Chinese medicine as its surface is linked to the *Zhang-fu* organs and, therefore, is the cornerstone of the diagnostic process.
2. Auscultation—an analysis of particular sounds, such as shouting, laughing, singing, weeping, and groaning. Auscultation also extends to olfaction, that is, the smell of body order, even though this is not a sound.
3. Palpation—an analysis by feeling, particularly the wrist pulse but also the abdomen and the meridian points.
4. Inquiry—asking the patient questions about their past health and habits. There are traditionally ten questions that the practitioner must ask ranging from diet to sleep.

Tongue and pulse examinations are considered especially important in traditional Chinese medicine diagnosis [1, 4, 8] because of the integral connection, through the meridians, of the interior and exterior [4].

Once the practitioner finishes the examination, they determine the syndrome that is causing the patient's illness. This syndrome is referred to as the *zheng* and is the basic unit and key term in traditional Chinese medical theory [4]. This will determine the treatment for the patient.

Theoretical Foundation of Treatments

The traditional Chinese practitioner treats the pattern/syndrome, the *zheng*, not the symptoms. There is a Chinese proverb of "different diseases, same treatment; same disease, different treatments." This is an important part of traditional Chinese medicine [10]. The traditional Chinese practitioner has several treatment modalities in their armamentarium [8]:

1. Acupuncture, which is the insertion of small needles at the meridians to restore the flow of *qi* from the body's *Zhang-fu* organs to the body's framework on the presumption that the illness is from an imbalance of *qi* due to blocked meridians.
2. *Tui na*, which is a type of message therapy to restore balance to *yin* and *yang*.

3. Herbal and other naturally sourced therapies. As previously mentioned, there is a large pharmacopoeia of herbal, mineral, and animal/insect, fungi products and supplements from which practitioners can choose. These can be classified by their four "natures" and five "flavors." The four natures include hot, warm, cool and cold, with the hot and warm natures used to treat *yin* or cold conditions and the cool or cold natures used to treat *yang* or hot conditions.

   The five flavors are as follows: (a) Acrid (aids lungs and stimulates moisture production); (b) Sweet (aids the spleen, particularly digestion, and is associated with calming properties and producing fluids); (c) Sour (aids the liver's functions and has moistening and softening effects, particularly in regard to tendons and ligaments. It also helps reabsorb fluids that have left the body); (d) Bitter (aids the heart and has heat removing properties, such as drying): and (e) Salty (aids the kidneys and has properties of dryness, which can help in removing moisture and softening hardness).
4. Nutritional therapy. Traditional Chinese medicine classifies food according to its effects on *yin* and *yang*. *Yang* energy and support warming, including activating bodily functions. *Yang* deficiency can include cold hands and lower back pain. *Yin* energy is responsible for cooling and moistening. *Yin* deficiency includes night sweats and hot flashes. Good nutrition is a balance of *yin-yang* through the five flavors, and the right diet will vary from person to person and season to season, since weather can affect *yin-yang* balance.
5. Moxibustion. This is a form of heat therapy where a bundle of dry herbs (moxa) is burned near the surface of the skin to stimulate the flow of *qi* in the body.
6. Cupping. This is another form of heat therapy where heated cups are applied to the skin at meridian points to stimulate *qi*.
7. *Qigong*. This is a form of exercise therapy that combines mediative, static, and dynamic body movements to balance the flow of *qi*.

8.2.4 Traditional Chinese Medicine, the Illative Core of Argumentation and Persuasion

Admittedly, this is a very brief overview of the vast subject of traditional Chinese medicine, which has a history spanning thousands of years. However, I believe that it still establishes that traditional Chinese medicine has a theoretical foundation and that its practices are based on this foundation. It determines a causal sequence that is used for therapeutic targeting. Moreover, practitioners of traditional Chinese medicine during their diagnostic process create an argument pertaining to a diagnosis, which places the patient in a diagnostic category for which the practitioner will match a treatment that is appropriate for patients in that category. The actual process is similar to what was presented in Chap. 7; it is just that the theoretical framework and premises used are from different sources.

The traditional Chinese practitioner follows a similar, but not exactly the same, clinical flow as presented in Fig. 1.1. Specifically, the diagnosis is based on the patient's symptoms and signs, with no objective testing done. However, the practitioner's cognition and metacognitions are the same as those in Fig. 1.1, just specific to how knowledge is obtained and determined to be true enough for application based on the theoretical foundation of traditional Chinese medicine passed down through a specific educational process. Although research into traditional Chinese medicine continues (for example, there is the *Journal of Traditional Chinese Medicine* that publishes research presenting new knowledge of traditional Chinese medicine) and such new knowledge will need to be assessed by practitioners using the analysis put forth in Chap. 6, much of the canon for traditional Chinese medicine has been in place for centuries and is taught as accepted knowledge. This forms the parts of the meta-cognition of Fig. 1.1.

With traditional Chinese medicine steeped in classical Chinese philosophy for thousands of years, it is certainly part of the cultural and social umwelt of the Chinese people. Given the intense focus of traditional Chinese practitioners on the patient with questions and careful "hands-on" examination (it appears that traditional Chinese practitioners use little, if any, mechanical, optical or other technological aids in their examinations), the patient *is* the center of the practitioner's attention, not the patient's data. One study showed that traditional Chinese practitioners spent approximately 9 min longer with their patients compared to Western allopathic practitioners, with a high degree of patient satisfaction [11]. Through this process, one can see how a reservoir of trust is filled between the practitioner and patient. Therefore, the opportunity for manifest rationality and persuasion is embedded in the practice.

Because of the nature of the traditional Chinese practitioner's interaction with the patient and their determination of the patient's syndrome (*zheng*), the development and application of practical wisdom is an essential feature.

The diagnosis and treatment recommendations are presented to the patient. Certainly, how much exchange there is between the patient and traditional Chinese practitioner may vary. There may be mutually assumed cultural knowledge that does not have to be made explicit, a version of an Aristotlean enthymeme. Nevertheless, the patient probably persuaded in a manner similar to what was presented in Fig. 4.2.

8.3 Defining Traditional Indigenous Medicine

The next sections will present examples of traditional indigenous medical practices. It is worth providing this definition from the World Health Organization [12]: Indigenous health systems are

> the sum total of the knowledge, skills, and practices based on the theories, beliefs, and experiences indigenous to different cultures, whether explicable or not, used in the mainte-

nance of health as well as in the prevention, diagnosis, improvement or treatment of physical and mental illness.

Quite frankly, if one takes the words "indigenous to different" out and replaces them with "of Western," the very same definition can be used for Western allopathic medicine. This is my point, medicine, no matter what form, exists within a culture and society. Medical theory conforms to the predominant "theory of reality" of that culture or society. The practices of medicine will attempt to alleviate affliction based on the perceived causal sequence attribution, and criteria for success will be dictated by the values of that culture or society. For example, in Western medicine, the predominant criterion for success is eliminating the causal agent or pathology of the disease; no attempt (or, perhaps, no great attempt) is made whatsoever in emotionally, spiritually, or psychologically reintegrating the patient back into their community, culture or society. We will find in the next sections that the focus of indigenous healers is exactly what Western allopathic physicians do not do.

8.4 Traditional North American Indigenous Medicine

This section will discuss the most basic tenets of the medical theory and practices of the North American indigenous peoples. The first caveat is that there are over 700 different tribes of indigenous peoples in North America and each have their own particular concepts and practices [13], so to make any claim that what follows is an exact representation of all of these customs and practices is foolish to say the least. Therefore, I will discuss these people's concepts in only the broadest terms. As with the last section, I claim no expertise on this subject, which is immense. There is no doubt that I will have glossed over much nuance and many important elements. I will apologize for this now. It is also important to acknowledge that much of these indigenous people's way of life was disrupted and suppressed by Europeans and their progeny, as both American and Canadian settlers and governments expanded into these indigenous people's ancestral lands.[1] Nevertheless, traditional medicine is an important part of the lives and health of indigenous people [14]. I do think that this example of human universals and a theoretical foundation of a non-Western medical tradition that illustrates trust and persuasion.

Of course, a complete and thorough account of native North American cultures would require several volumes and would probably still not do the subject justice, but there are certain concepts that are common that will help inform the below account of traditional North American indigenous medical practices. The first is that much of the knowledge of indigenous culture, tradition and practices comes from an oral tradition. There is no single book or books that have codified any particular laws that all tribes follow [15]. Moreover, native beliefs are not intrinsically linked

[1] An excellent book on this subject is William Brandon's *The Rise and Fall of North American Indians: From Prehistory to Geronimo.*

to politics or economics [15]. North American indigenous beliefs do not separate the spiritual world from the "real" world of daily experience. These worlds are viewed as the same thing, in that every supposed division between the spiritual and real worlds is permeable and people can easily access everything spiritual [15]. There is a general sense of the connectedness of all things, living and inanimate, and, in particular, of a person and other members of their tribe or community [15]. In this sense, a North American indigenous person is "one with nature," and spirituality is integrated into everyday life [15]. These, albeit very general, beliefs are the theoretical structure on which North American indigenous medical practices are secured.

8.4.1 Traditional Indigenous Medicine within Nature

A common feature in the belief system of indigenous North American people is spirituality [16–20]. A general belief among North American indigenous peoples is that there is a universal spiritual force, which has many different names depending on the community, with a "life force" or spirit that is within all things [21]. Therefore, all objects have a spirit that should be respected [21, 22]. Moreover, spirituality is an integral component in indigenous traditional medical practices.

Traditional North American indigenous medicine is recognized by governmental authorities both in the United States [23] and Canada [14] as a whole medical system that encompasses a range of holistic treatments used by indigenous healers for a multitude of active and chronic conditions, as well as general well-being. Although there are differences among the various peoples and tribes, they generally share a health belief that health promotion has a biopsycho-sociospiritual basis, although it may not be described in that manner [13, 19].

It is inappropriate to assume that there is a "pan-indigenous" way of understanding traditional indigenous medical practices among all of the different North American indigenous peoples [18]. Additionally, knowledge of traditional healing practices or medicinal substances was, and still is, passed on through a strong oral tradition that involves ceremonial practices. Therefore, academic scholarship may not reflect the actual medical knowledge within a specific indigenous community [18]. For example, healers follow the Red Path (described below) as healing practices and ceremonies taught to them by wise and experienced mentors [24]. Therefore, another caveat to this section is that the level of published scholarship is not reflective of the actual depth of knowledge by traditional healers.

Wellness and Disease

Wellness from an indigenous North American perspective considers the communal context for individuals as well as seeking out a balance of mental, spiritual, and physical aspects of living [25]. While the Western medical view typically equates healing with "curing," from an indigenous perspective, healing is more akin to "recovering one's wholeness" [13] or reestablishing harmony with nature [26, 27]. Traditional North American indigenous healers see a person as a whole being with body, mind and spirit that is connected to other people, families, communities, the Earth and the Universe [18]. Disease may be the result of disharmony with nature, offending natural forces, violation of taboos, or chance actions or circumstances that disturb wellness and cause illness [21].

Types of Indigenous Medical Practice

Traditional medical healing is intended to bring the being of the patient into "harmony" with their natural environment [28]. North American indigenous healers include the "nonmaterial" in their healing processes [29]. This healing approach places value on recovering a focus on quality of life through an intentional, compassionate, and relationship-oriented approach, enhancing the types of "energies" that exist in relationships between people, their spiritual connections, and their connections with the Earth [17]. Many traditional healers say that most of the healing is done by the patient and that every person has a responsibility for their proper behavior and health. Although one must be careful of ascribing too much uniformity in North American indigenous medical concepts [18], many tribes subscribe to the "pan-Indian" outlook, which include the practices of pow-wow, music, smudging, storytelling, sweat lodge, tobacco/pipe and other ceremonies and use of herbs [16, 17], to bring healing energies into the healing space and focus the efforts of the healers [16].

Ceremony

Ceremony is an essential part of traditional North American indigenous healing. This is related to the belief that physical and spiritual health are intimately connected and that the body and spirit must heal together [16]. Ceremonies promote wellness by reflecting native conceptions of the Spirit, the Creator, and the Universe. Ceremonial practices for healing include sweat lodge ceremonies, traditional tobacco ceremonies, birth and birthplace ceremonies, puberty ceremonies, relatives' deaths, or trauma [16]. Ceremonial practices are intended to lead to spiritual transformation and an improvement in the patient's medical illness [30]. Although these ceremonies can be held anywhere, they are often held in special structures and are only conducted by traditional healers and spiritual facilitators because of their sacred nature [16].

The Red Path (Road)

The Red Road describes a path to wholeness and harmony with nature. This results in a feeling of belonging, a sense of mastery, respect for independence, and promotion of generosity and unselfishness [31].

Pow-Wow

A pow-wow is a social and sacred coming together of North American indigenous peoples [17].

Drum and Drumming

The drum holds a special and/or sacred significance because it is round, representing the entire world, and the beat represents the heartbeat of the world [17].

Smudging

Smudging is a purification with smoke of burning sage, cedar or sweetgrass over individuals, including healers and those seeking healing. Cedar and sage dispel negative energies, and sweetgrass attracts positive energy, both of which promote the healing process [17].

The Sweat Lodge

The *Inipi* ceremony or sweat lodge is a means of purification leading to emotional and spiritual well-being [17]. The sweat lodge ceremony honors transformation and healing [32], improving spiritual and emotional well-being.

Herbal Medications

The beneficial effects of herbal medicine are not only in their pharmacological effects but also in the spiritual connection healer has with the plants. Healers will address the plant's spirit and engage with it [33]. Synthetic pharmaceuticals are not the equivalent, as healers do not have such a spiritual connection with them. Healers view herbs, however, as just one means to bring back balance for an individual with respect to emotional, intellectual, and spiritual dimensions, as well as a physical dimension [34].

The Medicine Wheel

The Medicine Wheel or Sacred Hoop is an object or structure used for health and healing. It is a circle that can take many forms and can be constructed with a variety of materials or places on land, which embodies the four directions (north, south, east and west), Father Sky, Mother Earth, and Spirit Tree [16]. Because it can take on specific details depending on the people and tribes, the depiction in Fig. 8.4 shows its barest form of four colors. The wheel can also be depicted with the quadrant designated north at the top. Some wheels also have a center circle depicting central cultural concepts of the particular peoples. The movement of the medicine wheel as well as typical North American traditional ceremonies is clockwise to align with the forces of nature [16]. The directions are represented by different

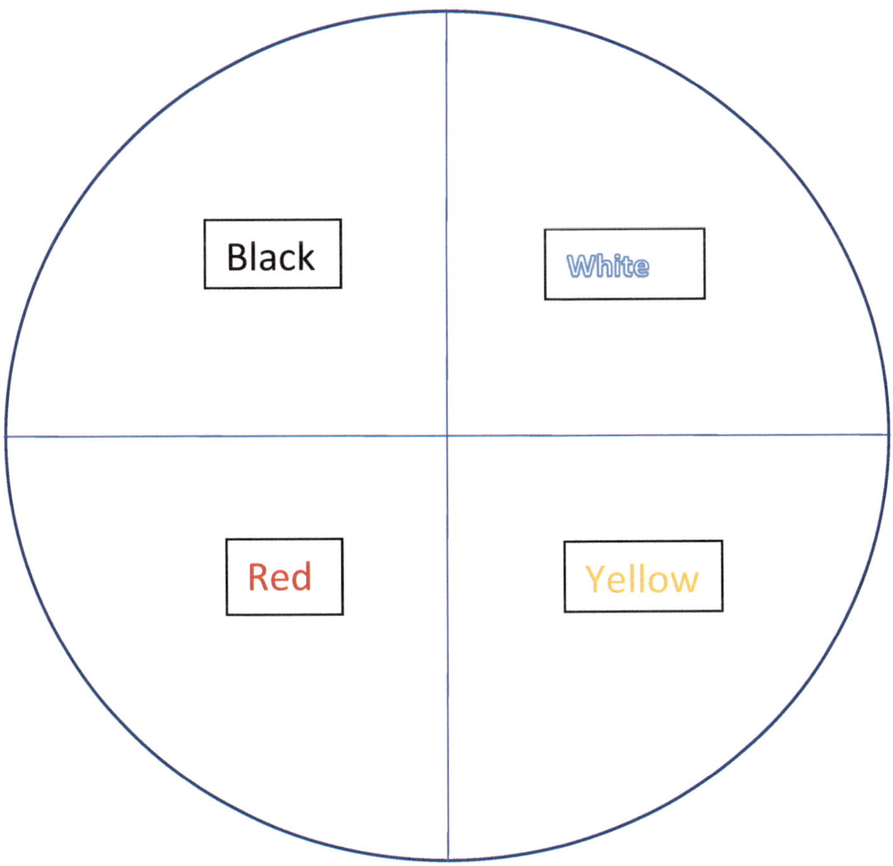

Fig. 8.4 A stylized representation of the North American indigenous people's medicine wheel. There are many variations of this wheel among the many tribes in North America. Some include a center circle as well. The quadrants (as well as the center circle) can represent directions, animals, seasons, stages of life, elements of nature, and ceremonial plants, among other concepts

colors that can represent the cardinal directions of the compass, the human races, stages of life (birth, youth, adult/elder, death), seasons of the year (spring, summer, fall, winter), aspects of life (spiritual, emotional, intellectual, physical), elements (fire or sun, air, water, earth), animals (eagle, bear, wolf, buffalo, and many others), and ceremonial plants (tobacco, sweetgrass, sage, cedar) [16].

8.4.2 Traditional North American Indigenous Medicine, the Illative Core of Argumentation and Persuasion

The underlying theoretical foundation of much of traditional North American indigenous medicine is the concept that everything in the universe has a spirit and that all spirits connect everything in the universe. Illness is a result of disharmony, and wellness is one's spirit being in harmony with their people and environment. These then become the premises for how traditional North American healers create the illative core of their arguments for determining the cause of the illness and what the appropriate treatment is. There is a causal sequence that leads to disharmony, which provides a therapeutic target for treatment.

I had previously discussed in Chap. 4 the importance of trust in accepting an argument as being persuasive. Traditional North American indigenous medicine practices reflect a deep understanding of their culture's human universals as elucidated by Brown [35], especially storytelling and music. In this setting of the indigenous community, the traditional healer, due to their education through the oral passing down of knowledge and through public ceremonies, has a position of trust. This trust is the basis of persuasion in this tradition, although this may not be explicitly expressed.

It appears that many of these practices, especially public ceremonies, enhance group cohesion. In Chap. 3, I asserted that the human brain and mind evolved to have a strong affinity to their group as a "default" setting. It is not surprising, therefore, that many afflictions are viewed, perhaps not overtly, as illnesses of an individual losing connection to the group.

Because of the nature of the traditional North American indigenous practitioner's interaction not only with the patient but also with their community, the practical wisdom of the practitioner is essential. The categories that the traditional North American indigenous practitioner places a patient are based not on pathologic changes in homeostasis but on the disharmony of the patient with their natural and social environment.

These practices are consistent with the physician's cognition and metacognition (Fig. 1.1). The traditional healer assesses the patient in the manner described in the "flow of the clinical encounter" in Fig. 1.1. As no objective testing is part of their theory of medicine, only their observations and interactions are used for a diagnosis. Once the cause is determined, then this places the patient in a diagnostic category for which there will be the most appropriate treatment. Traditional healers do have corresponding meta-cognitions with a theoretical framework, with evidence for their theory that is acceptable to them, and a way to appraise the evidence for their theory that is valid for them. They are able to achieve causal attribution, which is then used to target a therapeutic intervention.

This is communicated in some way to the patient, their family and, perhaps, the community. This becomes the basis for persuasion; whether there is an exchange between the patient and the traditional healer in the form of manifest rationality is probably variable among the many traditions of practice. However, in the Aristotlean sense of enthymemes, because of the deep level of common cultural knowledge, a type of argument still occurs but may not be as overt as in Western allopathic medicine (Fig. 4.2).

8.5 Traditional African Medicine

Africa is a vast continent of 54 countries, over 1.4 billion people, and hundreds, if not thousands, of ethnic groups and tribes. Therefore, claiming that there is a single, traditional African medical heritage is *prima facie* wrong. However, there are some commonalities among these peoples. To understand traditional African medicine, one needs to have some concept of traditional African culture.

Importance of Spirituality in African Culture Again, this is an immense topic, and it would be impossible to even give the briefest of outlines. Nevertheless, to understand the theoretical foundations of traditional African medicine, understanding the centrality of spirituality in African culture is essential. Professor Jacob Olupora of the Harvard Divinity School and a native of Nigeria provides a nice overview in an interview in the *Harvard Gazette* [36], from which the following is paraphrased. Indigenous African religions are by nature plural, varied and usually informed by one's ethnic identity and where one's family came from in Africa. Because all knowledge was passed down through an oral tradition, there are no permanent codified rules or tenets. This makes spirituality somewhat flexible, changing with the needs of the people.[2] Nevertheless, a basic idea in African spirituality is simply that spiritual beliefs and practices touch on and inform every facet of human life; therefore, African religious beliefs cannot be separated from everyday life or mundane activities. African spirituality is holistic (and I interpret this in the sense that it encompasses the entire universe) and informs everything in traditional African society, including politics, art, marriage, health, diet, dress, economics, and death.

Specifically, in regard to health and illness, sickness in the indigenous African worldview is not only an imbalance of the body (to use my term, dysfunctional

[2] Professor Olupora further goes on the say that approximately 40% of present-day Africans are either Christian or Muslim but still retain some of their regions' and cultures' traditional beliefs.

homeostasis of the corporal body) but also an imbalance in one's social life, which can be limited to a breakdown in one's kinship and family relations or even to one's relationship with one's ancestors. The role of ancestors in African cosmology is significant and ever-present. Ancestors are believed to occupy a higher level of existence than living humans. These deceased progenitors are believed to still play a role in the lives of their descendants. These ancestors can offer advice and bestow good fortune but can also make demands, and if not met, misfortune can befall the one who ignores such demands. The role of deceased ancestors in spirit form will be shown to be an important part of the theoretical structure of traditional African medicine.

8.5.1 African Culture and African Medicine

As stated above, there is no single doctrine of traditional African medicine, so the account given in this section will be necessarily incomplete. However, what I hope to show with the examples I have gathered is that overall traditional African medicine is consistent with the basic themes of this book. Namely, medical practices have a rationale that is based on specific social and cultural norms, which are derived from human universal traits [35] as developed in those cultures. Within these practices, diagnoses and treatments are based on developing an argument with an illative core stemming from an underlying theory of how the universe affects the human condition. Patients will be persuaded to accept a treatment as long as they can come to some form of manifest rationality with their caregiver based on their social and cultural umwelt. Moreover, the practitioners themselves will have a professional umwelt in how they approach their professional practice.

As with the indigenous peoples of North America, we must acknowledge that the peoples of Africa were subjected to colonial rule by European powers for centuries.[3] To say that this had and still has wide-ranging effects on Africans would be trite comment to say the least. From the standpoint of this book, the misunderstanding and dismissal of traditional African medicine was one of its egregious effects, leading to the suppression, and in some jurisdictions, the outright outlawing, of many of the traditional medical practices in various parts of Africa [37]. Given that much of the knowledge of medicine in Africa was preserved and passed down through an oral tradition, thus lacking written documentation [37], there may be aspects of these practices that are lost. In addition, Okpako [38] feels that this oral transmission of traditional African medical knowledge has hindered the development of a coherent theory of this medical corpus of knowledge. The information that is used

[3] There are numerous books and articles on this subject that will give the reader a good understanding of European colonialism and its lingering effects on Africa. One such book is *The Palgrave Handbook of African Colonial and Postcolonial History* edited by Martin S. Shanguhyia and Toyin Falola.

in this section is what is known and documented now, so I will emphasize the caveat that this information may be incomplete.

As with African spirituality, or perhaps more correctly, as a result, traditional African medicine is a holistic health care system, where healers provide services based on culture, religious background, knowledge, attitudes and beliefs that are prevalent in their community [37]. In other words, what is acceptable medical theory and practice is a result of the accepted corpus of knowledge of the society. Although African traditional health systems vary across the continent, there are many commonalities among them. One such commonality is that the theory goes beyond "naturalistic" conceptualizations (i.e., not solely viewing disease in only its physical pathological or pathophysiological sense) to explain disease but also encompassing individuals' social, physical, religious and spiritual environment [39]. Because spirituality pervades all aspects of African life, spiritual and religious elements are interlinked and involve metaphysical forces and the group's ancestors [40]. For example, the belief that ancestors play an important role in the traditional African medical theoryx of pathogenesis.

Theoretical Foundation of Traditional African Medicine

According to Okpako [38], traditional African medicine can be characterized by the following attributes: (1) belief in the supernatural as a cause of illness; (2) divination as a diagnostic procedure; and (3) ritualized use of plant- and animal-derived preparations in the treatment of illness. Others have also identified that in traditional African medicine, illness is considered a disorder that can have natural or supernatural causes [37, 41]. There appears to be an understanding that there are diseases that do not have supernatural causes and those that do. Nevertheless, this concept of supernatural causes of illness is relatively common throughout Africa [42, 43]. I interpret this concept of supernatural causes, such as ancestor anger, as an attempt at coming to a causal sequence of the pathogenesis of disease, as outlined in Chap. 5, just using a different theoretical framework.[4] Horton [44] asserts that this has rationality within the cultural context of the belief. That is, recalling my definition of rationality from Chap. 2, "a human mental framework that leads to the adoption of processes that result in well-founded beliefs and practices," in the context of the world viewpoint of someone who "sees" the actions of spiritual forces everywhere, such a belief is rational. These ideas have generally formed in small-scale societies [44], which was the majority of African tribes for millennia.

[4] I am not going to argue about whether this theoretical framework is "scientific" or not as that would be both disrespectful and unhelpful in the present discussion. However, I will say that much of what in the West is consider "scientific" smacks of the mystical with only a few "high priests" claiming understanding—for example, quantum entanglement, or what Einstein called "spooky action at a distance," is nearly incomprehensible to anyone but those with advanced education in physics.

Another view is that such beliefs use different words for the same concept. For example, Okapko [38] suggests that ancestor anger can be understood as a metaphorical reference for emotional stress of an individual or group, which may be related to hidden guilt. As should be noted, the ancestral spirits do not act at random but only afflict individuals who have offended them [38]. Alternatively, Okapko [38] suggests that the emotional stress endured by the individual can result in a deteriorated physical condition in the patient who eventually makes the individual susceptible to a disease. Because the disease can have either or both physical or spiritual (i.e., emotional stress) causes, it must be treated with physical and/or spiritual means. That is, a therapeutic target is identified in the sequence of causal attribution (see Chaps. 5 and 6). These means are based on culture, religious beliefs, accepted knowledge and community beliefs [37]. Because the determination of causal attribution can contain a spiritual component (something that Western allopathic medicine rarely, if ever, has), traditional African medicine answers not just the "what" of illness, but importantly, the "why has this happened to me?" [45]. That is, it provides causal clarity to the afflicted.

8.5.2 African Medical Practices

The use of traditional African medicine is widespread and is used even if patients have access to Western-trained allopaths [39]. This is because traditional African healers occupy a prominent position in their community [37]. The different African peoples, of course, have their own ancestral practices to heal using different methods [46]; therefore, there is variation from community to community. Nevertheless, the traditional healer is someone recognized by the community as competent to provide such care [47]. They utilize plant, animal and mineral substances based on the social, cultural and religious background of the community, incorporating the prevailing knowledge, attitudes and beliefs for the physical, mental and social well-being of the community [47]. Traditional African medical healers are able to provide culturally relevant care because their conceptualization of illness and well-being matches that of the communities they serve, which makes them respected members of their community [39].

Types of Traditional African Medical Practitioners

There seems to be some variability in the types of traditional African medical healers depending on the author. Chaitanya et al. [37] assert that there are three levels of specialization: divination, spiritualism, and herbalism. Practice concepts include herbal medication, surgery, bone setting, spinal manipulation, psychotherapy, hydrotherapy and occultism, among others [37]. Herbalism includes plants and other vegetable matter and animal and mineral substances [37]. Spiritualism includes prayers, invocations, incantations, divination, sacrifice, libation and exorcism consistent with the belief system of the community. Jolles and Jolles [48] identified two broad categories of practitioners in the Zulu community of South Africa: diviner-diagnostician (or diviner-medium) and healer/herbalist. On the other hand, in rural KwaZulu-Natal, South Africa, Zuma et al. [49] identified three types of practitioners: (1) diviners, (2) those who focus on traditional medical remedies (i.e., herbalists), and (3) faith healers. Moreover, the government of South Africa registers traditional healing practitioners, although many are not, as herbalists, diviners, traditional surgeons (who mainly do circumcisions), and traditional birth attendants [50].

Education and Training of Traditional African Medical Practitioners

The training of traditional African healers is generally an apprenticeship model, either through a mentor or a family member. They are called by their ancestors to become healers and/or go through an intensive process of learning [49]. In some communities, much of traditional medical knowledge is kept secret by practitioners as a "hidden treasure" to be passed down from father to his favorite or "most beloved" son [37]. In a study of 34 traditional healers from the Limpopo Province of South Africa, Semenya and Potgieter [51] interviewed 34 healers. Of these, 23 were male. These practitioners received their education in their region's traditional medical practices through mentoring from another healer, their parents or grandparents. For herbalists, the profession is open to anyone, although it does tend to run in families [47]. Herbalists in South Africa tend to be male and are selected and mentored by established herbalist practitioners [52]. Moreover, herbalists, as a whole, typically do not claim occult or supernatural powers [51]. On the other hand, no one can become a diviner by personal choice [53]; they are called by the ancestors to become so and, therefore, view themselves as servants to the ancestors [47].

Most traditional African healers practice across different categories. They also fill roles that are not specific to healing *per se*, such as custodians of traditional African religion and customs, educators about culture, counsellors, mediators and spiritual protectors, using similar, generic methods and practices to focus on the physical, spiritual, cultural, psychological, emotional and social elements of illness [49]. In this regard, it seems to me that they foster group cohesion within their communities.

8.5.3 Traditional African Medical Practices

The underlying theory of traditional African medicine is that disease can have either or both a physical and spiritual cause. Hence, the theoretical assumptions that traditional African medical practitioners make about the origin of an illness are consistent with their methods of treatment of the illness [38]. Because of the importance of spirituality in African cultures, these practices are not only directed at the ill person but are also ritualized in a way that appears to enhance group cohesion. I have previously asserted that the human mind evolved to favor group cohesion, and it seems to me that these practices also aim to restore the connection of the afflicted back into the group.

Herbalists and Herbal Remedies

Many illnesses do not require a spiritual explanation. These are treated with herbal medications. In most African communities, commonly known plant remedies are available to treat minor ailments, such as headaches, fever, aches and pains. There is no need for spiritual evocations with such ailments, as the cause appears clear [38]. When the illness is more serious, a traditional African medical practitioner is consulted.

Herbalists are expected to diagnose and prescribe medicines for everyday ailments and illnesses, prevent and alleviate misfortune or evil, provide protection against witchcraft, and bring prosperity and happiness to the individuals of the community [54]. Nearly 4000 medicinal plants have been documented in Africa [12]. Obviously, this will vary by region. In a study of community members in a rural Ethiopian town, community members identified 73 plants and were knowledgeable about recognition of the plants and their usage to treat common ailments, and they continued to use these plants. These community members were actually willing to share their knowledge with the researchers [55], which was somewhat unusual. Nevertheless, even with herbalists, these healers perform rituals subsequent to harvesting plants as a means of expressing gratitude toward the ancestors [51]. Because African medicinal plants tend to have few, if any, adverse events, plant use is then based on physical characteristics (e.g., aroma, texture, shape, taste, etc.) and rituals attending the preparation administration of plant compounds, such as incantation or song, are more important than its pharmacological constituents. Additionally, because they are safe, rules of dosing generally do not apply [38]. Poisonous plants, which are the source of many manufactured pharmaceuticals, are not used by African herbalists because of their potential ill effects [38]. Plant remedies appear to be used for their synergy with other rituals [38] that enhance belief in the efficacy of treatment, rather than pharmacological entities. Okapko [38] suggests that there may be a placebo effect, although some plants have immunomodulation and nutritional properties.

In Limpopo Province, the traditional healers surveyed claim to treat 52 different ailments, including chlamydial infections, diabetes mellitus, diarrhea, epilepsy, erectile dysfunction, eye infections, gonorrhea, HIV/AIDS, hypertension, malaria, menstrual disorders, mental illness and tuberculosis. These are also commonly treated by healers in other communities and cultures [51]. In other words, when an effective herbal treatment exists for a relatively common illness, it is used as the primary treatment.

Unlike day-to-day herbal remedies, appeals to supernatural causes occur in more serious circumstances or in circumstances where the cause is unknown. Spiritualism includes such things as (1) spiritual protection because an unknown illness may be due to an attack by evil spirits. The spiritual healer prescribes talismans, charms, amulets, body marks and/or a spiritual bath to drive away evil spirits [56]; (2) sacrifices that are made at the request of the spirits, gods, or ancestors of the afflicted; (3) spiritual cleansing, i.e., a spiritual bath; exorcism, which is done to expel demons or evil spirits from the ill person and is only performed by the traditional leader or priest of the community; and (4) libation, which is the offering of some specific type of liquid at the request of the spirits or ancestors.

Traditional African practitioners who are the intermediaries between the spiritual and physical world are diviners. In divination, the diviner contacts the spiritual world for guidance to heal [57]. This is generally used for ailments that are not clearly understood and, therefore, are considered spiritual [37]. Diviners are considered experts at applying diagnostic criteria for such sicknesses [58] and determining the cause of the ailment in terms of the particular African belief system [53]. Diviners can identify the origin and reason for the sickness and then prescribe an appropriate plant- or animal-based treatment for the ailment using spiritual means [52]. In Zimbabwe and elsewhere, diviners communicate with spirits when in a state of "possession" and convey the demands of the ancestors and the reason for their dissatisfaction [59]. It is then required of the patient to fulfill their demands.

Divination is used by members of the community when the illness is not understood in obvious physical terms, when Western-type allopathic medicine has failed, or if supernatural causes are suspected. In a survey of traditional healers in Ghana, these healers were consulted for obstetric complications rather than routine pregnancy and delivery. They claimed expertise in those complications that were thought to be related to witchcraft and other culturally defined syndromes, and in areas that patients thought Western medical practitioners lacked expertise [60]. It requires following the ancestor's instructions and sacrifices to the spiritual world. It may include activities such as dream, nightmare and/or omen interpretations [37]. After communication with the spiritual world, treatment may include a secret recipe of herbal baths, herbal decorations, sacrifices, incantations, and wearing of herbal talismans [61, 62]. The healer, in general, will not reveal the recipes of their herbo-magical remedies to other people. Moreover, traditional healers rarely, if ever, refer a patient to a fellow traditional healer for additional treatment [51]. Determining the effectiveness of the treatment has more to do with the spiritual world rather than the patient. Most (67%) traditional healers in Limpopo Province determined efficacy by consulting with their ancestors (90%) [51].

In chronic illness with an unknown cause that does not respond to common treatments, ritual treatment of hidden guilt becomes the major therapeutic consideration [38]. Okapko [38] comes close to providing a non-supernatural explanation for the effectiveness of spiritual healing practices with the suggestion that such illnesses are derived from emotional stress over hidden guilt. Moreover, in serious, life-threatening illness, diffusion of emotional tension in the patient, family and community seems to be the primary goal [38]. Treatment of this emotional stress includes exposition of the reason for the guilt and offering propitiatory sacrifices to the offended spirits [38]. The importance of this in the cohesion of the community is obvious. Therefore, it is not surprising that traditional healers in the Limpopo region work in close proximity and in association with their community members to treat a variety of diseases and ailments [51]. In traditional African medicine, every procedure is elaborately ritualized to optimize the placebo contribution to healing. Both practitioners and patients believe in the rituals [38].

8.5.4 Traditional African Indigenous Medicine, the Illative Core of Argumentation and Persuasion

How does this fit with the physician's cognition and metacognition (Fig. 1.1)? Clearly, the traditional healer assesses the patient and determines whether the presentation is a physical illness or spiritual one. With diviners, they also employ the diagnostic tests of contacting ancestors from the spiritual world to determine a cause. In other words, traditional healers will gather premises to develop their arguments. Once the cause is determined, then this places the patient in a diagnostic category for which there will be the most appropriate treatment. Traditional healers do have corresponding meta-cognitions with a theoretical framework, evidence for their theory that is acceptable to them, and a way to appraise the evidence for their theory that is valid for them. They are able to achieve causal attribution, which is then used to target a therapeutic intervention.

Such a diagnosis is presented to the patient and perhaps their family and even the community. The patient, family members or community members must judge whether the premises used in the argument are true or true enough to make the argument presented valid (Fig. 4.2). The patient will then come to a mutual understanding, that is, a manifest rationality, and either will or will not be persuaded by the traditional healer. However, given the healer's prominence in the community and their understanding of its cultural beliefs, there will be a strong desire of the patient to maintain group cohesion by accepting the diagnosis and treatment.

8.6 American Faith Healing

I realize that I am not a member of either the North American or African indigenous communities, and, therefore, I may be prone to error on my analysis above. However, for readers who may believe that because these people did not have the luxury of a scientific tradition, such as the West, is the reason for their beliefs in the spiritual nature of some illnesses, I would like to point out the popularity of faith healing in America. I do not intend to provide an analysis of American faith healing, my purpose is to say that faith healing, and other forms of spiritual healing, is not simply a consequence of a lack of a culture of science.

In 2008, a survey of Americans reported that approximately one-third of respondents said they either experienced or witnessed divine healing of an illness or injury [63]. The only difference between these individuals and those of indigenous African and North American people may only be the proportion who believe so. In many Christan denominations, "speaking in tongues" as a way to communicate with divine spiritual beings is accepted as actual communication with these beings [64]. I am not sure how much this is different than what African traditional medicine diviners do. Last, it is common in many places of worship that prayers are offered for the recovery of ill members [65]. In my view, this is another form of creating group cohesion, similar to the public ceremonies of the indigenous peoples of North America and Africa.

To be clear, my point here is not to cast dispersions on the individuals who hold these beliefs, because if reviewed carefully, there is a rationale to them, but rather, merely to aver that such beliefs are more universal, most likely as a result of how our mind evolved and the need to maintain group cohesion (see Chaps. 3 and 4), in light of these individuals' social and cultural umwelt, than, perhaps, some "scientifically" minded professionals would like them to be.

8.7 Alternative/Complementary Medicine: Homeopathy

Unlike the previous three examples of traditional medicine from China, North America and Africa, which have deep roots spanning centuries within their cultures, the modern notion of "alternative" or "complementary" medicine is relatively new. Certainly, much traditional indigenous medicine has been incorporated into the alternative and complementary medicine rubric, but I view these traditional medical practices as organic developments within the cultures and societies of their people. On the other hand, modern ideas of alternative and complementary medicine have their origins in a general dissatisfaction of modern, Western allopathic medicine. Although I am sympathetic with this dissatisfaction (e.g., Western medicine's almost singular focus on anatomic or physiologic pathology and almost complete indifference to emotional or social well-being), I am not going to debate this point. My purpose here is to contend that the alternative medical paradigms will have an underlying theory and that practice will stem from that theory. Again, I will make the same caveat I made before—I am not a practitioner of this type of medicine, and I have limited space, so there will be no doubt omissions and loss of nuance. Moreover, I will make no judgments about the efficacy of this type of medicine, as that is not my purpose in presenting it. However, I do think that this account will support my thesis in this book.

One such alternative medical paradigm is that of homeopathy. Homeopathy was conceived and developed by the German physician Samuel Hahnemann (1755–1843) due to his disappointment with the prevailing medical practice at the time, which he felt relied on "heroic," but "harsh," treatments of bleeding, cupping, purging, blistering and large doses of substances, which caused significant adverse events and very little cure [66, 67]. This led Hahnemann to assess why the prevailing practice of medicine at the time, the late eighteenth century, was failing its patients. At approximately the same time (1798), Edward Jenner successfully produced immunity to smallpox with the use of a small amount of cowpox virus [68]. Therefore, the idea of achieving medical success with small doses had evidence in support of it. Hahnemann ultimately developed the theory of homeopathy in the 1790s and ultimately codified it tenets in his book *Organon of the Art of Healing* published in 1810, with subsequent editions retitled *Organon of Medicine.* These books formed the basis of the practice of homeopathy.

8.7.1 Theory of Homeopathy

In explaining homeopathic theory, Morrell [67] makes the distinction between "theory" and "method", with the method being more important than the theory. He asserts that the "primary goal of homeopathic philosophy is not theoretical, but pragmatic," that is, to guide good practice. I interpret this as what he means by "method" is clinical practice. This being said, there is a theory that underlies homeopathy.

Hahnemann's concept of illness is that "illness is the destruction of the life force," and a cure would be "to return the reduced life force to its original state of tuning" [69].

The principles of homeopathy (i.e., its theoretical basis) are as follows:

1. The *Principle of Similarity*, which apparently has its roots from ancient times [70]. This principle is a teleological-anthropocentric concept in which the external similarities of things occurring in nature are "sensuously" related to corresponding human categories. How it is used in homeopathy is that substances that trigger a disease or its symptoms can be used to treat the disease [70]. This principle of similars is the basis of homeopathy's name—from Greek, "homo" = similar, "pathy" = disease [66, 71].
2. The *Principle of Provings*, which is the testing substance on healthy people. Hahnemann developed the concept that to determine if a substance would trigger a disease or symptoms (i.e., would it fit into the principle of similarity), it would be tested on a healthy person [70]. In fact, Hahnemann devised and executed the first so-called "provings" by experimentally administering substances to healthy individuals and recording their reactions [66]. These provings formed the basis of the homeopathic pharmacopoeia, *Materia Medica Pura*, first published by Hahnemann in 1821 [71].
3. The *Law of Infinitesimals* states that because larger doses could aggravate symptoms (i.e., produce a disease), diminishing the size of the dose could alleviate the aggravation of the symptoms and yet still provide the curative effect. This is intended to bring an "out-of-tune" spiritual life force back into a "normal state" by causing an "artificial disease" [70]. Typically, the dose would be diluted by

"centesimals" (i.e., 1 part to 100) until the 30th centesimal was reached, although the dilution could be much more [66].

The notion of reducing the concentration of a toxic substance was first proposed by Paracelsus in the sixteenth century,[5] although Hahnemann asserted that his concept was different than that of Paracelsus [67].

When a substance is diluted, it is shaken vigorously, a process known as "succussion," which leads to the "potentiation" of the medical potency of the liquid. The preparation that is then prescribed is called a "similimum." Paradoxically by common sense, in homeopathic theory, the more dilute the medication is, the more potent its effects [71]. Because of the very dilute nature of these treatments, theoretical concepts were created to explain this potentiation phenomenon. One concept was that "water retains a 'memory' or 'enduring imprint' of the original substance through the series of dilutions and succussions" [68]. Drofenik [69] listed a number of other proposals, including quantum mechanical entanglement, quartz crystals and the structural concept of glass, electromagnetic activities, biological signaling, nonlinear dynamics of complex systems, biopsychosocial models, thermodynamic models, and his own "thermodynamic principle of chemical equilibrium" after Le Chatelier's chemical equilibrium principle.

4. The *Theory of Miasms* (from the Greek *mianein* = to polute), in which Hahneman averred the "miasm" as a residual of disease that leads to a chronic condition, was put forth in his book *Chronic Diseases* published in 1828 [71, 72]. The three miasms are (1) syphilis, which are called veneral chronic diseases, (2) sycosis, which are the "fig wart" diseases, and (3) psora, which are the chronic diseases related to eruption of itching [72].
5. *Hering's*[6] *Laws*. Constatine Hering further developed additional ideas to further refine homeopathic disease theory. These include the following: (1) the body seeks to externalize disease, noting that symptoms will surface as part of the curative process; (2) a person's symptoms will appear and disappear in reverse order of their appearance upon the body; and (3) the body heals from the top to bottom and from more vital to less vital organs [73].

These principles are the basis of the homeopathic treatment convention of the use of a single drug in very small doses based on the law of similarity.

Montegomery [74] provides an interesting analysis of the rationale concerning alternative and complementary medicine in general and homeopathy in particular.

---

[5] Paracelsus was a Swiss physician who lived from 1493 to 1541. He was involved in several aspects of the "medical revolution" of the Renaissance. He is considered the father of toxicology and made the important contribution of relating dose to effect, especially toxic effects—"Only the dose makes the poison" (See Borzelleca JF. Paracelsus: Herald of modern toxicology. Toxicol Sci 2000;53:2–4.) This concept of dilution to lessen the toxic effects is similar to those of Hahnemann—and some say, therefore, this was not an original idea of Hahnemann's.

[6] Constantine Hering was a German physician who eventually moved to the United States and is generally considered the founder of homeopathy in America. Interestingly, he became involved in homeopathy to debunk it but, instead, became an adherent.

These medical paradigms have a foundation that each individual is their own "archetype." Allopathic medicine views variability among humans as variability of a specific human archetypal form, while homeopathy views each human as ontologically distinct, with just a diversity of these distinct types; that is, each human is their own archetype [74]. Therefore, the lack of consistency among treatments is present only if one views it from the standpoint of a particular disease within a patient but is completely consistent if one views it from the standpoint of a particular patient with a disease.

8.7.2 *Practice of Homeopathy*

Types of Physicians and Training

Homeopathic medical professionals come from the ranks of physicians (medical, osteopathic, naturopathic and chiropractic), dentists, veterinarians, nurse practitioners, physician assistants, pharmacologists, and pharmacists with additional training in homeopathy from various educators [71, 75, 76]. Although having licensure for one's respective profession is mandatory for membership in the American Institute for Homeopathy [71], it is certainly not required for practice [75]. In addition, the American Institute for Homeopathy encourages, but does not require, certification in homeopathy from one of the three existing certifying bodies [71]. In a survey of 42 homeopathic physicians, Lee and Kemper [75] found that 57% held a medical doctor's license.

The American Institute of Homeopathy promotes a "Standard of Practice" [71], which includes the following:

1. A medical history was taken, and any necessary physical examination was completed.
2. Obtaining appropriate laboratory and diagnostic studies.
3. Interpreting diagnostic studies and reviewing medical records.
4. Assessing the urgency of the medical conditions being treated and referring to appropriate specialists in a timely manner.
5. The patient was diagnosed and treated in accordance with the licensure of the practitioner.
6. The progress of the patient's condition was monitored, and the treatment plan was modified as needed.
7. Maintaining appropriate medical records.
8. Acquiring further training as required to maintain respective licenses in the form of continuing medical education courses and seminars.
9. Practicing in accordance with the professional codes of ethics and confidentiality.

In surveys by Jacobs et al. [76] and Lee and Kemper [75], most homeopathic physicians provide both homeopathic treatments and conventional, allopathic or osteopathic treatments. Most homeopathic physicians, therefore, do not see a conflict with conventional, allopathic or osteopathic medicine. This provides the professional basis, or rather, the professional umwelt, of homeopathic medical practitioners.

Typical Diagnoses Treated

In a survey by Jacobs et al. [75], the most common ailments treated in a homeopathic manner were asthma, depression, otitis media (ear infections), allergic rhinitis (congestion from airborne allergens), headache/migraine, neurotic disorders (anxiety), nonspecific allergies, arthritis and hypertension. In the United Kingdom, according to the National Health Service [77], the most common conditions treated by homeopathy are asthma, ear infections, hay fever, mental health conditions, such as depression, stress and anxiety, and allergies, such as food allergies, dermatitis, allergic skin conditions, arthritis, and hypertension [77]. These, for the most part, are common afflictions that affect quality of life but are usually, although not always (e.g., status asthmaticus or suicide-inducing depression), life-threatening.

Medication Preparation and Regulation

Homeopathic medications are recognized by some regulatory bodies, including the United States Food and Drug Administration (FDA) [78]. This was mandated by the *Food, Drug and Cosmetic Act* of 1938. This also produced the *Homeopathic Pharmacopoeia of the United States,* which is a repository of homeopathic medical preparations [71]. The FDA does not "approve" homeopathic medical preparations in the manner that they approve allopathic drugs but monitors the preparations for possible adverse events. This has led to several preparations being recalled [78].

In practice, to achieve increased potency according to homeopathic theory, a medication must be diluted. When the proper dilution is achieved, it is prescribed as a "similimum." This is done through the process of "centesimals," that is, diluting a solution containing the medication (i.e., the solute) 1 part to 100 consecutively, with each solution being shaken vigorously, i.e., "succussion." Figure 8.5 gives an example of a solution containing 1 mole (i.e., 6.02214×10^{23} particles/molecules/atoms/etc.) of solute. After 12 centesimals, the solution will contain <1 particle per given volume on average. In fact, the original solution would have to have at least 10^{60} solute particles to have 1 particle left in the solution after a standard 30 centesimal dilution. It is recognized by homeopathic practitioners that many of these dilutions reach a point that the original "active substance" no longer exists in the solution [71]. In this form, the potential for side effects is eliminated, or nearly so, but the potency through the process of potentiation through succussion maximized [71].

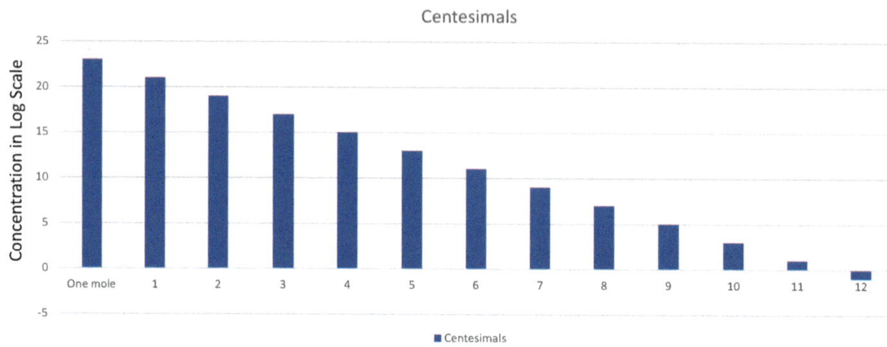

Fig. 8.5 Change in concentration of a solution containing 1 mole of solute (6.02214×10^{23}) diluted in the standard homeopathic manner of centesimals, i.e., 1 part per 100. By the 12 centesimal, there will no longer be any solute particles left in the solvent

8.7.3 Homeopathy, the Illative Core of Argumentation and Persuasion

The above account demonstrates that homeopathy has an underlying theoretical foundation and that its practice is based on this foundation. The theory accounts for the causal attribution of disease, which is then used to identify treatment targets (as analyzed in Chap. 5). It is also clear that the practitioners of homeopathy have a professional umwelt with which they view their practice. As most practitioners of homeopathy have some type of allopathic or osteopathic education, the "standard of practice" espoused by the American Institute of Homeopathy fits nearly perfectly with the physician's cognition of Fig. 1.1. These practitioners' meta-cognitions also fit nearly perfectly with the meta-cognitions of Fig. 1.1. As there is ongoing research into homeopathy, these practitioners must also judge whether any new knowledge should be accepted (as analyzed in Chap. 6) or incorporated into their practice (as analyzed in Chap. 7). The actual practice itself shows the potential for the experienced physician to develop a modicum of practical wisdom in the application of homeopathic theory.

These practitioners, similar to Western allopathic practitioners, must create an argument for both the diagnosis and treatment. The premises used come from the practitioner's examination, coupled with the overarching framework of homeopathic theory. Just reviewing the standards of practice of the American Institute for Homeopathy, it appears that the illative core of the diagnostic argument will be constructed very much like a typical allopath. Reviewing the commonly treated diseases by homeopathy, these practitioners also determine if the patient fits into a particular diagnostic category and then determine which treatment option is appropriate for that category.

These practitioners will present this illative core to the patient. Depending on the exchange and ultimate manifest rationality between the patient and physician, the patient may or may not be persuaded to accept the treatment (Fig. 4.2). This will be based on both the logical validity of the practitioner's argument and the social/cultural umwelt of the patient.

8.8 Conclusions

What I believe that I have demonstrated with these examples of traditional Chinese medicine, traditional indigenous North American and African medicine, American faith healing and the alternative/complementary homeopathic medicine is that the concepts of a theoretical foundation as a basis for practice, with rules for the acceptance of knowledge and their implementation in practice as similar despite widely different medical paradigms. Moreover, the relationship between the practitioner and the patient still requires persuasion, although in indigenous practices, more emphasis is placed on the patient's family and community. These practices are accepted by patients and their communities based on how the human mind evolved to prioritize group cohesion based on human universals. What is different is what is accepted as evidence, which premises are believed, and how much value is placed on the predictability of an anatomical/physiological compared to a social/emotional outcome.

I would like to end this chapter by once again reiterating that by selecting and presenting these particular examples, I am neither endorsing or condemning either these medical paradigms or the paradigms I did not choose to review. I am making no assertions as to the efficacy, either good or bad, of any of these paradigms. Although I am acutely aware that these accounts are truncated and incomplete, if I have made any egregious errors, I apologize.

References

1. Eigenschink M, Dearing L, Dalander TE, et al. A critical examination of the main premises of traditional Chinese medicine. Wein Klin Wochenschr. 2020;132:260–72.
2. Izzo AA, Hoon-Kim S, Radhakrishan R, Williamson EM. A critical approach to evaluating clinical efficacy, adverse events and drug interactions of herbal remedies: efficacy and safety of herbal remedies. Phytother Res. 2016;30:691–700.
3. Sun Y, Zhao Y, Xue SA, Chen J. The theory development of traditional Chinese medicine constitution: a review. J Trad Chin Med Sci. 2018;5:16–28.
4. Lu A-P, Jia H-W, Xiao C, Lu Q-P. Theory of traditional Chinese medicine and therapeutic method of disease. World J Gastroenterol. 2004;10:1854–6.
5. Shi J, Yang Y, Zhou X, et al. The current status of old traditional medicine introduced from Persia to China. Front Pharmacol. 2022;13:953352.
6. Chinese Pharmacopoeia Commission. People's Republic of China Pharmacopoeia. 2015.
7. World Health Organization. Index of pharmacopoeias. Geneva: World Health Organization; 2002.

8. Wang C. Health and illness in traditional Chinese medicine (TCM). https://www.amcollege.edu/blog.
9. Schaffner KF. Discovery and explanation in biology and medicine. Chicago: University of Chicago Press; 1993.
10. Zhai X, Wang X, Wang L, et al. Treating different diseases with the same method—a traditional Chinese medicine concept analyzed for its biological basis. Front Pharmacol. 2020;11:946.
11. Michlig M, Ausfled-Hafter B, Busato A. Patient satisfaction with primary care: a comparison between conventional care and traditional Chinese medicine. Complement Ther Med. 2008;16:350–8.
12. World Health Organization. Traditional medicine. 2003. https://apps.who.int/gb/archive/pdf_files/WHA56/ea5618.pdf.
13. Cohen K. Honoring the medicine. The essential guide to native American healing. New York: Ballatine Books; 2003.
14. First Nations Health Authority. Traditional medicine and traditional healers gathering report. n.d. https://www.fnha.ca/pages/traditional-medicine.aspx.
15. Native American Religion and Spirituality—Common threads, unique beliefs, and too many misconceptions. https://www.powwow.com. Last accessed 12 Oct 2022.
16. Native Voices. Healing ways. https://www.nlm.nih.gov/nativevoices/exhibition/healing-ways.
17. Rybak C, Decker-Fitts A. Understanding native American healing practices. Couns Psychol Quart. 2009;22:333–42.
18. Redvers N, Blondin B. Traditional indigenous medicine in North America: a scoping review. PLoS One. 2020;15(8):e0237531.
19. Koithan M, Farrell C. Indigenous native American healing traditions. J Nurse Pract. 2010;6:474–8.
20. Johnston SL. Native American traditional and alternative medicine. Ann Am Acad Pol Soc Sci. 2002;583:195–213.
21. Vemireddy R. The role of native American healing traditions within allopathic medicine. Inquiries J. 2020;12:1.
22. Matheson L. Valuing spirituality among native American populations. Couns Values. 1996;41:51–9.
23. NIH National Center for Complementary and Alternative Medicine. CAM Basics. Publication 347. 27 Feb 2010. http://nccam.nih.gov/health/whatiscam.
24. Lewis TH. The medicine men. Lincoln, NB: University of Nebraska Press; 1990.
25. Weaver H. Perspectives on wellness: journeys on the red road. J Sociol Soc Work. 2002;29:5–15.
26. Rybak C, Lakota Eastin C, Robbins I. Native American healing practices and counseling. J Hum Couns Ed Dev. 2004;43:25–32.
27. Thomason TC. Counseling native Americans: an introduction for nonnative American counselors. J Couns Dev. 1991;69:321–7.
28. George J, MacLeod M, Graham K, et al. Use of traditional healing practices in two Ontario first nations. J Commun Health. 2018;43:227–37.
29. Peat FD. Lighning the seventh fire: the spiritual ways of healing and science of the native American. New York: Birchland Press; 1994.
30. Maingay B, Pickren M, Mehl-Madrona L. Relationships between level of spiritual transformation and medical outcome. Adv Mind Body Med. 2013;27:4–11.
31. Thin Elk G. Walking in balance on the red road. J Emotion Behav Probl. 1993;2:54–7.
32. Garrett MT, Torres-Rivera E, Brubakei M, et al. Crying for a vision: the native American sweat lodge ceremony as therapeutic intervention. J Couns Dev. 2011;89:318–25.
33. Lame Deer J, Erdoes R. Lame deer, seeker of visions. New York: Touchstone; 1972.
34. Null G. Secrets of the sacred white buffalo: native American healing remedies, rites and rituals. Paramus, NJ: Prentice Hall; 1998.
35. Brown DE. Human universals, human nature and human culture. Daedalus. 2004;133:47–54.
36. Chiorezzi A. The spirituality of Africa (interview with Jacob Olupora). The Harvard Gazette. 6 Oct 2015.

37. Chaitanya MVNL, Baye HG, Ali HS, Usamo FB. Traditional African medicine. In: El-Shemy HA, editor. Natural medicinal plants. London: Intech Open; 2022.
38. Okpako DT. Traditional African medicine: theory and pharmacology explored. Trends Pharmacol Sci. 1999;20:482–5.
39. Oseni Z, Shannon G. The relationship between indigenous and allopathic health practitioners in Africa and its implications for collaboration: a qualitative synthesis. Glob Health Action. 2020;13:1.
40. Fokunang C, Ndikum V, Tabi O, et al. Traditional medicine: past, present and future research and development prospects and integration in the national health system of Cameroon. Afr J Trad Complement Alt Med. 2011;8:284–95.
41. Horton R. The problem of the rationality of magic. In: Wilson BR, editor. Rationality. 1st ed. Oxford: Blackwell; 1970.
42. Janzen JM. The quest for therapy: medical pluralism in lower Zaire. Berekeley, CA: University of California Press; 1978.
43. Twumasi PA. Medical Systems in Ghana. A study in medical sociology. Accra: Ghana Publishing Co. Ltd.; 1975.
44. Horton R. Patterns of thought in Africa and the west. Cambridge: Cambridge University Press; 1993.
45. Mpofu E, Peltzer K, Bojuwoye O. Indigenous health practices in sub-Saharan Africa. In: Mpofu E, editor. Counseling people of African ancestry. Western Cape: Cambridge University Press; 2011.
46. Dawit A, Ahadu A. Medicinal plants and enigmatic health practices of Northern Ethiopia. 1993. https://agris.fao.org/agris-search/search.do?recordID=XF. 2015013726.
47. Van Rensberg HCJ, Fourie E, Pretorius E. Health Care in South Africa. Pretoria: Academia; 2002.
48. Jolles F, Jolles S. Zulu ritual immunization in perspective. J Int Afr Inst. 2000;70:229–48.
49. Zuma T, Wight D, Rochat T, Moshabela M. The role of traditional health practitioners in rural KwaZulu-Natal, South Africa: generic or mode specific? BMC Complement Alt Med. 2016;16:304.
50. Peltzer K, Preez NF, Ramlagan S, Fomundam H. Use of traditional complementary and alternative medicine for HIV patient in KwaZulu-Natal, South Africa. BMC Public Health. 2008;8:255.
51. Semenya SS, Potgieter M. Bapedi traditional healers in the Limpopo Province, South Africa. Their sociocultural profile and traditional healing practice. J Ethnobiol Ethnomed. 2014;10:4.
52. Gumede WM. Traditional healer: a medical practitioner's perspective. Cape Town: Blackshaws; 1990.
53. Karim ASS, Zigubu-Page TT, Arendse R. Bridging the gap: potential for health care partnership between African traditional healer and biomedical personnel in South Africa. Report of the South African Medical Research Council. S Afr Med J. 1984;84:1.
54. World Health Organization. WHO traditional medicine strategy, 2002–2005. Geneva: World Health Organization; 2002.
55. d'Avigdor E, Wohlmuth H, Asfaw Z, Awas T. The current status of knowledge of herbal medicine and medicinal plants in Fiche, Ethiopia. J Ethnobiol Ethnomed. 2014;10:38.
56. Johnson KS, Elbert-Avila KI, Tulsky JA. The influence of spiritual beliefs and practices on the treatment preferences of African Americans: a review of the literature. J Am Geriatr Soc. 2005;53:711–9.
57. Larson P, Leeming DA, editors. Encyclopedia of psychology and religion. 1st ed. Boston: Springer; 2014.
58. Last M, Chavunduka GE, editors. The professionalism of African medicine. Manchester: Manchester University Press and the International Africa Institute; 1986.
59. Chavunduka GL. Traditional medicine in modern Zimbabwe. Harare: University of Zimbabwe Press; 1994.

60. Aborigo RA, Allotey P, Reidpath DD. The traditional healer in obstetric care: a persistent wasted opportunity in maternal health. Soc Sci Med. 2015;133:59–66.
61. Omonzejele PF, Maduka C. Metaphysical and value underpinnings of traditional medicine in West Africa. Chin J Integr Med. 2011;17:99–104.
62. Wiginton P. Methods of divination. 2019. https://www.learnreligions.com/methods-of-divination-2561764.
63. Stoddard E. A third of Americans report divine healing: pew. Reuters. 23 Jun 2008.
64. Smith Z. Speaking in tongues. New York Review. 26 Feb 2009.
65. Dossey L. Spirituality, prayer, and medicine: what is the fuss truly about? Virtual Mentor. 2005;7:390–4.
66. Grand Delusion? Center for the History of Medicine at Courtway Library. https://collections.courtway.harvard.edu/onview/exhibits/show/grand-delusion. Last accessed 13 Oct 2022.
67. Morrell P. Homeopathy—theory and method. https://www.homeoint.org/morrell/articles/pm_theor.htm. Last accessed 13 Oct 2022.
68. Nelson DH, Perchaluk JM, Logan AC, Katzman MA. The bells toll for homeopathy: time for a change in the training and practice of north American naturopathic physicians. J Evid Based Integr Med. 2019;24:1–11.
69. Drofenik M. Thermodynamic aspects of homeopathy. In: Akram M, editor. Alternative medicine. London: Intech Open; 2020.
70. Grams N. Homeopathy—where is the science? EMBO Rep. 2019;20:e47761.
71. The American Institute of Homeopathy. Regarding the practice of homeopathic medicine. https://homeopathyusa.org. Last accessed 14 Oct 2022.
72. Suvarna BS. Hahnemann's three miasmas: Theory of miasms. https://www.homeopathy360.com. Last accessed 13 Oct 2022.
73. Constantine Hering. https://www.wholehealthnow.com/homeopathy_info/constantine_hering.html. Last accessed 13 Oct 2022.
74. Montgomery EB. Medical reasoning: the nature and use of medical knowledge. New York: Oxford University Press; 2019.
75. Lee ACC, Kemper KJ. Homeopathy and naturopathy: practice characteristics and pediatric care. Arch Pediatr Adolesc Med. 2000;154:75–80.
76. Jacobs J, Chapman EH, Crothers D. Patient characteristics and practice patterns of physicians using homeopathy. Arch Fam Med. 1998;7:537–40.
77. Homeopathy. National Health Service. https://www.nhs/uk/conditions/homeopathy. Last accessed 13 Oct 2022.
78. United States Food and Drug Administration. Homeopathic products. www.fda.gov/drugs/information-drug-class/homeopathic-products. Last accessed 13 Oct 2022.

Chapter 9
Quantitative Calculation in Medical Decision-Making and Human Persuasion: Decision Sciences, Big Data, Computer Decision Aids, Medical Calculators, and Artificial Intelligence

9.1 Introduction: Medical Information Is Expanding and Changing

The prior chapter provided examples of argumentation based on a specific underlying theory of reality. This provided the foundational framework used by medicine in persuasion for traditional medical practices and alternative/complementary medical practices around the world. This chapter will address the same issues but in the fields of informatics and computer programs in medicine. Everything up to now had at its center the physician performing the tasks of containing within their mind the theoretical foundation and factual information of their medical knowledge, gathering information (data) pertaining to a particular patient, structuring an argument as to the diagnosis, matching that diagnostic category to appropriate treatment recommendations, presenting the illative core of that argument to the patient (and perhaps others), and ultimately achieving an agreed manifest rationality with the patient, which persuaded the patient and the physician as to which treatment options (if any) will be pursued (Fig. 1.1).

This is how medicine has been practiced since time immemorial. The physician was the repository of knowledge, wisdom and action. Although this paradigm, not only in Western allopathic medicine but also in traditional medical practices and even alternative and complementary medical practices, has produced a quantum of success in curing and preventing disease as well as alleviating suffering,[1] there have been an untold number of failures. Much medical research is devoted to reducing the number of these failures.

[1] The nineteenth century physician, Edward Trudeau (it is sometimes ascribed to William Osler or Edward Livingston), is ascribed this quote: "To cure sometimes, to relieve often, and to comfort always—this is our task." Which profound for both its humanity and humility. It was a recognition of the limits of what medicine can do and the vastness of what humans can do. One can easily imagine a traditional healer saying the same.

V. Velanovich, *Medical Persuasion*, https://doi.org/10.1007/978-3-031-30371-5_9

9.1.1 Growth of Medical Information

Medical knowledge continues to grow at an accelerated rate. In a study from 2011, Densen [1] asserted that the rate of doubling of medical knowledge was 50 years in 1950, 7 years by 1980, 3.5 years by 2010, and projected (as of 2011) to be 73 days by 2020. Although I do not have additional information as to how true his 2020 prediction turned out to be, I am comfortable believing it is close to this number. There are apparently approximately 30,000 medical journals worldwide [2] publishing original research, as well as other types of articles, most likely numbering in the 100s of thousands, if not millions.[2] This does not even touch on the unbounded information space of the internet. This is a very daunting amount of information indeed.

This, of course, begs the question of "How can a practicing physician keep up?" This answer is "*No one can keep up*"! Physicians, at least in the Western allopathic tradition, have responded to this limitation in a number of ways. The most consequential of which, at least in my view, has been the increase in specialization. It was common in the early twentieth century that one could go into "general practice" after a 1-year internship following medical school, which would include medicine, surgery, pediatrics, obstetrics and gynecology, and just about everything else. Even now, in the state of Florida, the requirements to obtain a medical license are to "Be a graduate of an allopathic U.S. medical school of a school recognized and approved by the U.S. Office of Education (AMG) and completed at least 1 year of approved residency training," with the additional requirements that the training was completed within the last 2 years and all parts of a national examination were passed [3]. Although this is the bare minimum for obtaining a medical license, most healthcare facilities and practices will require additional training for privileging and credentialing.

Medical specialization started in the twentieth century and accelerated in the late 20th and early 21st centuries. Presently, the Association of American Medical Colleges lists over 160 medical specialties and subspecialties [4]. All of these require residency training beyond the mandatory intern year (additional 2–8 years), most require additional "fellowship" training (additional 1–3 years), and a few require post-fellowship advanced training (additional 1–2 years). It is not unusual for a subspecialist to have an additional 10 years of medical training *after* receiving a 4-year bachelor's degree and a 4-year medical degree (i.e., approximately *18 years* of education!). Most of these specialties have their own professional societies, and many have their own certification boards. The consequence is that these physicians are very well trained in a quite narrow area of medicine, reducing the "breath" of

[2] How much actual useable knowledge or information is published is another matter, which I will not address. I will occasionally say that there is much "info-trash" out there.

medical knowledge they need to know to increase the "depth" of knowledge they need to know of their speciality.[3]

This increased specialization was a method of making the amount of knowledge that an individual physician has in their corpus of knowledge more manageable and retrievable. However, because of this, there is very much the potential that a physician may not have in their retrievable knowledge base the potential disease category that is afflicting the patient. If a physician does not know that a potential disease exists, then that physician cannot diagnose it (see the discussion of this in Chap. 7). Sadly, it is not unusual for patients to be referred from doctor to doctor until a physician actually has knowledge of the disease afflicting the patient. This is a problem of readily retrievable knowledge. The same can also be said for treatment recommendations. That is, doctors are more likely to recommend the treatments that they know,[4] not necessarily what would be best for the patient.

The "Beethoven String Quartet" Dilemma

In the mid-1960s, the economists William J. Baumol and William G. Bowen [5] put forth a theory to explain rising wages in occupations that did not have rising productivity. The general idea is that as workers become more productive, wages rise accordingly.[5] However, there have been some occupations in which there can never be an increase in productivity. The example that Baumol and Bowen used was the performing arts—specifically, it requires exactly the same number of musicians to play a Beethoven string quartet now as it did in the eighteenth century. That is, there can never be an "increase in productivity" for these musicians. Similarly, the present model of medicine requires (at least) one physician to interact with one patient for a period of time. Although technological advances have made some aspects of medical care more efficient, this underlying paradigm has not changed.

[3] I will give the example of myself. I graduated medical school in 1987 and then did a 5-year general surgery residency—all very common for the time. I passed the written and oral board examination as administered by the American Board of Surgery, which is a certificate of endorsement by that body attesting to my competency to practice general surgery. This certification included treatment of the following surgical disease categories (along with their medical management) of the head and neck, breast, thoracic cavity, abdominal cavity, skin, extremities, vascular system, endocrine system, certain aspects of gynecology, cancer care and trauma, as well as certain aspects of critical care medicine. In addition, for a time, that was my practice. However, over the years, due to developing a more focused interest, plus the increased number of other surgical specialists, I voluntarily narrowed by practice to a specific group of surgical diseases. Because I no longer needed to "keep up" with knowledge in these other disease processes, I could know more about my areas of interest. As I would say to the medical students and residents, "I know more and more about less and less."

[4] This calls to mind the aphorism: What you have a hammer, the whole world looks like a nail.

[5] I am not asserting that this is always still true, especially in an era of increasing productivity due to technological advancement, but the underlying point still holds.

One of the potential ways it could become more efficient—and what I mean here it that the physician can more quickly and accurately come to the correct diagnosis—is with application of decision sciences, especially computer decision aids. This poses its own dilemmas, namely, will such aids help or hurt persuasion.

9.2 Decision Sciences in Medicine

9.2.1 What is Decision Science?

Decision science is a field of study of how individuals, groups, and organizations actually make decisions [6]. Decision sciences are applicable to a number of activities, including business, government, education, and, of course, medicine. According to Kleindorfer et al. [6], there are two categories of analyzing decisions: descriptive and perspective. Descriptive analysis is how people actually make decisions, while prescriptive analysis is how people should make decisions according to a set of well-defined criteria. Prescriptive analysis requires understanding the context and descriptive realities of the situation in question [6]. This is a very important point, and one that is related to medical argumentation and decisions in the previous chapters, the premises involved in any logical argument related to a decision have to be relevant to that decision. Moreover, it is essential to have identified *all of the relevant premises*, not just the obvious ones (or, more likely, the ones that one likes).

In this sense, the decision process is a network of contexts and processes [6]. These include:

1. The context of the problem, that is, the environment in which the problem exists. For example, the social context, institutional constraints, and available information, among others.
2. Finding the problem, that is, identifying if, in fact, a decision opportunity exists. There may be problems that are simply "out of one's control," while other perceived problems are not those that truly have an effect on the decision maker.
3. Solving the problem, that is, devising a solution and executing it.
4. Process of legitimation, that is, determining what impacts of potential choice outcomes are on the relevant stakeholders' interest and articulating the choice in such a way as to persuade those stakeholders [6].

All these are interrelated and connected. A viable decision is based on all. There is no doubt that physicians and patients make decisions compatible with this framework.

The question is, will this give the correct decision in the medical context? Previous chapters discussed how humans perceive the world and how this perception (human universals, the social/cultural/and professional umwelt, etc.) can affect what type of arguments or conclusions are acceptable to any one individual or group. This will consistently lead to bias, such that arguments that are clearly *non sequiturs* will be accepted and those that are clearly valid will be rejected.

First, we must accept that everyone has biases. Although "bias" has a negative connotation, it is probably better to think of it as seeing a problem from a particular viewpoint [7]. Humans have many limitations that can affect decision-making. People do not have unlimited ability to store information mentally; they cannot necessarily perceive all the relevant quanta of information required for the decisions to be made; and they have relatively limited (compared to a large computer) ability to process these datapoints within a rules-based decision algorithm[6] [6]. Schulkin [7] identifies four biases in medical decision-making:

1. Omission bias is the tendency to choose not to do something because it could cause harm.
2. Proportionality bias is the tendency to over- or undervalue risk.
3. Ambiguity avoidance is a perception that the outcome is misleading or unclear.
4. Naturalistic bias, which is the notion that just because something is "natural," it must be "good" and, oppositely, those which are made by human manufacturing methods are "bad."

Schulkin [7] is certainly correct that these are bias, and, I would aver, that there are many other biases and fallacies in human reasoning. Gilovich filled a whole book of them [8]. However, as Kleindorfer et al. [6] note, "It is one thing to know a decision is faulty, it's another to know the cause of the fault."

9.2.2 *Quantification of the Consequences of Medical Decisions*

Decisions have consequences. This is an axiomatic truism. However, unlike many decisions in life that are decidedly qualitative, many, if not all, clinical decisions can be quantified. Was the patient cure? How much longer is the patient expected to live? How much did their pain improve? Was their quality of life improved? Did they suffer any adverse events? How much out-of-pocket cost did the patient have to pay? How long were they out of work? Was the patient satisfied with the care received? These questions, as well as many others, could be quantified either by Boolean algebra (yes = 1, no = 0) or an actual number (e.g., the patient is expected to live 10 years after this treatment for this disease).

It is just that these outcomes can be quantified, but we can also quantify the probabilities of these outcomes occurring using known frequencies as point estimates, as discussed in Chaps. 6 and 7. By combining the probability of the outcome with the value of the outcome, we can then determine which decisions would be expected to

[6] The fact that chess grandmasters are routinely bested by chess playing computer programs such that there is suspicion that other grand masters are cheating by using these programs in matches proves the point about the limitations of the human mind (see Keener G. Report accuses chest grandmaster of understating the extent of his cheating. *New York Times*, October 14, 2022).

yield the best results. This is the basis of the following methods of more "objective" medical decision-making.

9.3 Decision Analysis

Formal decision analysis was developed in the 1960s as a way to quantify the consequences of decision choices [9]. Since that time, it has been used extensively in the medical research setting to analyze a variety of medical decision problems [10]. Many have applied decision analysis for specific patient care decisions [11].

Decision analysis has four basic steps [12]:

1. Identify and bound the decision problem.
2. Structure the decision problem over time.
3. Characterize the information needed to fill the structure.
4. Choose a preferred course of action.

Although it is not my intention to give a formal primer on decision analysis, some explanation is required to understand how it quantifies a decision choice.

9.3.1 Basic Decision Tree

A decision is a choice among options. Returning to Fig. 1.1, once the diagnosis is reached, the physician will place the patient in a diagnostic category for which they will have one or more treatment options. There are some diagnostic categories for which there may be only one viable diagnostic option; for example, a complete bowel obstruction requires surgical intervention. However, most diagnostic categories will have two or more appropriate "standard of care" options. In Fig. 1.1, as well as the discussions on persuasion in Chaps. 4 and 7, the physician will then present the patient with these options, the risks and benefits, expected outcomes, potential adverse events, etc., to allow for the patient to have all the information the patient needs to make an "informed" decision. What decision analysis does is make all of these decisions with their probable outcomes explicit.

To make a decision, there must be a problem for which a decision has to be made. This may sound trite, but the important point is that the problem has to be defined in such a way that an *actionable* decision can be reached. As an extreme example, since we cannot control the occurrence of sunspots, thus making a decision on whether we should control sunspots is useless. Moreover, there are some problems that are very large or vague such that it would be impossible to define a single starting choice. For example, "I want my children to be happy." This is what Weinstein and Fineberg [12] mean when they assert that the decision problem needs to be "identified and bound."

In the clinical vignette presented in Chap. 1, the patient is presented with the options of medical management with PPIs or surgical intervention with a Nissen fundoplication. So now, the problem is identified and bound—namely, the physician and the patient have identified that the patient's symptoms of GERD are such that intervention is both warranted and desired and that the decision is bounded to the choice of either medication or surgery. From here, a *decision tree* is constructed.

A decision tree must always start with a choice. This choice between these options is represented in the decision tree by a "choice node," represented by a box in the decision tree (□). Once the decision is made, consequences occur. The branches of the tree that lead from this stem to the possible consequences, which are represented by a "chance node," depicted as a circle (○) in the decision tree (Fig. 9.1). When constructing a decision tree, the decision-maker must decide to what endpoints the decision pertains; how are these endpoints going to be quantified; how does the endpoint stem from the decision; and what are the probabilities that these endpoints will occur. Let us address these issues.

Values, Preferences and Utilities

It almost goes without saying that people want long life and good health.[7] For the most part, quantifying longevity is fairly straightforward. This is done through life-tables; for example, the Centers for Disease Control and Prevention produces yearly life tables [13]. For specific diseases, life expectancy can be either directly obtained or calculated from the relevant epidemiological or interventional studies [14, 15]. However, determining what constitutes "good health," although intuitively clear, is nevertheless difficult to quantify.

These estimates of placing a numeric value one's health is an area of interest, especially to those interested in outcomes. "Outcomes," in a broad sense, are the end-results of medical care. Although, yet again, intuitively easy to grasp, precision in what actual is an "outcome" can become problematic. It is problematic because there are numerous definitions and ways to measure outcomes [16]. Such issues as which outcome(s) is of importance, how will it be identified, and at which time point are all relevant, but I will not address these issues here. Moreover, one needs also to specify when the "end" is reached in order to define the "end-result." For my purposes, a definitive, well-defined outcome at a specific, agreed end will be assumed. Having said this, how are we to value this outcome?

This is done through understanding a patient's values and preferences [17]. Schwartz and Bilsky [18] state that values are (1) concepts or beliefs, (2) about desirable end states or behaviors, (3) that transcend specific situations, (4) guide the selection or evaluation of behaviors or events, and (5) are ordered by relative importance. This is consistent with what was previously presented in Chaps. 3 and 4

[7] I am found of telling the medical students and trainees that we do only two things in medicine—we either get people to live longer or we make them feel better, and hopefully both.

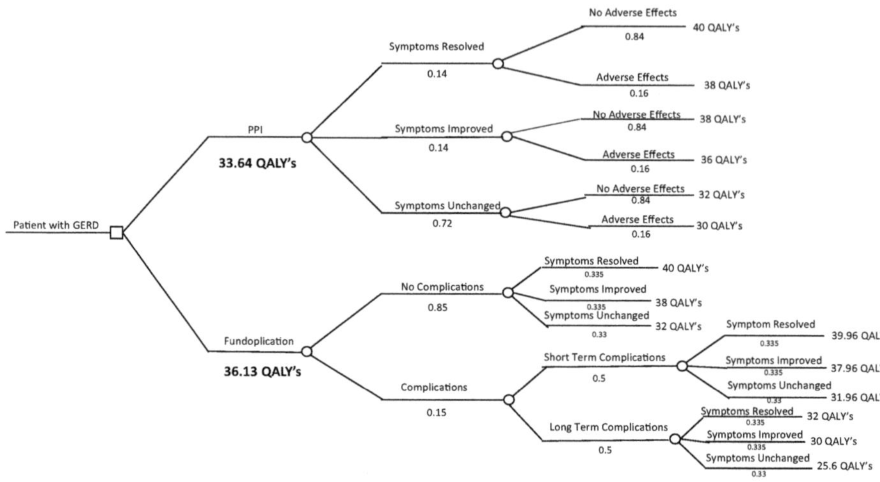

Fig. 9.1 Basic decision analysis tree for the treatment of refractory GERD. I used the data from Spechlar et al. [27] with additional assumptions to make the following valuations. I assume that the patient for whom the decision is to be made has a life expectancy of 40 years. If the symptoms of GERD are completely resolved, they have a utility of 1.0 (i.e., perfect health); if their symptoms are improved but not completely resolved, their utility is 0.95; if their symptoms are unchanged, their utility is 0.8. Spechler et al. [27] reported that 72% of PPI patients had treatment failure, which means no change in symptoms; therefore, 28% had treatment success. For the sake of the example, I will assume half (i.e., 14%) of the patients will have had complete resolution of symptoms and half symptom improvement. They reported that 16% of PPIs had "serious adverse events"; for these patients, I assigned a utility of 0.95. They reported that 15% of surgical patients had serious adverse events. For the sake of the example, I assumed that half of the complications were short-term, meaning complete resolution after a period of time, for which I assigned a short-term morbidity discount of 0.04 years (approximately 2 weeks), and half were long-term complications, meaning that they would affect the patient's quality of life for the rest of their life expectancy. I assigned a utility of 0.8 for this outcome. The box (☐) presents the choice node, while the circles (○) represent the chance nodes. The frequencies (probability estimates) of each event occurring are under the named branch

pertaining to the evolution of the human mind, human universals, the primal worldview, and the cultural and social umwelt. For humans, their value system is a "meaning-producing superordinate cognitive structure, and this cognitive structure can be affectively changed" [19]. The structure of the human value system is universal, and there are a finite number of universally important value types [17]. Additionally, quite obviously, people differ in their value priorities [20]. These values are converted to numeric quantifies, which are utilities.

In the context of a decision analysis, *utility* is a composite measure of the extent to which each outcome of each choice option achieves each of our ultimate goals [21]. The extremes of a utility scale are easily defined as 1 being perfect health and 0 being death (or something as bad) [10]. It's the in-between values which are more difficult to assign. There are several methods to do this, one being determination of patient *preferences*. "Preferences" are "statements made by individuals regarding the relative desirability of a range of health experiences, treatment options or health states" [22]. Preferences are related to values [22] but are object-focused and relate to specific options, or attributes of options, in a specific decision context [17]. Health-related preferences are described in different domains, for example, choice among treatment options, treatment aspects, health professionals, the desirability of procedural aspects of screening or treatment, desirability of resources, amount or kind of information, and the desirability of participating in health-related decision-making [17]. These utilities have a value placed on them by whomever the stakeholder(s) in the decision being considered, either as an individual or as a group.

There are many ways these utility values can be obtained. The two basic approaches are holistic and decomposed [17]. In the holistic method, participants assign values to each possible health state, where the state represents a combination of many attributes. In the decomposed method, the values for all health states are assigned without requiring the judge(s) to assign values to each one, such that the value expresses the overall value as a decomposed function of the attributes [17].

Holistic valuations encompass valuations of the quality of life of those states. This can be done through a variety of quality-of-life instruments [23]. Another method is the "standard gamble" [17], where a person would be willing to accept a risk of obtaining good health if the present state is undesirable. A person would be offered a choice between a certain outcome (the health state to be valued for one's remaining life expectancy) and a gamble with a certain probability of perfect health and the opposite probability of death. At the probability point where the person accepts the gamble is the utility. The "time trade-off" method requires participants to trade life time remaining in their present health state for perfect health. For example, an individual may have a life expectancy of 20 years in their present health. They may be willing to give 2 years of life to live 18 years in perfect health. The utility is then (time in optimal health)/(time remaining in present health) [24]. Last, with the visual analog scale, the person is asked to place a mark between 0 and 100, where 0 is defined as death and 100 as perfect health, although some do not consider this a preference-based or utility score, as there is no trade-off or risk [25].

The decomposed methods to value treatments express the overall value as a decomposed function of the health state or treatment attributes. One such method is multi-attribute utility theory (MAUT). In this method, each attribute of a health state or intervention is given an importance weight and then scored on how well each health status (or treatment) does on each attribute. These scores are weighted by the importance of the attribute and summed to give an overall multi-attribute score for each state [17]. Last, "conjoint analysis" is used to assess preferences participants judge hypothetical cases that are described in terms of combinations of attributes. Statistical analysis then reveals the attribute level utilities [26].

Quality-Adjusted Life Years

Regardless of how these utilities are determined, how they are used in a decision analysis (or observational and interventional studies for that matter) is the numeric fraction as expressed by the utility score is multiplied by the life expectancy (usually in years, but does not have to be) to give the "quality-adjusted life year" or QALY [14, 15]. This then becomes a standard unit of measure for decision analysis, but not the exclusive one. Other outcome measures may be appropriate depending on the circumstances.

Frequency Determinations

Each of the potential outcomes of a decision has a certain probability of occurring. The probabilities, as discussed in Chaps. 5 and 6, are estimated by the frequencies of their occurrence as determined by observational or interventional studies. If there are no published frequency point estimates, the probabilities can be estimated by the decision-maker's best judgment.

Decision Tree Construction

A decision tree is generally constructed from left to right, with the first node being the first (and many times, the only) choice that has to be made. As an example, I constructed a tree based on the clinical vignette presented in Chap. 1 (Fig. 9.1). The basic choice for the patient was either treatment for their GERD symptoms using a PPI medication or surgery with a Nissen fundoplication. With each choice, the consequences invariably follow. If treatment with PPIs was chosen, the patient's symptoms could have resolved, improved, or remained unchanged. The patients could then have either suffered some adverse events related to the medication or not. The sequence of consequences is somewhat arbitrary in this case, as the tree could have been constructed with the adverse events coming before the treatment resolution, but this would not have changed the QALY calculations. The consequences for surgical treatment, however, are different. As with any operation, there is a possibility that the patient could suffer some type of surgical complication. These complications could be either short-term, meaning that after a period of time, these complications will resolve and no longer impact the patient, or long-term, meaning that there would be a long-term or possibly permanent detriment to the patient. Similar to medical therapy, surgical therapy can lead to complete symptom resolution, symptomatic improvement, or no change in the patient's symptoms.

For the sake of this example, I used the data pertaining to these consequences from Spechler et al.'s [27] trial. I acknowledge that this does not fit exactly with the clinical scenario of Chap. 1, but it does have the virtue of being discussed previously. The frequencies of the outcomes are generally placed in the tree under the corresponding consequence branch. For example, Spechler et al. [27] had specific definitions for treatment success and failure. I used their reported treatment failure rate to correspond in the decision tree as the "no change" consequence branch. They did not specifically report the rates of complete symptom response and partial response (i.e., symptomatic improvement), so I made an assumption that half the patients in the treatment success group had complete responses and the other half had symptomatic improvement. This is arbitrary but does not change the effectiveness of the example as a decision tree illustration. Similarly, surgical adverse events were not reported as short-term or long-term complications, so I arbitrarily made half of them short-term and half long-term.

It is easy to assign a utility of 1 for a patient who is completely asymptomatic and suffers no adverse events, as this is the definition of a "perfect" outcome. However, it is somewhat more difficult to assign utilities to "less than perfect" outcomes. Therefore, again somewhat arbitrarily for illustration's sake, I assigned living long-term with a medical adverse event of 0.95, long-term surgical adverse event of 0.8, symptomatic improvement of 0.95, and no change in symptoms of 0.8. For a short-term complication, I will cut approximately 2 weeks (0.04 years) from a patient's QALY. This then gives the decision tree illustrated in Fig. 9.1.

The decision solution in QALYs is calculated by multiplying the outcome QALY by the probability of its occurrence and then adding the result to the other branch after the chance node. For example, the last chance node at the top of the decision tree has two branches, the "no adverse effects" branch and the "adverse effects" branch. The QALY for the "no adverse effects" branch is 40, while the QALY for the "adverse effects" branch is 38. The probability of the "no adverse effects" branch occurring is 0.84, while the "adverse effects" branch is 0.16 (Note that these must add up to 1, i.e., one or the other must happen). When one multiplies the QALY by the probability, this gives that branch's contribution to the preceding branch, in this case, the "symptoms resolved" branch. Thus, $[(40 \times 0.84) + (38 \times 0.16)] = 39.68$. When one does the same for the "symptoms improved" branch, one gets 37.68, and for the "no change" branch, one gets 31.68. When one multiplies these QALYs with their respective occurrence probabilities, the contributions of each for the choice of PPIs are $[(39.68 \times 0.14) + (37.68 \times 0.14) + (31.68 \times 0.72)] = 33.64$ expected QALYs for the choice of PPI therapy. When one does the same for fundoplication, the expected QALY's is 36.13. That is, in this choice, fundoplication has an expected outcome of approximately 2.5 QALYs more than PPI treatment, which, reassuringly, is consistent with the randomized trial [27].

Depending on the complexity of the decision problem, additional choice and chance nodes can be added. For example, I made the assumption (again, for simplicity's sake) of ending with the outcome of "no change" and "adverse effects." It is very unlikely that a physician would do nothing further for this patient. At this point, an additional choice node could be added, e.g., changing to another medication or considering surgical intervention. It is only in the cases of ideal outcomes or death that decisions stop for the patient.

Sensitivity Analysis

Of course, this decision analysis, nor any other for that matter, is immune to criticism. One can argue about the tree's construction, but most commonly, the criticisms have to do with disagreements about either the probabilities used or the determinations of the utility scores. The way to address such concerns is with sensitivity analysis. In sensitivity analysis, one is free to change any of the parameters of the tree. One could say that instead of the probability of complete symptom relief being 0.14, it was actually 0.2; or instead of the utility of symptomatic improvement being 0.95, it was 0.99; or what if the life expectancy was 6 years or 60 years? Changing these parameters and recalculating the expected QALY outcome can easily be done. For example, for the sake of simplicity, Fig. 9.2 shows the sensitivity analysis of two treatments for a particular disease. Treatment 1 has superior longevity and quality of life results compared to treatment 2. However, when adverse events occur, they are much more severe in treatment 1 than in treatment 2. At low probabilities of adverse events for both treatments, treatment 1 is superior to treatment 2. However, as the probabilities of adverse events increase for both, at some point, treatment 2 becomes superior. This is called the threshold rate for a change in treatment outcomes.

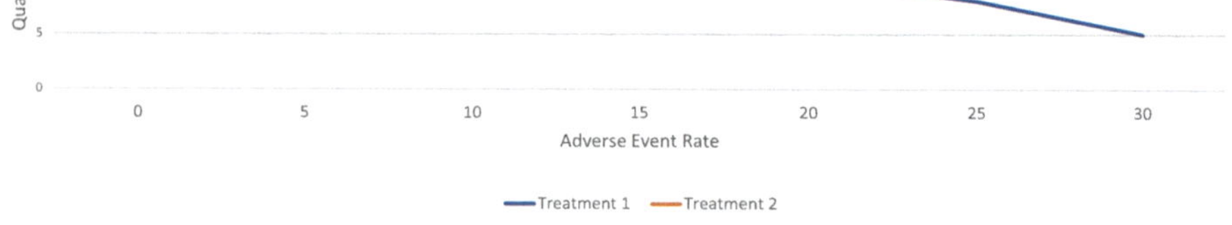

Fig. 9.2 Sensitivity analysis of two hypothetical treatments for the same disease. I will make the assumption that treatment 1 overall leads to a longer survival and better quality of life, but when adverse events occur, they tend to be more severe. On the other hand, treatment 2 has a shorter survival and somewhat poorer quality of life, but when adverse events occur, they are far less severe. The sensitivity analysis shows the change in QALYs based on the complication rate. At lower rates of complications, treatment 1 produces longer QALYs than treatment 2. However, at a rate of 10%, treatment 2 produces longer QALYs than treatment 1. This rate is the "threshold" for choosing treatment 2 over treatment 1

9.3.2 Markov Analysis

The above decision tree is relatively static. That is, it is a single choice for a single clinical problem, with a fixed, permanent outcome, for a specific time horizon. This is true for many diseases where the treatment definitively resolves the disease process and the patient returns to their normal state of health. However, there are many diseases for which there is no definitive treatment, and the patient may follow a waxing and waning course, for example, systemic lupus erythematosus or multiple sclerosis. In these circumstances, a static decision tree with a single endpoint will not do.

Markov models are useful when a decision problem involves risk that is continuous over time, when timing of events is important, and when important events may happen more than once [28]. The Markov models assume that a patient is always in one of a finite number of discrete health states (referred to as a Markov state), and all events represent a transition from one state to another [28]. For example, good health can be considered a health state that an individual is in; when that person becomes sick, they have transferred from the state of good health to the state of sickness (Fig. 9.3). Some transition relationships are bidirectional; for example, the patient can transition back to a good health state. Other transitions are unidirectional; for example, when a patient dies, that transition to death is permanent. In the parlance of the Markov process, this is called an "absorbing" state [28], and in medicine, death is the only absorbing state.

A Markov model may be evaluated by matrix algebra, as a cohort simulation, as a Monte Carlo simulation, and as a Markov cycle tree [28]. I am not going to delve the technical details of this, but a basic description would be clarifying. As with a basic decision tree, each Markov state will have a utility, for example, 1 for well, 0.7 for sick and 0 for death. The time in each state is fixed at whatever is appropriate for the given problem, for example, 1 day or 1 year. Therefore, a Markov time cycle will be quality-adjusted, similar to the quality-adjusted life expectancy of a decision tree, but as a summation of the quality-adjusted cycles. For example, if an individual

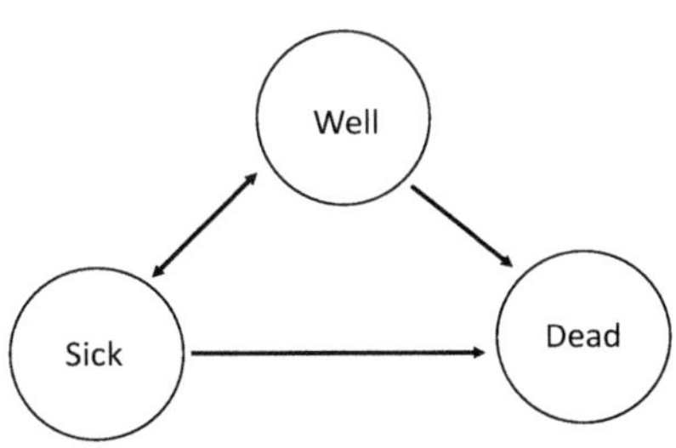

Fig. 9.3 Basic Markov health state transitions. In this particular example, there are three health states: Well, Sick and Dead. The transition from Well to Sick is bidirectional; that is, a well person can become sick, and a sick person can become well. There is one absorbing state, and that is death. Either a well or sick person can transition into death. Of course, additional states can be added depending on the particular problem

spends 1 year being well, that would be 1 QALY, and 2 years sick, that was be 1.4 QALYs and died in the fourth year; their QALYs were 2.4. A Markov cohort is a cohort of patients where the QALE is summation of the fraction of the cohort in the given states and is then added to the running total to give a cumulative utility.

Monte Carlo Simulation

One of the most common methods of simulation using the Markov methodology is the Monte Carlo simulation. A Monte Carlo simulation uses random sampling and statistical modeling to estimate mathematical functions and mimic operations of complex systems [29]. The key points in defining a model are as follows: (1) what are the desired outputs? (2) What will these outputs be used for? (3) How accurate/precise must the outputs be? (4) How exactly can/must we model? (5) How exactly can/must we define the inputs? and (6) How do we model the underlying process [29]? These types of models are most useful when the model requires time-dependent parameters (e.g., recurrence probability after cancer treatment), time to an event (e.g., disease-free survival) or repeated events (e.g., a second myocardial infarction) [30].

A Monte Carlo simulation simulates the outcomes of a large number of patients, usually in the thousands. The basic method of Monte Carlo simulation is that each "patient" in the simulation is assigned to the next state by a random process based on the probability of transitioning to a particular state. For example, the probability of transitioning from state 1 to state 1 in the following cycle may be 50%; therefore, the patient has a 50–50 chance of this transition. If the chances of transitioning from state 1 to state 2 are, say, 25%, that patient has a one in four chance of this transition. However, a patient must transition to some defined state in the next cycle. Figure 9.4 shows an example of a Monte Carlo simulation of 4 patients in the well state but at risk for sickness. By the end of the simulation, one patient was in the well state, one in the sick state and two in the dead state. The amount of time each patient "spends" in a given state is multiplied by its utility to obtain a distribution of quality-adjusted time outcomes.

9.3.3 Difficulties and Impracticality of Decision Analysis

There are many difficulties with decision analysis. While it certainly helps one to think critically and in an organized manner about the potential consequences of each choice, it is far more appropriate as a research tool than a clinical tool. Because only outcomes that can be quantified can be used, qualitative preferences are not addressed overtly, perhaps, at best, in the global assessment of utility.

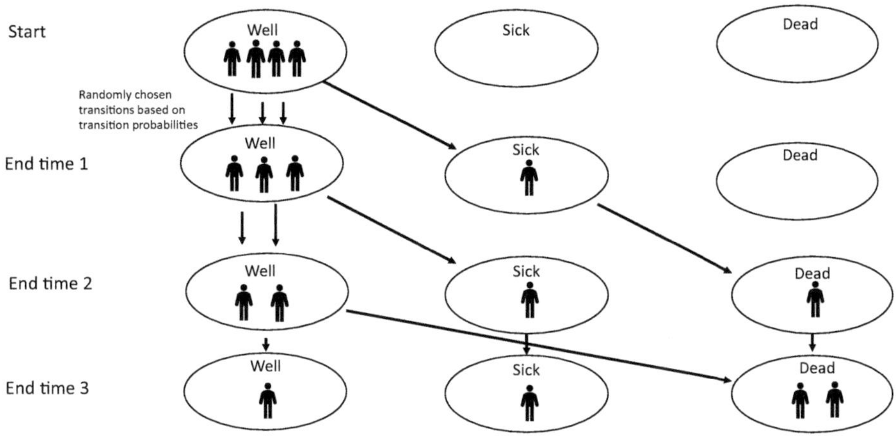

Fig. 9.4 A basic Monte Carlo simulation. This particular example is a simulation of four individuals through three time periods. Each transition has a particular probability of occurring. The transitions are from well to well, well to sick, well to death, sick to sick, sick to death, and death to death. In this particular example, there is no sick to well, but this can be included in the model if appropriate. Each patient is randomly assigned to a transition based on the probability of the transition occurring by usually a computer program. At the end of the third time period, in this example, one patient is in the well state, one in the sick state and two in the dead state

Multiple Objectives

It is not uncommon that medical decisions must be made when the decision maker has multiple objectives, some of which may be in conflict. For example, a patient certainly would like to increase their longevity and quality of life but also reduce the cost of their care and the burden on their family. This is very difficult to capture in a single utility score. Some, but not all, of these potential conflicting issues can perhaps be addressed formally with multicriteria decision analysis [31], but this also adds another layer of decision complexity.

Difficult to Implement Clinically

Decision analysis is probably completely unnecessary for routine decisions. To expect a busy clinician to construct a decision tree or run Markov chains while seeing patients in the clinic is just impractical. Perhaps a dedicated clinical service with experts who are facile in decision analysis may be useful in particularly difficult cases, but this cannot be done in real time.

The Problem of Gradation in Outcome

Decision analysis requires distinct outcomes, or rather, health states. Not all such states are distinct (e.g., cured, not cured). Many have gradations of symptomatic or quality of life improvement. For example, in the example of GERD (Fig. 9.1), I used three health states: symptom resolution, symptom improvement, and no symptom change. This is clearly an oversimplification. Although symptom resolution is a distinct health state, what does symptom improvement mean? A little bit or a lot? Enough that the patient is satisfied? What about if the symptoms are worse? What if the symptoms improved, but there was another bothersome problem for the patient? This makes some modeling difficult.

9.3.4 Decision Analysis in Medical Persuasion

Although decision analysis was quite a useful research tool and such research can certainly be used in constructing the illative core of an argument, for the clinician, its practical uses are limited. In other words, the results of such decision analysis studies can be used as premises in an argument that the physician constructs for determining how to proceed with diagnostic testing and/or treatment recommendations, using similar criteria that they would use for the acceptance of new information as outlined in Chap. 6.

Nevertheless, it may be useful in persuading a patient as to what can potentially lie in the future for that patient, but it would probably be done in a more qualitative than quantitative way. Nevertheless, there may be some patient who would be keen to see the consequences of a decision laid out in a decision tree to visualize. Perhaps this would stimulate a discussion to achieve manifest rationality.

9.4 Big Data

9.4.1 What Is "Big Data"?

"Big Data" has become one of the magical buzzwords of the twenty-first century. It certainly seems that everyone is talking about it with giddy excitement. This is no question that the amount of information that is being generated, gathered, stored and used has increased beyond all reasonable imagination compared to before the computer era. This volume of data is astronomical in all fields, including healthcare. For example, in 2013, there was an estimated 153 exabytes[8] of health data produced

---

[8] An exabyte is 2^{60} or approximately 10^{18} bytes of data. One byte of data contains 8 bits of data. A bit of data is a single unit of data that a computer program can manipulate. By comparison, there

worldwide. This was projected, at the time, to increase to 2314 exabytes of data by 2020 [32]. I do not think anyone would dispute that this volume has been exceeded in our present day. In genomics alone, researchers deposited 4.5 petabytes[9] of data into the United States National Cancer Institute's Genomic Data Common from 2016 to 2017 [33]. Even routine activities can generate data. A typical hospitalization generates approximately 150,000 discrete pieces of data [34]. By any measure, these are colossal numbers. Therefore, this begs the question: Is this what "Bid Data" is?

There are many definitions of "big data" as, although stimulating the imagination, it is otherwise a fairly imprecise term. One definition from Banks [33] is that big data, as opposed to "small data," is too complex and varied to be contained on a spreadsheet or sometimes even on a computer. Shilo et al. [35] define big data as data with the size and complexity such that it cannot be analyzed by traditional data analytic methods. DeMauro et al. [36] state that big data are information assets characterized by high volume, velocity, and variety that require specific technology and analytic methods for its transformation into use. These are referred to as the three "Vs" of big data [37], but some also include a fourth V, which is veracity [38]. In my opinion, the last one is the quite important because large amounts of untrustworthy data will not be persuasive.

Although the amount of data is huge, the variety of data is equally impressive. Almost anything that can be stored digitally is data—numbers, words, images, and codes—in all languages. If it can be placed into a computer, it can become big data. This can be done with great speed. Almost at the moment of its inception, the data can be stored for later analysis. Of course, this poses various challenges with each step of handling big data, which can only be addressed by using high-end computing solutions for big data analysis [38]. One of the major challenges is the credibility and accuracy of the data. Data science has emerged to address various aspects of data, including data management and analysis, to extract deeper insights for improving the functionality or services of a system and to understand the functioning of complex systems.

9.4.2 Big Data and Healthcare

At present, big data is used primarily in health care research, particularly health services research. Big data is being used particularly in the private sector to analyze health care markets and insurance needs. However, there are numerous initiatives to use big data in a way that is specifically actionable for individual health care decisions. In this setting, Burton [39] points out that health is not a single state but a dynamic process of different states in different points in time that together assemble

are an estimated 7.5×10^{18} grains of sand on Earth.

[9] A petabyte is 2^{50} or approximately 10^{15} bytes of data.

a health trajectory. The goal of medicine is to understand and predict this trajectory for the individual patient, with the aim of redirecting the trajectory in the patient's favor. This trajectory can be considered a more continuous form of the health states with transitions that was discussed in the last section pertaining to decision analysis, Markov models and Monte Carlo simulations. Analyses of large-scale medical data may have the potential to identify new and unknown associations, patterns, and trends in the data that may pave the way for new scientific discoveries in the pathogenesis, classification, diagnosis, treatment, and progression of disease [35].

The Data

The data in big data come from numerous sources. These sources produce many types of data, such as administrative health data, biomarker data, biometric data, and imaging data, which can originate from many different sources [35]. Longitudinal population studies and biobanks represent two sources of big data [35]. Medical data can be characterized by certain properties: (1) structured vs unstructured, (2) patient-care-oriented vs research-oriented, (3) explicit vs implicit, and (4) raw vs ascertained (i.e., data without processing vs data after standardization and validation processing) [35]. Other sources and characteristics of big data include those from biological sources (e.g., hospital laboratory specimens, national/international biobanks, industry-collected samples), biometric sources (e.g., pulmonary function, exercise tolerance, cardiovascular function, neural activity), electronic sources (e.g., electronic health/medical records, DNA/RNA sequences, insurance-sourced data, smartphone medical applications), biological/biometric overlap sources (e.g., health fair specimens), biological/electronic overlap sources (e.g., imaging diagnostics), and electronic/biometric overlap sources (e.g., wearable medical devices) [40].

Special mention should be made of the electronic medical record. Electronic health or medical records are computerized medical records of a patient for any information relating to the past, present or future physical/mental health or condition of an individual which resides in an electronic system(s) used to capture, transmit, receive, store, retrieve, link and manipulate multimedia data for the primary purpose of providing healthcare and health-related services [41]. Electronic medical records contain a vast, valuable and varied amount of information, which is both structured and unstructured. Structured information is that data which is relatively easy to quantitize, such as laboratory values, or even ordered, "drop-down" descriptions. Unstructured information includes items such as the physician's or nurse's clinical note, which provides descriptions that are qualitative. How big data analytical tools handle unstructured data is still progressing.

A potential future source of continuous data may come from the devices around us. The "Internet of Things" is the concept that devices that can gather data are linked to the internet and can send and receive information [38]. This is envisioned as a system of wireless, interrelated, and connected digital services that can collect, send, and store data over a network without requiring human-to-human or human-to-computer interaction [42]. Such resources can interconnect various devices to provide reliable, effective and smart healthcare services to elderly individuals and patients with chronic conditions [43]. It has the potential to improve the accessibility of preventative public health services and transition our current secondary and tertiary care to be a more proactive, continuous and coordinated system [42]. However, issues with respect to confidence and acceptability, privacy and security, interoperability, standardization and remuneration, data storage, control and ownership remain to be solved [42].

Because of the variety of data, attempts have been made to define their properties more precisely. Shilo et al. [35] introduced the concept of "axes of data," which have the following quantitative properties: (1) number of participants, (2) depth of phenotyping, (3) length of longitudinal follow-up, (4) interactions between subjects included in the data, (5) heterogeneity and diversity of the cohort population, (6) standardization and harmonization of data, and (7) linkage between data sources.

Data Analytics

Of course, it is of no use to have data by itself; it must be analyzed for meaning. The volume and breadth of the data require advanced data analytics. These analytics come under the rubric of "data science" [44]. Data science has been divided into three distinct tasks: descriptive, prediction, and counterfactual prediction. Descriptive analysis uses data to provide a quantitative summary of certain features of the world [45]. Prediction analysis aims to learn a "mapping" from a set of inputs to some outcome of interest, such that the mapping can later be used to predict the outcome from the input in a different, unseen set [46]. This, using data computer science parlance, is what any medical research program hopes to accomplish. Namely, identifying information to enhance the predictability of an outcome. Much of Chaps. 5–7 were devoted to this concept. Last, counterfactual prediction aims to construct models that address limiting flaws inherent to observational data for inferring causality. This is essentially the same as the concepts of counterfactual causation discussed in Chap. 5.

There are many ways big data can be studied. There are several types of study designs specifically developed for big data [40], as well as a variety of data analytical techniques [47]. The details of which are more than what is required for this book, although I will discuss some aspects below in the "Artificial Intelligence" section. However, big data accumulation and analysis follow a basic four-step process (Fig. 9.5). What is distinctly missing from Fig. 9.5 is the *interpretation*—data, no matter how big—still requires an interpretation, let alone implementation, by at least one, usually more, human.

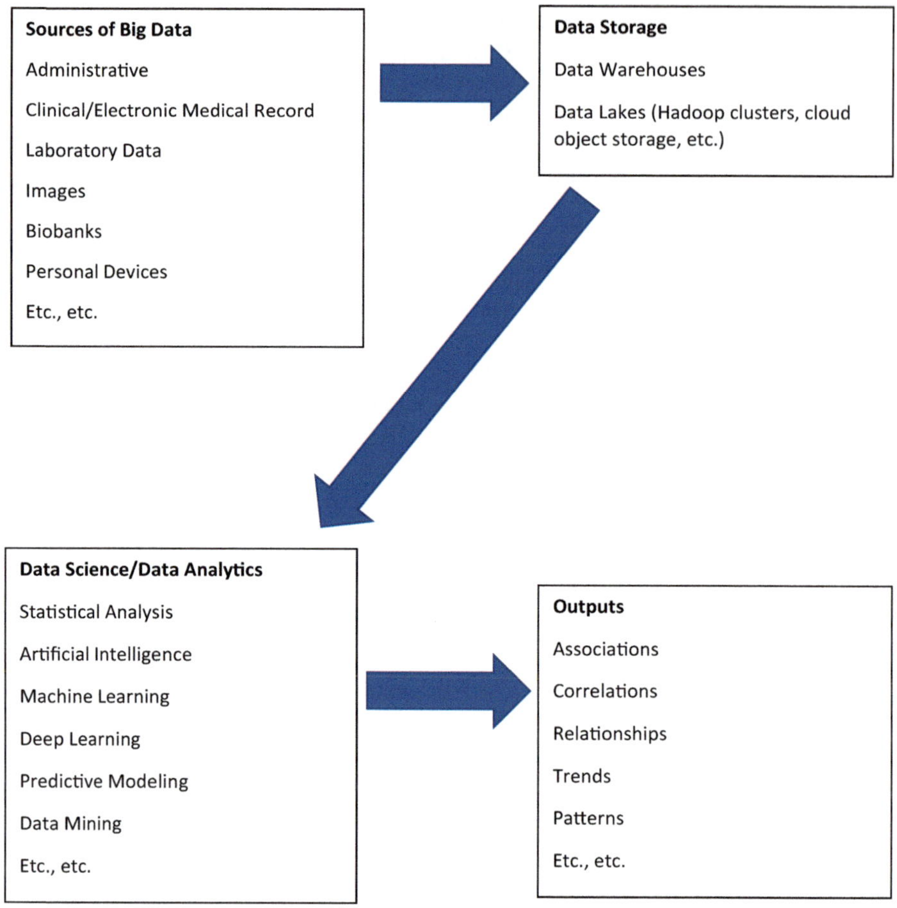

Fig. 9.5 Inputs, storage, analysis and outputs of big data

9.4.3 Strengths and Weaknesses of Big Data

The promise of big data is that we will be able to find solutions to intractable problems by using the large volume of data analyzed using computer analytics, which surpasses the computational and analytical capabilities of humans. Therefore, hidden or rare relationships may be revealed. Specifically, for healthcare, big data may be able to reveal health patterns and provide solutions to previously intransigent dilemmas [40]. There has certainly been much published in the medical literature using what had been characterized as "big data."

There are, however, limitations to these models. For use in actual clinical medicine, predictive models need to be continuously updated, accurate, well-calibrated and delivered at the individual level with adequate time for early and effective intervention by clinicians [35]. These are both theoretical and practical concerns. The point about being "continuously updated" harkens back to previous discussion about induction. That is, how reliable are past data in predicting future events? Although we have no other resources but to use past data, the problem remains. Furthermore, the induction problem of going from specifics (albeit a great number of specifics) to a general law or principle remains.

Another problem is that of "model interpretability," that is, understanding the mechanism by which the model works [48]. We will further discuss the "black box" nature of machine learning below. However, the point pertaining to the lack of transparency of the model, as well as a post hoc explanation of the model, leads to confusion and a lack of understanding [48]. When there is lack of understanding, persuasion fails. Moreover, it also appears that instead of going from hypothesis to data to conclusion, big data goes from data to conclusion to hypothesis. This is especially true for the "data-driven" models. This is quite reasonable as a "hypothesis-generating model" that identifies potential hypotheses to be tested. However, big data is touted as "actionable" analysis.

There are other practical issues. For routine clinical practice, the model should be cost-effective and broadly applicable [35]. In addition, as these models are entirely based on the data inputs, if these inputs are systematically in error or biased, the outputs will also be biased. For example, it has been identified that there are instances of big data models that produce racial biased outputs [49]. Mallappallil et al. [40] bemoan the fact that the murkiness of international laws, questions of data ownership, public ignorance and privacy and security concerns are "slowing the progress" of big data implementations. Others would disagree that this "slowing of progress" is problematic, but rather a recognition that abuse potential exists and safeguards against such potentials are needed.

Mallappallil et al. [40] listed other issues. Big data is heterogeneous in nature such that information may not be readily accessible. To that I would add that the information may be irrelevant. There may be limited insight into content and procedure, such that there could be an imbalance in power between the large, complex systems of international technology firms and a lone individual in the public. The data systems may not be compatible or integrated with other systems, such that an information silo is created where the data remain isolated within a dataset and are not adequately shared. Big data is vast and regulated under privacy laws, such that there is a risk of loss of privacy for participants, providers, and biological relatives. In some instances, there has been an insufficient vetting process of the technology, which has led to its premature introduction into the marketplace. Artificial intelligence can predict patterns and associations; although this is the first step in determining causal attribution, it can be used in unethical ways by commercial actors. There are also potential problems with data ownership and finances.

There are several companies that now provide big data services, whose motivations are entirely pecuniary.

9.4.4 *Big Data and Persuasion*

Although big data has certainly enjoyed a mystic prestige since its conceptualization was introduced, it is actually no different than any other method of developing premises for an argument. Big data may produce information that may be judged as more reliable than other methods, but that is a judgment for the consumer of that information, just as with any other source. Issues of causation remain. With big data, all arguments toward causation are stochastic probabilities. By the very nature of the analysis, there is no attempt at creating deterministic mechanisms of causal sequences. Therefore, the issues surrounding knowledge generation and acceptance, as well as clinical application, remain exactly the same as those described in Chap. 5–7.[10]

9.5 Patient Decision Aids and Physician Decision Support

9.5.1 *Patient Decision Aids*

In any clinical encounter, the patient is usually confronted with some type of healthcare choice. In Fig. 1.1, the choices have to do with accepting the diagnosis and treatment recommendations as presented by the physician. These choices can be difficult, especially for patients with a relatively low level of medical literacy. The physician, as part of the decision-making process, should inform the patient of their rationale for coming to the decisions that they have, such as the diagnosis and treatment recommendations, as well as reviewing the benefits and risks, as well as any options, of any treatment choice. Unfortunately, this process can be somewhat inconsistent, leading to poor comprehension of these decisions by the patient [50]. To address this deficiency, patient decision aids were created.

A patient decision aid is a means of helping people make informed choices about their health care that take into account their personal values and preferences [51]. This is essential in the doctrine of "shared decision-making," which was discussed in Chap. 4. That is, clinicians and patients work together to decide about treatments based on clinical evidence and the patient's valued preferences [52]. These patient decision aids must inform the patient about the available options from an evidence-based perspective, encourage active engagement of the patient with the decision-making process, and help the patient think through what is important to them so that they can make choices that reflect their own values and preferences [51]. These aids

---

[10] It will also be very interesting if we get to the point where individuals must consent to having their "data" in these large datasets. Although much, if not all, of the data is deidentified by the time the researcher receives it, I can easily see a level of suspicion, especially for commercial and governmental agencies, having access to these data.

need to improve the quality of the decision-making process and the quality of the choices made, that is, the "decision quality" [53].

At a minimum, a decision aid should describe the decisions that need to be made, the options available, and the outcomes of these options based on the evidence [51]. Of course, this last requirement of "based on the evidence" implies that there is agreement upon "best evidence." I previously discussed in Chap. 7 that sometimes the best evidence is not the most appropriate evidence. The presentation of the options may use various formats. A review of these formats is not essential for my purpose here, but there are resources available that provide templates of these formats for the interested reader.[11] Another key goal in a decision aid is an explanation of risks and consequences. In addition, decision aids should help patients think about their values and possible trade-offs [54].

The International Patient Decision Aids Standards collaboration lists decision aid requirements as [54]:[12]

1. A systematic development process for the creation of the aid.
2. The provision of information about options and probabilities.
3. Clarification of values.
4. Disclosure of conflicts of interest.
5. A balanced presentation of options.
6. Use of plain language.
7. Information based on current evidence.

This produces a decision aid with the core attributes for the patient of (1) recognition that a decision needs to be made, (2) feeling informed about the options and about the risks, benefits, and consequences of the options, (3) being clear about what matters most to them for this decision, (4) discussing goals, concerns, and preferences with their health care providers, and (5) being involved in decision making. This will lead to a quality decision with the core attributes of (1) an informed patient and (2) a concordance between what matters most to the patient and the chosen option [53].

Decision aids have been used for some time now and have been shown to lead to more accurate risk perceptions, reduced decisional conflict and improved patient–physician communication [55]. Lists of patient-related decision aids have been compiled [56].

---

[11] For example, https://www.optiongrid.co.uk.

[12] Another source of information is the Informed Medical Decisions Foundation. https://informedmedicaldecisions.org.

Patients Decision Aids and Persuasion

How do these aids function in persuasion? By helping patients develop their responses to the illative core of the physician's arguments for diagnosis and treatment recommendations, these are simply aids and prompts to help achieve manifest rationality. The patient is able to better question the physician's argument, and therefore, the physician is able to revise the argument in a manner acceptable to the patient. Therefore, the patient will be more likely to be persuaded.

9.5.2 Decision Support Systems for Physicians

Whereas the previous section discussed decision aids for the patient, in this section, I will discuss computerized decision support systems designed to promote better decision-making by the physician. Decision support systems are computer programs that use as their inputs the patient's clinical data and have their output conclusions about the patient's diagnosis/physical condition and treatment options [57]. These systems use "targeted clinical knowledge, patient information, and other health information" with computer software designed to be a direct aid to clinical decision-making in which characteristics of an individual patient are matched to a computerized clinical knowledge base and patient-specific assessments or recommendations are then presented to the clinician for a decision [58]. These systems are primarily intended to be used at the point of care for the patient. Computerized clinical decision support systems make use of web applications or integration with electronic medical records and computerized provider order entry [57]. Another source of information for these systems is big data repositories [40]. These systems can be administered through desktop and/or laptop computers, tablets, smartphones, biometric monitoring devices, and wearable health technology devices [57].

The classification of computer decision support systems includes knowledge-based systems and nonknowledge-based systems [57]. In knowledge-based systems, "rules" are created for how the program should use the input data to logically construct and produce a conclusion output of a suggested action [58]. The rules can come from the extant medical literature, the rules that physicians use in practice, or rules about patient-directed decisions, which are then written into the code of the computer program [58]. That is, the patient data are premises in an argument that the computer constructs from the programs menu of relevant rules to come to a conclusion. On the other hand, a nonknowledge-based system requires a data source, but the decision process is an artificial intelligence, machine learning, or statistical pattern recognition program based on statistical patterns that the program identifies (e.g., see the section on big data above and artificial intelligence below) rather than expert medical knowledge [59].

Computer decision support systems have several functions. These can include diagnostics, alarm systems, disease management, medication prescriptions, drug control, etc. These are operationalized in an electronic medical record as computerized alerts and reminders, computerized guidelines, order sets, patient data reports, documentation templates and clinical workflow tools [57]. Although quite useful, there are potential disadvantages and risks to these decision support systems. Table 9.1 provides a comparison of the advantages/benefits and the corresponding disadvantages/risks.

Computerized decision support systems do not actually make decisions. Physicians and patients do. The outputs of these programs are simply premises that the patient and physician can choose to believe and use in the construction of their arguments or not. As with any computer program, the veracity of the data is vital in producing reliable results. Moreover, as with any new source of knowledge, there will need to be a level of trust in the programs. More on this below.

9.5.3 *Risk Calculators*

One of the most important activities of a physician is the determination of risk. That is, what is the likelihood that some event, x, will occur in patient P over some arbitrary time interval t. For example, what is the likelihood that a 50-year-old male patient will develop colon cancer over the next 10 years? The answer to this question has significant consequences because the recommended time interval between colonoscopies could be as long as 10 years for the "average" risk patient, 5 years for the moderate risk patient, 3 years for a high risk patient, or 1 year for a "very high risk" patient. Because of this need to quantize risk for more accurate patient disease categorization (see Chap. 7), risk scores were developed for a variety of treatment decisions.

Initially, these risk scores were manually calculated, and nomograms were created to allow the physician to determine risk. However, with the ubiquity of online resources, risk calculators can now be easily accessed for this purpose. This could

Table 9.1 Advantages/benefits and disadvantages/risks of computerized decision support systems

Advantages and benefits	Disadvantages and risks
Patient safety	Alert fatigue
Clinical management	Negative impact on user skill
Cost containment	Financial challenges
Administrative function/automation	System and content maintenance challenges
Diagnostic support	User distrust
Imaging, laboratory, pathology support	Transportability/interoperability
Better documentation	Inaccurate and poor-quality data/documentation
Patient decision support	Dependency on computer literacy
Workflow improvement	Disrupted/fragmented workflow

be as simple as determining body mass index as a measure of obesity[13] to far more complex ones. Medscape [60] lists 480 medical calculators in 33 different categories.

As an example, one such risk calculator is offered by the American College of Surgeons based on their National Surgical Quality Improvement Program (NSQIP) [61]. This calculator estimates the risk of 30-day morbidity and mortality based on the operation type. Table 9.2 shows the factors involved in the calculation. If we take

Table 9.2 American College of Surgeons-National Surgical Quality Improvement predictive factors

Factor	Variable categories
Operation	CPT code[a]
Age group	<65, 65–74, 75–84, ≥85 years
Sex	Female, male
Functional status	Independent, partially dependent, totally dependent
Emergency case	No, yes
ASA[b] class	Health patient, mild systemic disease, severe systemic disease, severe systemic disease-constant threat to life, moribund-not expected to survive surgery
Steroid use	No, yes
Ascites within 30 days prior to surgery	No, yes
Systemic sepsis within 48 h prior to surgery	None, SIRS3[c], sepsis, septic shock
Ventilator dependent	No, yes
Disseminated cancer	No, yes
Diabetes	No, oral hypoglycemics, insulin dependent
Hypertension requiring medications	No, yes
Congestive heart failure within 30 days prior to surgery	No, yes
Dyspnea	None, with moderate exercise, at rest
Current smoker within 1 year	No, yes
History of COPD[d]	No, yes
Dialysis	No, yes
Acute renal failure	No, yes
Body mass index	Height, weight

[a] All operations have a code assigned through the Current Procedure Terminology (CPT) published by the American Medical Association

[b] The American Society of Anesthesiologists (ASA) classification of a patient's general preoperative health status. This is designated preoperatively by the attending anesthesiologists

[c] SIRS stands for systemic inflammatory response syndrome, a syndrome frequently, but not always, associated with infection that causes a generalized inflammatory response

[d] COPD stands for chronic obstructive pulmonary disease

[13] For example, the Centers for Disease Control and Prevention has such a calculator. https://www.cdc.gov/healthyweight/assessing/bmi/adult_bmi/english_bmi_calculator/bmi_calculator.html, last accessed October 22, 2022.

an example of a 64-year-old female with a body mass index of 24 requiring a partial colectomy (current procedural terminology [CPT] code 44140) with no risk factors, Table 9.3 reports the predicted probabilities of the occurrence within 30 days of 15 potential adverse events. Table 9.3 also reports the predicted probabilities of a patient at the opposite end of the risk spectrum—an 86-year-old female with a body mass index of 44 and the most severe of every risk factor. The healthy 64-year-old has an overall risk of any complication of 10% and a risk of perioperative death so infinitesimal that it was calculated as 0. The 86-year-old moribund patient, on the other hand, has a near perfect chance of perioperative death at 99.8%. Clearly, this information can be used in patient counseling and decision making. The first patient can be offered an operation confidently, and she can feel secure that she will survive the procedure. The second patient should not be operated upon and should be counseled that hospice is the humane choice for her.

The value of these calculators is in providing actual probability data with which the physician and the patient can use and premises in their arguments pertaining to treatment options.

Table 9.3 Predicted 30 day adverse outcomes of two patients undergoing a partial colectomy with anastomosis

Outcome	64 year old female, BMI 24, no risk factors	86 year old female, BMI 44, all risk factors
Serious complication	6.8%	92.3%
Any complication	10.0%	95.5%
Pneumonia	0.3%	61.1%
Cardiac complication	0.1%	62.1%
Surgical site infection	5.7%	15.4%
Urinary tract infection	0.9%	7.7%
Venothrombolic event	0.8%	20.2%
Renal failure	0.1%	N/A (preoperative renal failure present)
Colectomy ileus	11.4%	76.3%
Colectomy anastomotic leak	2.4%	7.3%
Readmission	4.2%	58.5%
Unplanned return to the operating room	3.5%	34.3%
Death	0.0%	99.8%
Discharge to nursing or rehabilitation facility	1.1%	99.6%
Sepsis	1.3%	N/A (preoperative septic shock present)

9.6 Artificial Intelligence and Applications to Healthcare

9.6.1 What Is Artificial Intelligence?

Artificial intelligence has certainly received much attention and interest; however, it is poorly understood by the general public [62], including medical practitioners. It seems to engender a certain mystical or supernatural quality in the common mind, resulting in either giddy admiration or fearful loathing. The term "artificial intelligence" was coined by Stanford University professor John McCarthy in 1955 [63], and he provided the first definition—"getting a computer to do things which, when done by people, are said to involve intelligence" [62]. Since then, several other definitions have been proposed:

> Machines that respond to simulation consistent with traditional responses from humans given the human capacity for contemplation, judgment, and intention [62].
>
> The ability of a digital computer or computer-controlled robot to perform tasks commonly associated with intelligent beings [64].
>
> An intelligent entity created by humans [64].
>
> [A computer program] Capable of performing tasks intelligently without being explicitly instructed [64].
>
> [A computer program] Capable of thinking and acting rationally and humanely [64].

Such systems are said to have three qualities: intentionality, intelligence, and adaptability [62].

Functionally, artificial intelligence is computer software that codes a set of algorithms that can produce results without having to be explicitly instructed to do so [64]. The algorithm(s) is a crucial feature of the programs. An algorithm is a process or set of rules to be followed in calculations or other problem-solving operations, especially by, but not isolated to, a computer [65]. The goal of an algorithm is to solve a specific problem, usually defined by someone as a sequence of steps [65]. Fundamentally, any set of instructions can be viewed as an algorithm. For example, the steps described for a surgical procedure are a type of physical algorithm solving the patient's anatomic problem. However, for the most part, algorithms are thought of in a computational sense. In artificial intelligence, algorithms are designed to allow computers to learn on their own. These algorithms were initially written in computer codes (e.g., Python, Java, etc.) by programmers based on mathematical and/or statistical assumptions [65].

Categories of Artificial Intelligence

Artificial intelligence can be broadly categorized into three increasingly sophisticated classes [65]:

1. Narrow artificial intelligence, which are specialized programs dedicated to one area of interest, solving problems in that area. This type of program is currently available and solves problems in very controlled environments. For example, chess-playing artificial intelligence programs.

2. General artificial intelligence, which is machine intelligence that can be applied broadly in the same way humans can apply their intelligence across a breadth of tasks necessary for their existence. At present, there are no programs available that have achieved this (at least, none that are known to the general public).
3. Super artificial intelligence, which is a theoretical concept of a machine with superior intellectual capabilities compared to humans and, perhaps, a consciousness and sense of self-awareness. Again, at present, there are no known programs that have this capability.

Some also categorize artificial intelligence programs into weak and strong forms [64]. The weak forms are programs with narrow applications with limited scope, are good at a specific task, and use supervised and unsupervised learning to process data. The strong forms have wider applications with a more varied scope, have human-level intelligence, and use clustering and association to process data [64].

"Supervised" learning entails a process where a human programmer/user supplies specific rules that the program must follow, while in "unsupervised" learning, the program is allowed to revise its algorithms without human guidance. Supervised programs can also be referred to as knowledge-based, while unsupervised programs can also be referred to as data-driven. Knowledge-based artificial intelligence starts with information entered by humans to solve a query in a domain of expertise formalized by the software. Data-driven artificial intelligence starts with large amounts of data generated by human activity to make a prediction [66, 67].

Types of Artificial Intelligence

There is no one type of artificial intelligence program. There are several types of programs that are considered forms of artificial intelligence.

1. *Machine learning* programs teach machines how to make inferences and decisions based on past experience [64]. In reality, the "machine" (i.e., the computer) is not "taught" anything, but rather, as the programs run through the input data in its algorithms, it is able to revise the algorithms to achieve a better "fit" of the data to the identified patterns or associations. It identifies patterns and analyzes past data to infer the "meaning" of these data points to reach a possible conclusion without having to involve human experience [64]. To clarify, "meaning" in this usage is not an increase in understanding but a maximization of data fit into a particular pattern. In machine learning, a set of algorithms enables the software to update and "learn"[14] from previous outcomes without the need for programmer intervention. Structured data are downloaded for the program to complete a

[14] Use of such words by artificial intelligence enthusiasts such as "teaches," "learns," "meaning," etc., anthropomorphizes these programs in a way that implies that these hardware computers and software programs have a human-like quality that they do not. One should take such, perhaps unconscious, efforts at anthropomorphization with some healthy skepticism.

task without being programmed to do so [65]. Figure 9.6 shows the basic flow of a stylized machine learning program.
2. *Deep learning* programs are a subset of machine learning, such that the program teaches the machine to process inputs through multiple layers to classify, infer and predict the outcome [64].
3. *Neural networks* are programs that work on principles similar to those of human neural cells. These programs contain a series of algorithms that capture the relationship between various underlying variables by processing data similar to a human brain. The connections between the variables can be positive or negative through the neurodes and can be hidden in the architecture (Fig. 9.7).
4. *Natural language processing* is a program dedicated to reading, understanding, and interpreting a language by a machine [64].
5. *Computer vision* is a program containing algorithms that understand an image by disassembling the image and studying its different component parts [64].
6. *Cognitive computing* are programs that contain algorithms that mimic a human brain by analyzing text/speech/images/objects in a manner that a human does and tries to give the desired output [64].

We must also make the distinction between artificial intelligence and augmented intelligence. Artificial intelligence implies that the program replaces human input with its own and operates with a high level of accuracy; it replaces human decision-making; and, in the internet of things or robot form, it will replace all human in menial manufacturing tasks. On the other hand, augmented intelligence does not replace humans but creates systems that enhance human capabilities, enhances human decision-making, and, in the internet of things and robot form, works along with humans to ease tasks that are difficult or repetitive [64].

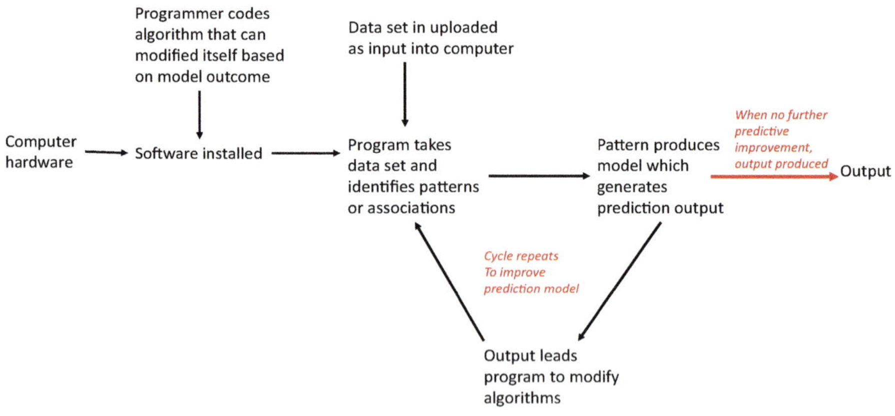

Fig. 9.6 The basic method of how a machine learning program learns from the output of its analysis is to adjust its algorithms until no further improvement is reached in its prediction model. Then, the final output is presented to users of the program

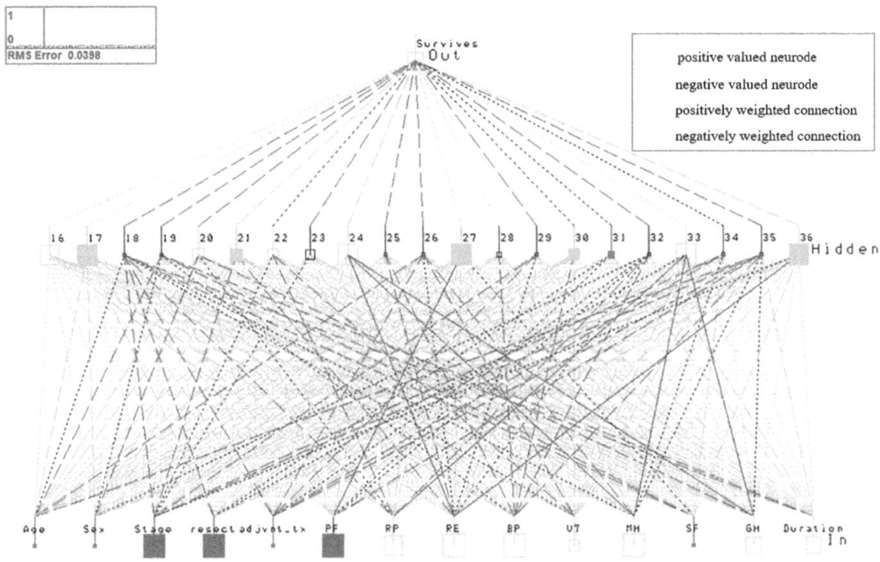

Fig. 9.7 An example of an artificial neural network with positive and negative neurodes that have positive and negative connections through one "hidden" layer of architecture. (From Walczak S, Velanovich V. Evaluation of artificial neural networks in predicting pancreatic cancer survival. J Gastrointest Surg 2017;21:1606–1612, Springer)

9.6.2 Machine Learning Programs/Tools

Machine learning programs, which are a subset of artificial intelligence, can further generate output data that are derived from input data [40]. That is, these programs contain algorithms that can come to some type of conclusion as an output. To some extent, in a manner of speaking, such artificial intelligence programs can create new knowledge from big data [40]. A distinction must be made between traditional and machine learning algorithms. A traditional algorithm outputs results, whereas a machine learning algorithm outputs a model that outputs results. A machine learning algorithm takes an input and an output and gives some logical structure that can be used to work with the new input to give one an output. The logical structure generated is to best fit the data into a pattern and revise the algorithms to do so—this is what makes it machine learning [40].

Data that the program uses can be structured or unstructured. Structured data have precise meanings, such as numbers or ordinally ranked descriptions. Unstructured data are natural language-based narrative descriptions. Approximately 80% of medical data are unstructured text (e.g., medical notes). Tools are needed to extract meaning from the natural language of the text [33], which may lead to misinterpretation and can affect the reliability of the output.

Ultimately, machine learning artificial intelligence programs seek patterns, associations and correlations within the data. The nature of the results is not different from any other method of data analysis. The results still require an interpretation—the real question is whether the computer is empowered to do the interpretation and act, or if this must be done by a human. The philosophical issues of determining causation, as discussed in Chap. 5, remain. That is, the output of a machine learning process is not a mechanistically deterministic causal sequence but a probabilistic causal association at best.

However, unlike a human, such knowledge will not enhance the understanding or wisdom of the program because the underlying code is not malleable (not to be confused for the algorithms, which are). The programs do not judge the inputs and outputs. The program never decides if the output "makes sense." It does not "know" if it is doing good or evil. On the other hand, whether such knowledge enhances the wisdom and understanding of a particular human reviewing the output would be exactly the same as that human reviewing any other medical information claiming new knowledge, as discussed in Chap. 6.

9.6.3 Artificial Intelligence-Possible Clinical Applications

Artificial intelligence programs are already in use in many applications in many fields of business, science and medicine, among other areas. In the medical fields, several types are being employed by payers and providers of care, as well as life science companies [68]. These programs are involved in diagnosis and treatment recommendations, patient engagement and adherence to health recommendations, and a variety of administrative activities [68]. Ameen et al. [69] list numerous examples of highly efficacious modeling capabilities of supervised machine learning programs, and I will not enumerate them here. Additionally, they have documented that unsupervised machine learning using a data-driven approach independent of human interference can successfully disentangle "meaning" out of complex data structures [69].

Predictions

The use of machine learning programs to generate predictions of outcomes based on extant datasets is one of its most common uses. For example, machine learning programs are used in precision medicine to predict which treatment protocols are likely to succeed on a particular patient based on various patient attributes and treatment contexts [70]. A machine learning analysis led by Google of 216,221 electronic health records for adult patients hospitalized for at least a day was effective at predicting in-hospital mortality, 30-day unplanned readmissions and all final diagnoses [57]. Figure 9.6 pertaining to an artificial neural network architectural structure is from a study predicting survival after pancreatic cancer treatment [71].

Diagnostic Dilemmas

Diagnostic dilemmas are those situations in which the patient has some illness that has evaded all attempts at diagnosis. The patient is clearly unwell, but all clinical evaluations and tests have failed to determine from what. Although this is a relatively unusual situation in modern Western medicine, it certainly has vexed nearly every physician at one time or another. Such a situation may be appropriate for artificial intelligence diagnostic programs.

Humans can be afflicted by legions of known diseases as well as an untold number of unknown diseases. The International Classification of Disease 10th Revision (ICD-10) contains over 69,000 diagnostic codes [72]. Although not each of these codes represents a unique disease, it is still fair to say that there are tens of thousands of diseases that can afflict humans. It is, of course, impossible for a single physician to know all of these possible maladies, let alone their diagnostic criteria and treatments. Many of these obscure diseases are quite rare, further pushing them out of the body of knowledge of the typical physician. Because of a computer's ability to store and retrieve vast amounts of data, these rare diseases or other diseases causing diagnostic dilemmas may be appropriate for artificial intelligence programs.

Rare Diseases

In fact, in a scoping review [73] of machine learning in the diagnosis of rare disease, 211 studies of 74 diseases were studied using machine learning methods. De La Vega et al. [74] showed that an artificial intelligence program could successfully identify rare genetic disease diagnostic candidates by genome interpretation in 90% of cases. Although certainly not ready for widespread clinical applications yet, Mirbabaie et al. [75] provide a path guiding future research in artificial intelligence diagnosis.

An Example of Early Sepsis Identification

Sepsis is usually, but always, caused by an infectious agent, usually a bacterial infection. It is well accepted that early treatment with antibiotics and/or other therapies directed at controlling the source of sepsis is the most effective method of reducing mortality and complications related to sepsis. To this end, Henry et al. [76] developed a machine learning program for the identification of early sepsis. This program was developed as a decision support tool that was trained on historical electronic medical record data to recognize sepsis early in its progression using a mixture model of several Cox proportional hazards models to account for patient heterogeneity. The developed program, the Targeted Real-Time Early Warning System (TREWS), was then installed in two academic and three community hospitals' electronic medical records systems. TREWS monitored each hospitalized patient's relevant data (vital signs, laboratory results, notes, medication history [excluding antibiotic history], procedure history and clinical history) as inputs. When the program identifies a patient who may possibly have sepsis, it sends an alert to that patient's providers through the electronic medical record to notify them that sepsis may be present.

In a trial of this system in the five hospitals of 173,931 patient encounters over a 26-month period, TREWS was shown to have 82% sensitivity for identifying septic patients [76]. Moreover, 89% of sent alerts prompted patient evaluations from one or more of the patient's providers, and of these evaluations, 38% of evaluated septic alerts were confirmed by the provider [76]. This is a false positive rate of 62%, with a positive predictive value of 27% [76]. Of the patients with provider-confirmed sepsis, there was a median reduction in the ordering of antibiotics by 1.85 h [76]. This resulted in an adjusted absolute reduction in mortality of 3.3% and an adjusted relative reduction in mortality of 18.7% [77]. That is, the artificial intelligence machine learning program monitoring hospitalized patients' data was able to identify many septic patients early, and the resulting actions by the providers reduced the mortality of these patients.

Image-Based Diagnosis

Most medical images, such as radiologic images and pathologic images, are now digitalized for storage in the electronic medical record. That is, these images are "pixelated" by the computer for storage. These images are therefore available for computer analysis using computer vision-directed artificial intelligence machine learning techniques.

There is evidence to suggest that artificial intelligence programs pertaining to image interpretation can perform better than humans in some radiological diagnostic tasks [68]. Moreover, computer vision can "see" these pixelated images better than humans. The field of "radiomics" studies features on an image that are beyond the perception of the human eye but not to the artificial intelligence program in pixelated form [68]. These types of artificial intelligence programs are being pursued commercially. The company Infervision has over 1 million radiological images as of 2019, which it is using to develop AI algorithms for imaging diagnosis [33].

Similar efforts are being put forth in pathological diagnosis [78]. However, at this point, there are few actual results to report.

9.6.4 Artificial Intelligence-Possible Research Applications

Hypothesis Generation

Artificial intelligence machine learning programs are essentially a type of statistical methodology that identifies associations, patterns and correlations, usually from retrospective datasets. In this sense, they are not different from other observational studies, as discussed in Chap. 6. Therefore, similar to observational studies, the results of research using machine learning programs can generate hypotheses to be tested with either prospective study designs or experimental/interventional study designs.

Drug Development

Drug discovery and development has been another fruitful area for artificial intelligence. Using machine learning programs, pharmaceutical researchers can better identify potential molecular candidates that may have pharmacological actions and reduce the time to develop these drugs [79, 80]. For example, an artificial intelligence program was able to predict with great accuracy the three-dimensional shape into which proteins fold based solely on the amino acid sequence [81].

9.6.5 Limitations of Artificial Intelligence

Artificial intelligence is just another method of generating premises that can be used in argumentation, like any other statistical method. However, it has its own limitations.

The Black Box

Because these programs are taken in inputs, process the inputs, and then produce outputs without the intermediate steps being transparent, there is difficulty in understanding the logic that these artificial intelligence programs use to produce recommendations. This has been referred to as the "black box" nature of machine learning [82]. Additionally, the outputs tend to be aggregate in nature, such as sensitivities and specificities are calculated for the entire machine learning process, so that physicians have difficulty in understanding how these conclusions can be used clinically [83]. This black box nature is philosophically not much different, *prima facie*, that traditional healers appeal to unseen spiritual forces or magic.

Problems with Data and Implementation

A theoretical concern is that artificial intelligence programs rely on forms of reductive reasoning and computational determinism that embed problematic assumptions about clinical decision-making and clinical practice, such that clinical autonomy, experience and judgment are reduced to inputs and outputs framed as binary or multiclassification problems benchmarked against a clinician's capacity to identify or predict disease states [69]. Ameen et al. [69] list the potential limitations and risks of artificial intelligence reductive reasoning as follows:

1. Artificial intelligence systems have inherent biases due to (a) the nature of the retrospective training datasets and (b) the embedded assumptions in the underlying artificial intelligence program's architectures and algorithms.
2. Limited evaluations of artificial intelligence systems prior to integration into clinical practice.
3. The marginalization of sociotechnical factors in the context-dependent interactions among clinicians, patients and the health system.

These authors caution that there should be a more nuanced and balanced approach to these systems. In other words, the inputs and outputs should not be taken at face value but should undergo the same judgment process that the healthcare professional would use for any other new knowledge.

With respect to clinical practice, health information technologies, although widely touted as indispensable, disruptive, and quantum leaps forward as a result of the research that developed these technologies, rarely achieve the touted claims in real-world clinical practice results [69]. There are also unintended and unanticipated consequences at the interface between new health information technologies and socio-organizational systems, such that there is the potential for the creation of more errors rather than a reduction of them [84, 85]. Over-optimism on the promise of medical artificial intelligence and haphazard consequences may arise if sufficient external evaluations of the impact on patient outcomes in varied settings prior to clinical integration do not occur [86].

Artificial intelligence systems have their own limitations that require attention, for example, problematic representational, temporal, and cultural biases embedded in end-data used to train the programs' algorithms [87, 88]. Issues related to the data include human-introduced errors in data collection and labeling and interobserver variability among labelers, which can affect the generalizability of the program's results because of its dependence on diverse and equitable data distribution, which may not always be achieved in big data [69]. Another potential issue is data availability [82]. Artificial intelligence program computations discretely frame problems of the real world independent of context. For example, IBM Watson has had difficulties in being taught to address particular types of cancers and integrating Watson into care healthcare processes and systems [68].

These challenges can be summarized as follows [68, 69]:

Dataset challenges: Representational bias, temporal bias, cultural bias, noise and artifacts, and class imbalances.

Epistemological challenges embedded in the training of machine learning models: Inability to appropriately learn context, inability to adapt outside model constraints, challenges of model drift, tendency to reinforce bias in data distributions, confined to problem frame preimposed by the human programmer.

Challenges to clinical decision-making: Automation complacency, confirmational bias, algorithmic bias, tendency to deflect accountability to the artificial intelligence program, limited interpretability of the models.

Broader conceptual challenges related to impact on modern medicine: Clinician autonomy, patient autonomy, changes in clinical interaction with the artificial intelligence program, accountability and insensitivity to the impact of artificial intelligence, diverse socio-organizational and sociocultural contexts.

Model adaptation in the presence of distributional data shift [89]: A mismatch between the training data and unanticipated and/or evolving patient/healthcare contexts that emerges at a later point in time, an inability of an artificial intelligence algorithm to accurately adapt to such a nonstationary clinical operational environment due to the way the model frames its assumptions of the world [90]; for example, when historical electronic medical record data are used to train a machine learning algorithm and new data are later recorded and captured by the electronic medical record due to new clinical practices, which then cause "model drift" [91–93].

Algorithms are unaware of situational context, where environmental factors may have a significant impact on the appropriateness of the predictions [69].

There are potential solutions to these issues, which may mitigate these adverse effects [69]. For example, in the patient context [94], missing data can be handled [95], untrustworthy alerts can be suppressed [96], and reliability and transportability can be improved [97, 98]. Healthcare professionals consuming the results of conclusions based on artificial intelligence programs should be cognizant of such issues and how they were mitigated.

9.6.6 Artificial Intelligence and Persuasion

Although it is clear that the present, and most likely the future, artificial intelligence programs are powerful statistical tools to analyze very large datasets to identify patterns, associations, and correlations, they are not a substitute for human intelligence. They provide premises for any eventual argument that the physician may wish to construct. There is nothing intrinsically more insightful about the data outputs of artificial intelligence than any other data analytic method. Because of the large datasets used, perhaps more of the associations and correlations will be statistically significant, but that does not infer clinical significance. They will be subject to the same methods of determining if the new knowledge created should be added to the physician's existing corpus of knowledge. The black box nature of the process may prove to be a barrier to some physicians. On the other hand, if these methods can be shown in an understandable way that the information provided is useful, they will be incorporated into the physician's practice.

It is unclear how persuasive the outputs of artificial intelligence programs will be for the patient. It will most likely be even more difficult for the patient to understand the outputs. This will require careful presentation of the illative core to the patient.

9.7 Non-Human Based Decisions and Human Persuasion

In the examples of computer-based and/or quantitazation of the decision process, one thing is very clear. *The only data a computer algorithm can analyze are those data that can be digitalized.* The "analog" data of what the physician observes and hears from the patient, which may greatly affect the physician's judgment and may not even be characterizable, cannot be made into "bits" of data for a computer algorithm. Perhaps there are correlations with other digitalized data, but this cannot be known for sure. The computer will have no intuition or understand the social and cultural context in which the patient perceives their illness, as depicted in Fig. 6.1, for example. Although this can change in the future, at the present time, the computer is disassociated from actually implementing any of its outputs. A person is required to review the output and proceed with its implementation. Perhaps at some point, an artificial intelligence robot may be able to implement treatments based on algorithmic treatment target identification, but this will certainly add a layer of complexity to ethical and accountability issues.

9.7.1 Computers and Wisdom

Computers produce calculated output, not wisdom or *phronesis*. One can say that this part of intelligence is completely absent from artificial intelligence. In fact, in this sense, the "intelligence" in artificial intelligence is a misnomer. The outputs dispensed by an artificial intelligence program are merely a premise, perhaps a very strong, reliable premise to be sure, but still a premise, to be used in an argument toward a conclusion. It is not a conclusion itself. It is left to the physician to determine its value.

9.7.2 Will Humans Be Persuaded by Computers?

The computer does not provide an argument; therefore, it cannot persuade. The outputs have to be used by a physician, and any conclusions made with manifest rationality with the patient. However, knowledge that some of the premise used in the physician's illative core came from computer output may affect the acceptance of those premises one way or another depending on the patient's social and cultural umwelt.

9.7.3 *The Beethoven String Quartet Dilemma Revisited*

I started this chapter with the Beethoven string quartet dilemma. That is, it takes the same number of musicians to play a string quartet piece of music now as it did in the eighteenth century. In other words, there was no increase in the productivity of these musicians. So now the question is, has computer-based health information technology improved the productivity of the physician? Certainly, access to information is easier as well as other aspects of ordering and communication. However, the essential interaction between the physician and patient, as well as the physician actually thinking about the patient, is unchanged.

References

1. Densen P. Challenges and opportunities facing medical education. Trans Am Clin Climatol Assoc. 2011;122:48–58.
2. Gower T. What are medical journals? WebMD, 12 May 2021. https://webmd.com. Last accessed 16 Oct 2022.
3. Florida Board of Medicine. Medical Doctor—Unrestricted. https://flboardofmedicine.gov/licensing/medical-doctor-unrestricted. Last accessed 16 Oct 2022.
4. Association of American Medical Colleges. Specialty profiles. https://www.aamc.org/cim/explore-options/specialty-profiles. Last accessed 16 Oct 2022.
5. Baumol WJ, Bowen WG. Performing arts: the economic dilemma. New York: Twentieth Century Fund; 1966.
6. Kleindorfer PR, Kunreuther HC, Schoemaker PJH. Decision sciences: an integrative perspective. Cambridge: Cambridge University Press; 1993.
7. Schulkin J. Decision sciences and evidence-based medicine—two intellectual movements to support clinical decision making. Acad Med. 2000;75:816–8.
8. Gilovich T. How we know what isn't so: the fallibility of human reason in everyday life. New York: The Free Press; 1991.
9. Howard JG. The foundations of decision analysis. IEEE Trans Syst Sci Cybernet. 1968;SSC-4:211–9.
10. Dobler CC, Guyatt GH, Wang Z, Murad HM. User's guide to medical decision analysis. Mayo Clin Proc. 2021;96:2205–17.
11. Clinical Decision Consultative Services. Tufts Medical Center. https://tuftsmedicalcenter.org/patient-care-services/Departments-and-Services/Clinical-Decision-Making/Clinical-Care-and-Services/Clinical-Decision-Consultative-Service. Last accessed 16 Oct 2022.
12. Weinstein MC, Fineberg HV. Clinical decision analysis. Philadelphia: WB Saunders Co; 1980.
13. Centers for Disease Control and Prevention. Life tables. https://www.cdc.gov/nchs/products/life_tables.htm. Last accessed 18 Oct 2022.
14. Beck JR, Kassirer JP, Pauker SG. A convenient approximation of life expectancy (the "DEALE"). I. Validation of method. Am J Med. 1982;73:883–8.
15. Beck JR, Pauker SG, Gottlieb JE, et al. A convenient approximation of life expectancy (the "DEALE"). II. Use in medical decision-making. Am J Med. 1982;73:889–97.
16. Lenderking WR, Revicki DA, editors. Advancing health outcomes research methods and clinical applications. McLean, VA: Degnon Associates, Inc.; 2005.
17. Pieterse AH, Stiggelbout A. What are values, utilities, and preferences? A clarification in the context of decision-making in health care, and an exploration of measurement issues. In:

Diefenbach MA, Miller-Halegoua S, Bowen DJ, editors. Handbook of health decision science. New York: Springer; 2016.
18. Schwartz SH, Bilsky W. Toward an universal psychological structure of human values. J Pers Soc Psychol. 1987;53:550–62.
19. Rohan MJ. A rose by any name? The values construct. Person Soc Psychol Rev. 2000;4:255–77.
20. Schwartz SH. Are there universal aspects in the structure and contents of human values? J Soc Issues. 1994;50:19–45.
21. Baron J. Thinking and deciding. New York: Cambridge University Press; 2008.
22. Brennan PF, Strombom I. Improving health care by understanding patient preferences: the role of computer technology. J Am Med Inform Assoc. 1998;5:257–62.
23. Velanovich V. Using quality of life instruments to assess surgical outcomes. Surgery. 1999;126:1–4.
24. Wakker P, Stiggelbout A. Explaining distortions in utility elicitation through the rank-dependent model for risk choices. Med Decis Mak. 1995;15:180–6.
25. Torrence GW, Feeny D, Furlong W. Visual analog scales: do they have a role in measurement of preferences for health states? Med Decis Mak. 2001;21:329–34.
26. Ryan M, Farrar S. Using conjoint analysis to elicit preferences for health care. BMJ. 2000;320:1530–3.
27. Spechler SJ, Hunter JG, Jones KM, et al. Randomized trial of medical versus surgical treatment for refractory heartburn. N Engl J Med. 2019;381:1513–23.
28. Sonnenberg FA, Beck JR. Markov models in medical decision-making: a practical guide. Med Decis Mak. 1993;13:322–38.
29. Harrison RL. Introduction to Monte Carlo simulations. AIP Conf Proc. 2010;1204:17–21.
30. Siebert U, Alagoz O, Bayoumi AM, et al. State-transition modeling: a report of the ISPOR-SMDM modeling good research practice task force 3. Value Health. 2012;15:812–20.
31. Frazao TDC, Camilo DGG, Cabral ELS, Souza RP. Multicriteria decision analysis (MCDA) in health care: a systematic review of the main characteristics and methodological steps. BMC Med Inform Decis Making. 2018;18:90.
32. EMC Digital Universe with Research and Analysis by IDC, Apr 2014.
33. Banks MA. Sizing up big data. Nat Med. 2020;26:5–6.
34. Esteva A, Robicquet A, Ramsundar B, et al. A guide to deep learning in healthcare. Nat Med. 2019;25:24–9.
35. Shilo S, Rossman H, Segal E. Axes of a revolution: challenges and promises of big data in healthcare. Nat Med. 2020;26:29–38.
36. DeMauro A, Greco M, Grimaldi M. A formal definition of big data based on its essential features. Lib Rev. 2016;65:122–35.
37. Laney D. 3D data management: controlling data volume, velocity, and variety, application and delivery strategies. Stamford, CT: META Group, Inc.; 2001.
38. Dash S, Shakyawar SK, Sharma M, Kaushik S. Big data in healthcare management, analysis and future prospects. J Big Data. 2019;6:54.
39. Burton-Jeangros C, Cullati S, Sacker A, Blane D. A life course perspective on health trajectories and transitions, vol. 4. New York: Springer; 2015.
40. Mallappallil M, Sabu J, Gruessner A, Salifu M. A review of big data and medical research. SAGE Open Med. 2020;8:1–10.
41. Reisman M. EHR's: the challenges of making electronic data usable and interoperable. Pharm Ther. 2017;42:572–5.
42. Kelly JT, Campbell KL, Gong E, Scuffham P. The internet of things: impact and implications for health care delivery. J Med Internet Res. 2020;22:e20135.
43. Yin Y, Zeng Y, Chen X, Fan Y. The internet of things in healthcare: an overview. J Ind Inf Integr. 2016;1:3–13.
44. Donoho D. 50 years of data science. J Comput Graph Stat. 2017;26:745–66.
45. Hernan MA, Hsu J, Healy B. A second chance to get causal inference right: a classification of data science tasks. Chance. 2019;32:42–9.

46. LeCun Y, Bengio Y, Hinton G. Deep learning. Nature. 2015;521:436–44.
47. Beinrohr L, Kail E, Piros P, et al. Anatomy of a data science software toolkit that uses machine learning to aid 'bench-to-bedside' medical research—with essential concepts of data mining and analysis explained. Appl Sci. 2021;11:12135.
48. Lipton ZC. Mythos of model interpretability. Commun ACM. 2018;61:36–43.
49. Obermeyer Z, Powers B, Vogeli C, Mullainathan S. Dissecting racial bias in an algorithm used to manage the health of populations. Science. 2019;366:447–53.
50. Hall DE, Prochazka AV, Fink AS. Informed consent for clinical treatment. CMAJ. 2012;184:533–40.
51. Drug and Therapeutics Bulletin. An introduction to patient decision aids. BMJ. 2013;346:f4147.
52. Coutler A, Collins A. Making shared decision-making a reality: no decision about me without me. 2011. https://www.kingsfund.org/uk/publications/nhs_decisionmaking.html. Last accessed 22 Oct 2022.
53. Sepucha KR, Borkhoff CM, Lally J, et al. Establishing the effectiveness of patient decision aids: key constructs and measurement instruments. BMC Med Inform Decis Making. 2013;13(Suppl 2):S12.
54. International Patient Decision Aids Standards Collaboration. Criteria for judging the quality of patient decision aids. 2005. https://ipdas.ohri.ca/IPDAS_checklist.pdf. Last accessed 22 Oct 2022.
55. Stacey D, Bennett CL, Berry MJ, et al. Decision aids for people facing health treatment or screening decisions. Cochrane Database Syst Rev. 2011;10:CD001431.
56. Patient Decision Aids. https://decisionaid.ohri.ca/AZinvent.php. Last accessed 22 Oct 2022.
57. Sutton RT, Pincock B, Baumgart DC, et al. An overview of clinical decision support systems: benefits, risks, and strategies for success. NPJ Digit Med. 2018;1:18.
58. Sim I, Gorman P, Greenes RA, et al. Clinical decision support systems for the practice of evidence-based medicine. J Am Med Inform Assoc. 2001;8:527–34.
59. Berner ES, editor. Clinical decision support systems. New York: Springer; 2007.
60. Medscape. Drugs & diseases. Calculators. https://references.medscape.com/guide/medical.calculators. Last accessed 22 Oct 2022.
61. American College of Surgeons National Surgical Quality Improvement Program. Risk calculator. https://riskcalculator.facs.org/RiskCalculator. Last accessed 17 Oct 2022.
62. West DM. What is artificial intelligence? Brookings Institute, 4 Oct 2018. https://www.brookings.edu/research/what-is-artificial-intelligence. Last accessed 23 Oct 2022.
63. McCarthy J. Encyclopedia Brittanica. https://www.britannica.com/biography/John-McCarthy. Last accessed 23 Oct 2022.
64. Great Learning. What is artificial intelligence? https://www.mygreatlearning.com/blog/what-is-artificial-intelligence. Last accessed 23 Oct 2022.
65. Gonfalonieri A. What is an AI algorithm? https://medium.com/predict/what-is-an-algorithm-aceeab80e7e3. Last accessed 23 Oct 2022.
66. Montani S, Striani M. Artificial intelligence in clinical support: a focus literature survey. Yearb Med Inform. 2019;28:120–7.
67. Magrabi F, Ammenwerth E, McNair JB, et al. Artificial intelligence in clinical decision support: challenges for evaluation AI and practice implications. Yearb Med Inform. 2019;28:128–34.
68. Davenport T, Kalakota R. The potential for artificial intelligence in healthcare. Future Healthc J. 2019;6:94–8.
69. Ameen S, Wong M-C, Yee K-C, Turner P. AI and clinical decision-making: the limitations and risks of computational reductionism in bowel cancer screening. Appl Sci. 2022;12:3341.
70. Lee SI, Celik S, Lodsdon BA, et al. A machine learning approach to integrated big data for precision medicine in acute myeloid leukemia. Nat Commun. 2018;9:42.
71. Walczak S, Velanovich V. Evaluation of artificial neural networks in predicting pancreatic cancer survival. J Gastrointest Surg. 2017;21:1606–12.

72. National Center for Health Statistics. International Classification of Disease (ICD-10-CM/PCS) transition—background. https://www.cdc.gov/nchs/icd/icd10cm_pcs_background.htm. Last accessed 24 Oct 2022.
73. Schaefer J, Lehne M, Schepers J, et al. The use of machine learning in rare diseases: a scoping review. Orphanet J Rare Dis. 2020;15:145.
74. De La Vega FM, Chowdhury S, Moore B, et al. Artificial intelligence enables comprehensive genome interpretation and nomination of candidate diagnoses for rare genetic diseases. Genome Med. 2021;13:153.
75. Mirbabaie M, Steiglitz S, Frick NR. Artificial intelligence in disease diagnostics: a criticial review and classification on the current state of research guiding future direction. Health Technol. 2021;11:693–731.
76. Henry KE, Adams R, Parent C, et al. Factors driving adoption of the TREWS machine learning-based early warning system and its effects on sepsis treatment timing. Nat Med. 2022;28:1447–54.
77. Adams R, Henry KE, Sidharan A, et al. Prospective, multisite study of patient outcomes after implementation of the TREWS machine learning-based early warning system for sepsis. Nat Med. 2022;28:1455–60.
78. Cui M, Zhang DY. Artificial intelligence and computational pathology. Lab Investig. 2021;101:412–22.
79. Hessler G, Baringhaus K-H. Artificial intelligence in drug design. Molecules. 2018;23:2520.
80. Paul D, Sanap G, Shenoy S, et al. Artificial intelligence in drug discovery and development. Drug Discov Today. 2021;26:80–93.
81. Jumper J, Evans R, Pritzel A, et al. Highly accurate protein structure prediction with AlphaFold. Nature. 2021;596:583–9.
82. Deo RC. Machine learning in medicine. Circulation. 2015;132:1920–30.
83. Velanovich V, Walczak S. Artificial neural networks in surgical research. Am J Surg. 2020;220:1532–3.
84. Harrison MI, Koppel R, Bar-Lev S. Unintended consequences of information technologies in health care—an interactive sociotechnical analysis. J Am Med Inform Assoc. 2007;14:542–9.
85. Ash JS, Berg M, Coiera E. Some unintended consequences of information technology in health care: the nature of patient care information system-related errors. J Am Med Inform Assoc. 2004;11:104–12.
86. Kelly CJ, Karthikesalignam A, Suleyan M, et al. Key challenges for delivering clinical impact with artificial intelligence. BMC Med. 2019;17:195.
87. Mori Y, Bretthauer M, Kalager M. Hopes and hypes for artificial intelligence in colorectal cancer screening. Gastroenterology. 2021;161:774–7.
88. Norori N, Hu Q, Aellen FM, et al. Addressing bias in big data and AI for healthcare: a call for open science. Patterns. 2021;2:100347.
89. Nestor B, McDermott MBA, Chauhan G, et al. Rethinking clinical prediction: why machine learning must consider year of care and feature aggregation. 2018. arXiv:1811.12583.
90. Yu K-H, Kohane IS. Framing the challenges of artificial intelligence in medicine. BMJ Qual Saf. 2018;28:238–41.
91. Challen R, Denny J, Pitt M, et al. Artificial intelligence, bias and clinical safety. BMJ Qual Saf. 2019;28:231–7.
92. Davis SE, Greevy RA, Fonnesbeck C, et al. A nonparametric updating method to correct clinical prediction model drift. J Am Med Inform Assoc. 2019;26:1448–57.
93. Duckworth C, Chmiel FP, Burns DK. Explovable machine learning was used to characterize data drift and detect emergent health risks for emergency department admissions during COVID-19. Sci Rep. 2021;11:23017.
94. Jordan MI, Jacobs RA. Hierarchical mixture of experts and the EM algorithm. Neural Comput. 1994;6:181–214.
95. Soleimani H, Hensman J, Saria J. Scalable joint models for reliable uncertainty-aware event prediction. IEEE Trans Pattern Anal Mach Intell. 2018;40:1948–63.

96. Schulman P, Saira S. Can you trust this prediction? Auditing pointwise reliability subsequent to training. In: Proceedings of the 22nd international conference of artificial intelligence and statistics, vol. 89; 2019. p. 1022–31.
97. Subbaswany A, Saria S. From development to deployment: dataset shift, causality, and shift-stable models in health AI. Biostatistics. 2020;21:345–52.
98. Finalyson SG, Subbaswamy A, Singh K. The clinician and dataset shift in artificial intelligence. N Engl J Med. 2021;385:283–6.

Epilogue: Can We Ever Get to a Normative Standard for Medical Discourse?

What I have presented is mostly a descriptive account of how physicians and patients make judgments about information received and what factors could be used in determining if arguments presented are persuasive by both physicians and patients. This included discussions of rationality, reasoning/logic, argumentation, and intuition, concluding that the most effective mode of coming to rational, agreed-upon conclusions is through manifest rationality. In this process, premises are vetted for truth, the logical structure for validity and the conclusion for soundness. However, understanding that no matter the validity of the argument, individuals may not ever reach a mutually agreeable conclusion. Understanding this requires some understanding as to how the human mind evolved, a process that prioritized survival over truth. This evolutionary prioritization led to a "default setting" for humans of maintaining social cohesion, accepting knowledge outside the norm of the group requires intellectual self-discipline and moral courage. The ability of the human brain to be persuaded is "hardwired" into it, with certain areas of the brain activated during the process, no doubt a consequence of our evolution. The human mind is set such that certain messages, delivered in a certain way, will be more persuasive. Into this hardwired brain, the "software" of cultural, social and professional training is "uploaded" such that the human mind will "sense" certain cues and be insensate to others, what I have referred to as the social umwelt.

With this background, I reviewed the various conceptualizations of causation. I have concluded that causation is a human construct for understanding regularities that occur and, more importantly, for predicting future events. This process identifies a causal attribution and creates a causal sequence. The importance of the causal sequence is the identification of target points in the sequence upon which to act to achieve a desired outcome. The causal sequence is essential in understanding how new knowledge is developed and accepted. This acceptance process uses the same tenets of argumentation and persuasion as with any other subject. Once accepted, this knowledge is then used as the theoretical basis for practical application. All practical applications have a theoretical basis in which the premises and conclusions

V. Velanovich, *Medical Persuasion*, https://doi.org/10.1007/978-3-031-30371-5

become coherent to the individual. The process of determining the best practical course of action requires not only valid argumentation but also *phronesis*, that is, practical wisdom.

Because the substrate of my analysis was Western allopathic medicine, it is appropriate to wonder if other medical traditions approach their tasks similarly or not. Using the traditional medical practices of Chinese, North American indigenous, African indigenous, and American faith healers, I have shown that these practices do have an underlying theoretical framework that is consistent with the cultural and social norms of their people. Homeopathy did arise within Western allopathic medicine as a response to its failings, and it also has an elaborate theoretical framework. Nevertheless, in all of these traditions, the processes of argumentation and persuasion are the same, with only the agreed-upon goals valued differently. Finally, I discuss the rise of a more "quantitized" approach to medical decision making, such that numerical calculations of quantifiable data are used. I have come to the conclusion for all its advantages, these techniques simply produce premises, perhaps more reliably, perhaps not, to be used in argumentation.

What I have not attempted in earnest is to produce a comprehensive normative proposition of medical argumentation, although I did touch on some normative aspects. There are several reasons for this lack of effort. First, just because one sets rules for "what is right" in no way dictates that others would accept such rules. Some disciplines, such as mathematics, are entirely rules-based and are not subject to cultural or social misinterpretation. Most other areas of human existence do, however. Next is that persuasion is not solely about the illative core of an argument but rather is the conclusion an acceptable one such that social cohesion is maintained. Last, even within a relatively homogenous profession such as medicine (homogenous in the sense that all Western physicians have an almost uniform medical education), consensus cannot be reached, so what are the chances that consensus can be reached elsewhere?

That leaves open the question of whether a normative account can ever be reached. This requires all participants to accept a body of rules governing the illative core of argumentation, as mathematicians and logicians have accepted rules of mathematical proofs and logical inference. I must confess that broadly speaking, these rules exist, but they exist in a form into which our human brains have evolved. This brings us back to my original thesis: The human mind evolved to survive, not to discern truth. Therefore, I am not sanguine on the prospect of ever coming to universally agreed upon rules of discourse to satisfy all. However, that does not mean that better argumentation cannot be achieved on a more individual level.

Medical persuasion is unlike other forms of persuasion. In other forms of persuasion, one person, A, is attempting to convince another person, B, of the correctness of A's belief that A wants B to adopt or an action that A wants B to do. Although this is certainly true when a researcher or other professional is trying to persuade a physician that the new knowledge that is being presented is true and should be accepted, this should not be the goal of the physician with the patient. What Western allopaths generally do is present diagnoses and treatments to rid the patient of the disease. However, this may not be the only thing patient wants. To that, I would add, the patient may not even know what they want. I would say that understanding what an acceptable conclusion for the patient is essential in knowing if an argument can be constructed to attain an acceptable conclusion. Again, this is a matter of *phronesis.*

There simply may be a mismatch, consciously or unconsciously, as to for which conclusions we should strive. The WHO definition of "well-being" is impossibly broad from a strict practice of Western, allopathic medicine. The allopathic physician is concerned with health in its most narrow definition of absence of disease. Although absence of disease is a desire of the patient, this is not their only desire. There are social relationships, financial considerations, spiritual strivings, intellectual pursuits, and cultural considerations that all affect well-being to which the allopathic physician (but perhaps not the traditional indigenous healer) is blind as a result of their professional umwelt. This potential mismatch of what conclusions should be made has great implications not only for the manifest rationality of the argumentation process between the physician and the patient but also for any normative analysis. The rules used depend on the conclusions desired.

Could a normative doctrine be made of such an approach? Most likely, not for all, but maybe for each patient encounter.

Glossary

Abductive logic A type of inductive logic in which a person infers an explanation for previously unexplained observations.

Accuracy of a test The frequency of correct test results in the entire number of tests administered.

Acupuncture In traditional Chinese medicine, the insertion of small needles at the meridians to restore the flow of *qi* from the body's *Zhang-fu* organs to the body's framework on the presumption that the illness is from an imbalance of *qi* due to blocked meridians.

Afferent nerves Nerves that carry stimuli/information from the body to the brain.

Alethic Denoting modalities of truth, such as necessity, contingency, impossibility, etc.

Allopathy/allopathic The system of medical practice which treats disease by the use of remedies which produce different effects from those with produced the disease, as distinct from homeopathy. Presently referring to scientific-based, conventional Western medicine.

Anatomically modern humans The human species that evolved into the *Homo sapiens* phenotype.

Anemia A condition in which the level of red blood cells and/or hemoglobin level is lower than normal.

Antrectomy Surgical removal of the antrum of the stomach, the most downstream part of the stomach.

Antrum The most downstream portion of the stomach.

Argument A language-product that reaches a conclusion that the arguer believes to be true.

Argumentation A fundamental method of communicating the rationality of one's position to someone else

V. Velanovich, *Medical Persuasion*, https://doi.org/10.1007/978-3-031-30371-5

Artificial intelligence Computer program software into which is coded a set of algorithms that can produce results without having to be explicitly instructed to do so, having the characteristics of intentionality, intelligence, and adaptability.

Attitude A relatively enduring predisposition to respond favorably or unfavorably toward something.

Augmented intelligence Computer programs designed not to replace humans, but to create systems than enhance human capabilities, enhance human decision-making, and to work along with humans to ease tasks which are difficult or repetitive.

Axon An extension from the neuron traveling to another cell which allows the neuron to signal to that cell.

Bayes theorem The conditional probability of an event related to any prior condition.

Bian Zheng The method for identifying the patterns of imbalances leading to disease in traditional Chinese medicine.

Bias A systematic error introduced into sampling or testing by selecting or encouraging one outcome or answer over others.

Big data Data with the size and complexity such that it cannot be analyzed by traditional data analytic methods, characterized by high volume, velocity, and variety that require specific technology and analytic methods for its transformation into use.

Bing A "disease category" or "diagnosis in traditional Chinese medicine.

Boomerang effect In persuasion, where a persuasive technique results in the opposite effect. That is, the person being persuaded will develop adverse feelings toward the subject of the persuasion effort.

Bootstrapping When an individual uses information delivered by a particular source to conclude that the source is reliable, without external confirmation of the source.

Bounded (with respect to data) The concept that the data coming from a particular groups of subjects is only logically applicable to that group from which the data was drawn.

Cause A condition or phenomenon which reliably produces the occurrence of another phenomenon.

Centesimals In homeopathy, the unit of measure of dilution of a medication in solution 1 part to 100 consecutively, with each subsequent solution undergoing succussion.

Central limit theorem The statistical theory that states that the distribution of a mean of a sample of values is approximately normal, whatever the distribution of the values used to calculate the mean, and grows closer to normal as the sample size increases.

Cerebellum Located in the lower, back part of the brain, and is associated with coordinating muscle activity as well as numerous other activities.

Cerebrum The largest part of the brain which includes the frontal, parietal, temporal and occipital lobes.

Confounder/confounding A factor(s) that influence(s) the results of an association spuriously, and, if unknown, can lead to data misinterpretation.

Conspecific(s) An animal belonging to the same species. In human society, members of the same group.

Cortex, cerebral (brain) The very outer layer of the cerebrum containing nerve cells (neurons) that perform brain functions.

Counterfactual A statement expressing the results of phenomenon if some condition(s) had been present if not been present, or had not been present if present.

Cupping In traditional Chinese medicine, a form of heat therapy where heated cups are applied to the skin at meridian points to stimulate *qi.*

Data analytics Mathematical, statistical and computer programming methods to analyze data.

Data science A field of study and application of advanced mathematics, statistics and computer programing to analyze complex data sets.

Decision A conclusion pertaining to an individual's state of mind or course of action.

Decision aid A means of helping individuals make informed choices that take into account their personal values and preferences.

Decision analysis A quantitative method to assess all possible consequences of a decision.

Decision science A field of study of how individuals, groups, and organizations actually make decisions.

Decision support system Computer programs that use as their inputs the patient's clinical data and have has their outputs conclusions about the patient's diagnosis/physical condition and treatment options.

Decision tree A formally construction flow diagram of the choices and outcomes of a decision.

Deductable In health care insurance, the initial costs of medical care for which the patient is responsible in paying.

Deduction/deductive logic A form of logic or reasoning which orders premises or proposition to support a conclusion such that if the premises are true, the conclusion must be true.

Deep learning A type of artificial intelligence program which is a subset of machine learning, such that the program teaches the machine to process inputs through multiple layers in order to classify, infer and predict the outcome.

Defensive medicine The practice of ordering tests or other procedure not necessarily because the doctor thinks it is necessary, but for the fear that if they did not, and the patient had a poor outcome, that they would be sued for malpractice

DeMeester score A scoring system of the amount and severity of acid reflux into the esophagus based on the results of pH monitoring.

Descriptive An enumeration of the characteristics, facts, qualities, etc. of a phenomenon with the purpose of educating someone about the phenomenon.

Determinism The concept that every phenomenon is necessitated by an antecedent phenomenon and condition that when taken together with a "law of nature" must be produced.

Disease An abnormal deviation of the homeostatically operational structure and function of a specific human body or mind, such that the individual will perceive adverse well-being or will have shortened survival, with or without intervention.

Diviner In traditional African medicine, a healer who is able to communicate with ancestors or other spirits.

Doxastic Relating to beliefs.

Duhem-Quine problem Any study used to test a claim is simultaneously testing many ancillary hypotheses about the study methodology and thus cannot be assured the observed results inform the causal hypothesis of interests.

Effectiveness A measure of the degree of beneficial effect under "real world" clinical settings.

Efficacy The extent to which an intervention produces a beneficial difference in patient outcome under "ideal" circumstances.

Endoscopy Any of a category of tests that can directly visualize the hollow internal organs (gastrointestinal tract, respiratory tree, and urinary tract) with specialized flexible instruments.

Enthymeme A premise in an argument in which is not explicitly stated but assumed known by the arguer and listener.

Epistemology The philosophical study of knowledge, including its nature, origin, generation and limits.

Esophageal pH monitoring A test using a device placed within the esophagus to monitor the pH (acid) level within the esophagus for a given period of time.

Esophagogastroduodenoscopy Direct visualization of the esophagus, stomach and duodenum with a flexible endoscope, a device which can be passed orally into the upper digestive tract.

Etiology The purported causative origin(s) or agent(s) of the disease.

Evidence-based medicine The conscientious, explicit, judicious and reasonable use of modern, best evidence in making decisions about the care of individual patients.

Explanadum The thing to be explained.

Explanation A language-based description of sequences in the occurrence of a phenomenon.

Frequency A mathematical expression of the number of times an event actually occurred divided by the number of times the event had the opportunity to occur.

Gastric acid The acid produced by the stomach.

Gastrinoma A neoplastic tumor of the gastrointestinal tract which produces a hormone which promotes excessive secretion of stomach acid, causing ulcers of the stomach and duodenum.

Gastrocutaneous fistula An opening or tract from in hollow space of the stomach to the surface of the skin.

Gastroduodenostomy Surgically connecting the stomach to the duodenum so that gastric contents can pass from the stomach to the duodenum.

Gastroenterostomy Surgically connecting the stomach to the any part of the small intestine (duodenum, jejunum or ileum) so that gastric contents can pass from the stomach to the small intestine.

Gastroesophageal reflux disease (GERD) A disease in which an abnormal amount of stomach acid moves from the stomach to the esophagus causing symptoms and/or damage to the esophagus.

Gastrojejunostomy Surgically connecting the stomach to the jejunum so that gastric contents can pass from the stomach to the jejunum.

Glial cells Supportive cells of the central nervous system that structurally support and insulate the nerve cells (neurons).

Helicobacter pylori A bacterial species that is now thought to be the cause of peptic ulcer disease.

Hemoglobin The protein in the red blood cells that contains the molecule heme which carries oxygen to the body.

Hering's laws In homeopathic disease theory, the principles of: (1) the body seeks to externalize disease, noting that symptoms will surface as part of the curative process; (2) a person's symptoms will appear and disappear in reverse order of their appearance upon the body; and (3) the body heals from the top to bottom and from more vital to less vital organs

Hermeneutics The study of how texts (i.e., words in a communication) are interpreted.

Hiatal hernia A condition in which the stomach and/or other abdominal organ protrude from the abdomen into the chest through an enlarged esophageal/diaphragmatic hiatus, which is a natural opening which allows the esophagus to enter the abdomen from the chest through the diaphragm.

High resolution esophageal manometry A physiological test which measures the pressures, and by extension muscle function, of the esophageal musculature. Specifically, the upper and lower esophageal sphincters, and esophageal body peristalsis.

Homeopathy A theory and practice of medicine based on the belief that "like cures like" and using very dilute dosing of medication, in conjunction with other holistic practices.

Homeostasis The self-regulating processing of living things to maintain healthy functioning.

Hominid The taxonomic group of all the modern and extinct great apes.

Hominin The taxonomic group of human species, and all immediate evolutionary ancestors.

Hominoid Any of a superfamily of primates including hominids and gibbons together with extinct evolutionary ancestral and related forms.

Human universals Those features of culture, society, language, behavior and mind that, so far as the record has been examined, are found among all peoples known to ethnography and history.

Implication A logico-linguistic relationship between two linguistic items (best thought of as propositions or premises) such that one of them follows the other(s).

Incidence How often the disease occurs within a given population over a set period of time.

Indigenous health systems The sum total of the knowledge, skills, and practices based on the theories, beliefs, and experiences indigenous to different cultures, whether explicable or not, used in the maintenance of health as well as in the prevention, diagnosis, improvement or treatment of physical and mental illness.

Induction/inductive logic The logical form using probability propositions, and/or the logical form where a set of particular observations are used to make a generalization.

Inference A movement of the mind from one item to another where the former serves as the basis for and leads to the later.

Interventional studies/controlled trails These are experiments, in which a group of patients with a particular disease is subjected to an intervention and the effects of that intervention on the disease process is measured as the outcome.

Intuition A recognition of a non-obvious phenomenon.

Law of infinitesimals In homeopathy, the law which states that because larger doses could aggravate symptoms (i.e., produce a disease), diminishing the size of the dose could alleviate the aggravation of the symptoms and yet still provide the curative effect.

Logic (1) A field of study which investigates and classifies the structure of statements and arguments, both through the study of formal systems of inference and through the study of arguments in a natural language, but is not concerned with the psychological processes connected with thought or emotions. (2) The structure of a reasoned argument.

Los Angeles classification A classification system measuring the severity of the inflammation of the esophagus as a result of acid reflux, from A (little inflammation) to D (most severe inflammation associated with ulceration).

Lower esophageal sphincter The sphincter mechanism at the bottom of the esophagus which prevents pathological acid reflux.

Machine learning A type of artificial intelligence program that "teaches" a machine how to make inferences and decisions based on past experience.

Markov analysis/model A type of decision analysis such that a subject is always in one of a finite number of discrete states (referred to a Markov states) and all events represent a transition from one state to another.

Medicine wheel (sacred hoop) An object or structure used for health and healing by many traditional indigenous North American peoples.

Meridian(s) (*jing-lua*) The "channels" through which *qi* and other fundamental substances flow in the body in traditional Chinese medicine.

Metaphysics The philosophical study of ideas outside material reality.

Miasm In homeopathic theory, a residual of a disease which leads to a chronic condition.

Modal logic A type of logic with features of necessity, possibility, impossibility and related concepts.

Model A mental representation of mechanisms of the occurrences of specific phenomena.

Monte Carlo simulation A type of simulation used in Markov analyses which use random sampling and statistical modeling to estimate mathematical functions and mimic operations of complex systems.

Moxibustion In traditional Chinese medicine, a form of heat therapy where a bundle of dry herbs (moxa) is burned near the surface of the skin to stimulate the flow of *qi* in the body.

Mucosa The inner most lining of hollow organs.

Necessary condition A condition that must be present for a phenomenon to occur.

Negative predictive value of a test The frequency with which the test is correctly negative in a patient without the disease.

Neural crest (cells) The neural crest with it associated cells is formed during the embryonic development of vertebrates. These cells are the origins of including peripheral and gastrointestinal neurons, glial cells, pigment cells, cartilage and bone of the skull and face, and smooth muscle.

Neural networks A type of artificial intelligence program that works on similar principles to human neural cells, contain a series of algorithms that captures the relationship between various underlying variables by processing data similar to a human brain.

Neuron A nerve cells that produces electrical impulses to lead to some action for the organism.

Neuropil The portion of the brain containing the axons which connect to other portions of the nervous system.

Nissen fundoplication An operation in which the top of the stomach (the fundus) is wrapped around the bottom of the esophagus (the lower esophageal sphincter) in order reduce the amount of reflux of the contents of the stomach into the esophagus.

Nociceptor A nerve receptor of painful or other noxious stimuli.

Non-steroidal anti-inflammatory agents/drugs A class of drugs, which are not steroids, but have the pharmacological property of reducing inflammation.

Normative Establishing the rules or standards on the most optimal way to do something.

Nosology A classification or list of diseases. The branch of medical science that deals with classification of diseases.

Nucleus, brain A cluster of neurons (nerve cells) in the brain that have shared functions.

Observational studies/data/articles These are studies generating new medical knowledge (data) in which a researcher "observes" phenomena, while not actively trying to control the environment in which the phenomena occur.

Occipital lobe The region of the brain located in the back part of the brain, primarily involved in the processing of visual information.

Odds ratio A measure of association between an exposure and an outcome which represents the odds that an outcome will occur given a particular exposure compared to the outcome occurring in the absence of that exposure.

Ontic Relating to entities and the facts about them.

Ontology The branch of metaphysics related to the study of being, including concepts of existence, becoming and reality.

Paralanguage The acoustic properties of speech, e.g., volume, pitch, timber, etc.

Parietal lobe The region of the brain located at the top and toward the back of the brain, primarily functioning to integrate sensory perceptions, among other activities.

Pathogenesis A description of how an etiological agent transforms the normal homeostatic mechanisms of the individual into the disease's pathological manifestations.

Peptic ulcer disease An ulcer involving the lining of the stomach or duodenum.

Percentile The value below which a percentage of data falls.

Peristalsis The muscle wave produced by hollow organs (the gastrointestinal tract and urinary tract) to propel material downstream.

Persuade To move by argument, entreaty or expostulation to a belief, position or course of action.

pH A measure of the concentration of acid (hydrogen ion, H^+) in a solution. The lower the number, the higher the concentration of acid, with 7 being defined as neutral.

Phenotype The set of observable characteristics of an organism as a result of its genetics.

Phronesis Practical wisdom derived from the learning of practical things that guides to achieve the good end of human flourishing, using prudence and the "right" means.

Positive predictive value of a test The frequency the test is correctly positive in a patient with a disease.

Potentiation In homeopathic theory, the increased medical potency of the liquid in which the medication is diluted and subsequently undergoing succession.

Pow-wow A social and sacred gathering of North American indigenous peoples.

Precision medicine The tailoring of medical treatment to the individual characteristics of each patient.

Predicate Descriptors of nouns used in declaratives statements in logic, especially having to do with number.

Preference(s) In decision sciences/analysis, statements made by individuals regarding the relative desirability of a range of health experiences, treatment options or health states.

Prefrontal cortex The most forward part of the frontal cortex associated with thinking and other executive function of brain activity.

Premise A statement or sentence used as a step in an argument to support or establish a conclusion.

Prevalence How many individuals within a population have the disease at a set time.

Principle of provings In homeopathy, the principle that allows the testing substances on healthy people.

Principle of similarity In homeopathy, the priniciple that substances that trigger a disease or its symptoms can be used to treat the disease.

Probability The description of the likelihood that event will occur, usually expressed as the number of times the event will occur divided by the number of opportunities for the event to occur.

Proposition The meaning of a statement, phrase or sentence.

Proton pump inhibitor A class of drugs whose primary function is to reduce the amount of acid that the stomach produces.

Pyloroplasty The cutting of the pylorus muscle between the stomach and the duodenum to allow for more easy passage of contents from the stomach to the duodenum.

Qi The vital life force in traditional Chinese medicine.

Qigong In traditional Chinese medicine, a form of exercise therapy that combines mediative, static, and dynamic body movements to balance the flow of *qi.*

Quality-adjusted life year (QALY) The product of the numeric fraction as expressed by the utility score multiple by the life expectancy (usually in years).

Rationality A human mental framework that leads to the adoption of processes that lead to well-founded beliefs and practices.

Reactance A conscious resistance to persuasion attempts.

Reason A proposition related to some fact, evidence, idea, item, observation, situation, intention, etc. used to infer some conclusion or belief.

Reasoning A mental process by which well-founded beliefs and practices can be determined.

Red Road (path) The path to wholeness and harmony with nature as practiced by many indigenous North American healers.

Risk calculators Programs designed to determine the probabilities of various outcomes dependent on patient clinical factors.

Semiotics The theory of signs and their meaning.

Sensitivity analysis In a decision analysis, changing the parameters used in the decision tree to determining how such changes affects the consequences of the decision.

Sensitivity of a diagnostic test The ability of a test to be positive (i.e., showing an individual has a disease) if, in fact, the individual has the disease.

Similimum A prescribed homeopathic medicinal preparation.

Smudging A purification with smoke of burning sage, cedar or sweetgrass over individuals, including healers and those seeking healing in traditional indigenous North American medicine.

Social influence The process by which one human individual or group affects a change in attitude or behavior in another conspecific individual or group

Specificity of a diagnostic test The ability of a test to be negative (i.e., showing an individual does not have a disease) if, in fact, the individual does not have the disease.

Stochastic The concept that the occurrence of a phenomenon is a random event dependent on the probability of that event occurring.

Structural rationality A property a person has when they have consistent beliefs and intentions, intend means to ends, etc.

Succussion When preparing a homeopathic medication, the process of after dilution of a substance, it is shaken vigorously, which, in homeopathic theory, enhances its medicinal properties.

Sufficient condition A condition that when present a phenomenon may occur.

Tacit knowing/knowledge Knowledge that is accumulated during the course of focused practice without consciously realizing that it is being accumulated.

Temporal lobe The region of the brain located in the lower, middle part of the brain, functioning in auditory and memory processing amount other functions.

The sweat lodge (*Inipi* ceremony) A ceremony occurring in a building that is heated as a means of purification leading to emotional and spiritual well-being in many traditional indigenous North American medical traditions.

Theory A coherent set of concepts that are a bounded set of propositions, which may include models, to explain and predict the occurrences of these phenomena, including causal attribution.

Tui na In traditional Chinese medicine, a type of message therapy to restore balance to the *yin* and *yang*.

Umwelt, social/cultural/professional The way an individual perceives the world because of the culture and social structure in which they were raised, educated and live related to human biological, social and cultural evolution.

Upper gastrointestinal series A radiological image using a contrast material, usually either barium or Gastrograffin, to visualize the esophagus, stomach and duodenum.

Utility In decision analysis, a summary measure of the extent to which each outcome of each choice option achieves each of the decision-maker's ultimate goals.

Vagotomy Severing of the vagus nerves.

Vagus/vagal A nerve with many pathways involved in a number of activities in the respiratory and digestive tracts as well as the heart.

Valid/validity The quality of being logically or factually sound; soundness and cogency.

White blood cells The immunologically active cells in the blood stream that fight foreign invaders in the body, particularly infectious agents like bacteria or viruses.

Wu Xing **cycle** The cycle followed by the *Zang-fu* organs having generating and restraining interactions in traditional Chinese medicine.

Yin/Yang The equal opposite portions of *qi* in traditional Chinese medicine.

Zang-fu **organs** A collection of organs that produce and regulate *qi* within the human body in traditional Chinese medicine.

Zheng The symptom pattern recognized in traditional Chinese medicine, which is a result of the disharmony of the functional entities.

Index

V. Velanovich, *Medical Persuasion*, https://doi.org/10.1007/978-3-031-30371-5

GPSR Compliance

The European Union's (EU) General Product Safety Regulation (GPSR) is a set of rules that requires consumer products to be safe and our obligations to ensure this.

If you have any concerns about our products, you can contact us on ProductSafety@springernature.com

In case Publisher is established outside the EU, the EU authorized representative is:

Springer Nature Customer Service Center GmbH
Europaplatz 3
69115 Heidelberg, Germany

Batch number: 10732076

Printed by Printforce, the Netherlands